YOU HAVE SAVED MONEY
BUYING THIS USED BOOK AT
C S U HAYWARD BOOK STORE

INTRODUCTION TO DIAGNOSTIC MICROBIOLOGY

A TEXT AND WORKBOOK

INTRODUCTION TO DIAGNOSTIC MICROBIOLOGY

A TEXT AND WORKBOOK

Maria Dannessa Delost, MS, MT (ASCP)

Associate Professor and Director of
Medical Laboratory Programs
The Department of Allied Health
College of Health and Human Services
Youngstown State University
Youngstown, Ohio

With 413 *illustrations*

Mosby

St. Louis Baltimore Boston Carlsbad Chicago Naples New York Philadelphia Portland
London Madrid Mexico City Singapore Sydney Tokyo Toronto Wiesbaden

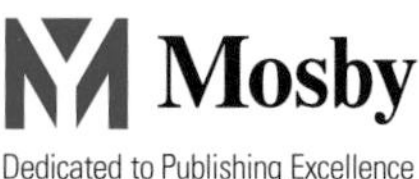

Dedicated to Publishing Excellence

A Times Mirror Company

Vice President and Publisher: Don Ladig
Editors: James F. Shanahan and Jennifer Roche
Developmental Editor: Sandra J. Parker
Project Manager: Patricia Tannian
Senior Production Editor: Ann E. Rogers
Manuscript Editor: Roger McWilliams
Layout Artist: Jeanne Genz
Design Manager: Nancy J. McDonald
Interior Designer: B.J. Crim
Cover Designer: Frank Loose Design
Manufacturing Manager: Tony McAllister

Copyright © 1997 by Mosby–Year Book, Inc.

All rights reserved. No part of this publication may be reproduced, stored in a retrieval system, or transmitted, in any form or by any means, electronic, mechanical, photocopying, recording, or otherwise, without written permission of the publisher.

Permission to photocopy or reproduce solely for internal or personal use is permitted for libraries or other users registered with the Copyright Clearance Center, provided that the base fee of $4.00 per chapter plus $.10 per page is paid directly to the Copyright Clearance Center, 27 Congress Street, Salem, MA 01970. This consent does not extend to other kinds of copying, such as copying for general distribution, for advertising or promotional purposes, for creating new collected works, or for resale.

Printed in the United States of America
Composition by Graphic World, Inc.
Printing/binding by Walsworth Publishing Company

Mosby–Year Book, Inc.
11830 Westline Industrial Drive
St. Louis, Missouri 63146

Library of Congress Cataloging in Publication Data

Delost, Maria Dannessa.
Introduction to diagnostic microbiology: a text and workbook/Maria Dannessa Delost.
p. cm.
Includes bibliographical references and index.
ISBN 0-8016-7853-6
1. Diagnostic microbiology. 2. Diagnostic microbiology—Problems, exercises, etc. I. Title.
QR67.D45 1997
616'.01—dc20 96-48334
CIP

96 97 98 99 00 / 9 8 7 6 5 4 3 2 1

To my
Mom and **Dad,**
Mary and **Amil Dannessa,**
for their unfailing guidance and support

PREFACE

Introduction to Diagnostic Microbiology: A Text and Workbook provides a concise study of clinically significant microorganisms for the clinical laboratory student and the laboratory professional. Although comprehensive textbooks on diagnostic microbiology abound, this text is unique in that it provides a focus on that material which is most essential for the beginning student. In fact, the concept of this text was suggested by some of my students who were frustrated by the length and depth of other microbiology textbooks.

Introduction to Diagnostic Microbiology: A Text and Workbook provides learning objectives, laboratory exercises, and review questions. Didactic and laboratory skills are also presented and reinforced in each chapter. Introductory chapters discuss the infectious process, specimen collection and processing, microscopic methods, antibiotic susceptibility testing, and laboratory safety. Overviews of laboratory instruments and serologic methods in clinical microbiology are also presented. Medically significant bacteria and introductions to clinical virology, mycology, and parasitology are covered in later chapters. The final chapter, Clinical Specimens, summarizes the medically important pathogens that are commonly found in clinical specimens with identification schemes.

This textbook/workbook will provide the clinical laboratory student with the skills necessary for entry into the medical laboratory profession. The information is organized into a format that facilitates learning through the use of integrated text, charts, figures, and instructions for laboratory practice. The format also provides quick reference to the most often utilized procedures and most frequently referred to topics in clinical microbiology.

Many reference texts in clinical microbiology are available with complex descriptions and highly detailed methods. Such texts can be intimidating to the beginning student. The purpose of *Introduction to Diagnostic Microbiology: A Text and Workbook* is to provide a condensed and practical approach for beginning clinical microbiologists. A mastery of the material and procedures in this text will provide students with a strong background to pursue higher levels in clinical microbiology.

ACKNOWLEDGMENTS

I would like to thank Roseann Baca of St. Elizabeth Health Center for her technical assistance, especially in the preparation of microscopic photographs. I would also like to thank Daniel Sahli of Youngstown State University for the preparation of cultures, specimens, and media.

My special thanks to the Media Department of Youngstown State University, and in particular to Carl Leet, for their expertise in photography used for figures in this book.

Finally, my sincere thanks to my family for their encouragement, and a special heartfelt thank you to my husband Raymond and children Gregory and Michael for their patience and support during this project.

CONTENTS

PROCEDURES

COLOR PLATES

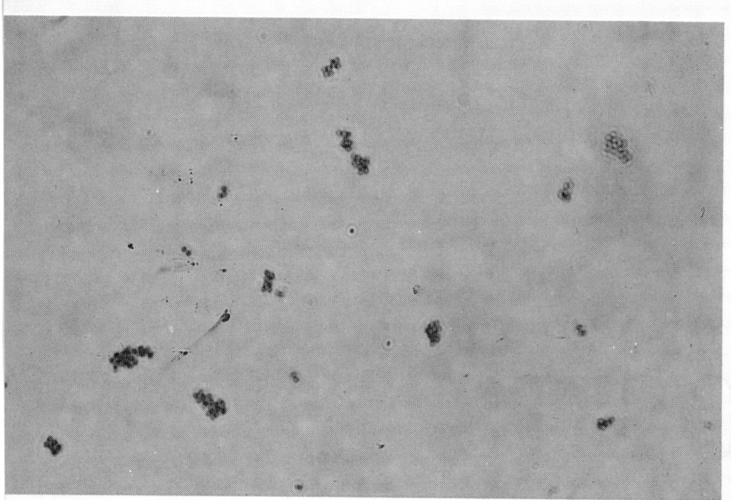

BACTEREMIA

CHAPTER OUTLINE

NORMAL FLORA
OPPORTUNISTIC PATHOGENS
ROUTES OF INFECTION
HOST DEFENSE MECHANISMS
EXOTOXINS AND ENDOTOXINS
- Signs of Infection

NOSOCOMIAL INFECTIONS

KEY TERMS

ACQUIRED IMMUNITY
ANTIBODY
ANTIGEN
ASYMPTOMATIC CARRIER
CELL-MEDIATED IMMUNITY
COLONIZATION
ENDOTOXIN
EXOTOXIN
HUMORAL IMMUNITY
IMMUNOGLOBULIN
IMMUNOSUPPRESSIVE
INFECTION
INFECTIOUS DISEASE
INFLAMMATORY RESPONSE
INNATE IMMUNITY
NORMAL FLORA
NOSOCOMIAL
OPPORTUNISTIC
PATHOGEN
PHAGOCYTOSIS

Introduction to Clinical Microbiology

AN INTRODUCTION TO THE INFECTIOUS PROCESS AND DISEASE TRANSMISSION

CHAPTER ONE

LEARNING OBJECTIVES

1. Define the following terms:
   a. Infection
   b. Infectious disease
   c. True pathogen
   d. Opportunistic pathogen
   e. Nosocomial infection
   f. Endogenous infection
   g. Exogenous infection
   h. Asymptomatic carriage (carriers)
   i. Colonization
2. Define normal flora and discuss its role in each of the following sites:
   a. Mouth and oral cavity
   b. Nasopharynx
   c. Stomach and small intestine
   d. Colon
3. List and describe the major routes of infection.
4. Describe the following host defense mechanisms:
   a. Innate (natural) immunity
   b. Inflammatory response
   c. Acquired immunity
   d. Humoral immunity
   e. Cell-mediated immunity
5. Describe the function of B and T cells in the immune response.
   a. List and summarize the characteristics of the human immunoglobulin classes.
   b. List and state the function of four populations of T cells.
6. Define and describe endotoxins and exotoxins.
7. List the signs of microbial infection.
8. List the laboratory procedures that might be requested to identify infectious disease.
9. List the major types of nosocomial infection and describe how such infections are acquired.

The purpose of clinical microbiology is to isolate and identify pathogenic microorganisms. Clinical microbiologists work with clinicians and other personnel to assist in the diagnosis, management, and treatment of infectious disease. The microbiology laboratory can provide the physician with information from direct smears and stains, cultures, and antibiotic susceptibility testing and from serological tests, including antibody titers. The physician also relies on the patient's medical history, physical examination, results of x-rays, laboratory tests, and epidemiological information (such as previous infections, travel, and illness in the family) to aid in the diagnosis.

An **infection** is the entrance and multiplication of a microorganism in or on a host. The microorganism may enter the host through many routes, including the respiratory tract, gastrointestinal (GI) tract, or breaks in the skin. The microorganism next establishes itself and multiplies. Infections can spread directly through tissues or through the lymphatic system into the blood. **Infectious disease** refers to an infection with functional and structural harm to the host that usually is accompanied by signs and symptoms.

Clinical microbiology begins when the patient presents signs of infection to the physician. An initial diagnosis is made, and the physician then orders diagnostic medical and laboratory procedures. A direct stain, culture, and antibiotic susceptibility test are typical tests that may involve the microbiology laboratory. The appropriate laboratory specimens are collected, labeled, and sent to the laboratory with a requisition (laboratory order form). The laboratory performs direct stains, plates the specimen on appropriate culture media, and incubates the plates at the suitable temperature and atmosphere. The plates are examined and interpreted for the presence of pathogens, most often at 24 and 48 hours. Subcultures are performed as needed, and any biochemical, serological, antibiotic susceptibility, and automated procedures are performed next. These tests are interpreted and the organisms identified. The final report of the identification and antibiotic susceptibility tests is sent to the physician. The physician interprets the report and treats the patient appropriately.

Early diagnosis is associated with early treatment and a better prognosis for the patient. Testing must be performed in a timely yet accurate manner. Often, a presumptive identification can be sent to the physician so that antibiotic therapy can be initiated. A final, definitive identification is then sent to update the report.

All **pathogens** in a specimen must be identified and reported to the physician. A pathogen is a microorganism, including bacteria, viruses, fungi, and parasites, that is capable of causing infectious disease. The identification of pathogens is difficult, since many microorganisms are present in the normal microbial flora. **Normal flora** refers to those microorganisms normally residing in a particular body site; they do not generally cause infection.

NORMAL FLORA

A limited number of organisms can be categorized as normal flora. The slightly acidic pH of the **skin** (5.5 to 6.0) results from the presence of acids produced by a number of bacteria. For example, *Propionibacterium acnes* produces large amounts of propionic acid. Other normal skin flora include *Staphylococcus epidermidis,* the viridans streptococcus, and enterococcus. In addition, a number of contaminating organisms may be found transiently on the skin, such as intestinal tract and soil contaminants.

In the **mouth and oral cavity,** the major normal flora is the viridans streptococcus, a collection of streptococcal species exhibiting alpha hemolysis or greening of sheep blood agar. In addition, *S. epidermidis,* nonpathogenic *Neisseria* species, *Moraxella catarrhalis,* lactobacilli, and diphtheroids may be present. Members of the anaerobic normal flora in this area include *Actinomyces, Veillonella,* and *Bacteroides* species.

The **nasopharynx** may serve as a site for **asymptomatic carriage** of several microorganisms. **Asymptomatic carriers** maintain a reservoir for the microorganism but do not have an infectious disease. Such individuals, however, may serve as an infectious source for others. Bacteria that may be carried asymptomatically in the nasopharynx include *Staphylococcus aureus* and *Neisseria meningitidis.*

The **stomach and upper small intestine** are usually sterile, containing less than 1000 organisms per milliliter. Organisms entering the stomach are usually killed by the hydrochloric acid and resulting low pH of the stomach, as well as by gastric enzymes. Other organisms are passed to the small intestine, where they may be destroyed by bile and pancreatic enzymes. When the gastric pH increases over 5.0, colonization from bacteria of oral, nasopharyngeal, or colon origin may occur.

The **colon** is heavily colonized and serves as a reservoir for infection for numerous body sites, including the urinary tract and peritoneal cavity. Major components of the normal bowel flora include *Bacteroides, Lactobacillus, Clostridium, Eubacterium,* coliforms such as *Escherichia coli,* aerobic and anaerobic streptococci, and yeast.

The normal flora of the distal **urethra** in both males and females may contain diphtheroids, alpha and nonhemolytic streptococci, *Peptococcus, S. epidermidis,* and *Bacteroides.*

Those sites considered to be sterile in the body, containing no normal flora, include the **blood, cerebrospinal fluid,** and **urinary bladder.** Normal flora can become pathogenic if they are removed to another site. Thus normal flora *E. coli* of the colon is an important cause of urinary tract infection (UTI) once it enters the bladder or kidneys. Likewise, although viridans streptococcus is considered to be normal flora of the oral cavity, the organism is a significant cause of subacute bacterial endocarditis when established in the heart.

OPPORTUNISTIC PATHOGENS

Opportunistic infections are infections in immunocompromised hosts that do not cause disease in individuals with a normal immune system. These infections are increasing due to a number of factors, including the widespread use of broad-spectrum antibiotics that can alter the normal flora, the increased use of immunosuppressive drugs to prevent organ transplant rejection, the use of chemotherapeutic agents to treat cancer, and the increased and prolonged use of urethral catheters. Thus an **opportunistic pathogen** is one that attacks an already debilitated host but usually presents no danger to an individual with an intact immune system.

In **immunosuppressive** conditions the host immune system is unable to effectively battle those microorganisms considered to be normal flora for the general population. Other individuals at risk for opportunistic pathogens include dialysis patients, individuals on heart pumps, burn victims, diabetics, and any individual who has chronic medical problems or who is undergoing invasive medical techniques. Those individuals with foreign body implants, including heart valves, prosthetic devices, and indwelling intravenous (IV) catheters, alcoholics, and IV drug users are also at increased risk of opportunistic pathogens.

By contrast, a **true pathogen** has the ability to infect those individuals with a healthy immune system as well as those with an immunosuppressed state.

ROUTES OF INFECTION

Infectious disease can be transmitted by several routes, which can be categorized as direct or indirect transmission. Types of **direct transmission** include congenital contact, sexual contact, hand-to-hand contact, and droplet infection.

Congenital contact may occur across the placenta or as the child passes through the vaginal canal during delivery. Rubella virus and syphilis may be acquired during pregnancy, whereas *Streptococcus agalactiae* and *Neisseria gonorrhoeae* are examples of bacteria that may be transmitted to the infant during delivery.

Sexual contact may be the route of infection for several sexually transmittable diseases, including gonorrhea *(N. gonorrhoeae)*, syphilis *(Treponema pallidum)*, chlamydia *(Chlamydia trachomatis)*, acquired immunodeficiency syndrome or AIDS (human immunodeficiency virus or HIV), and herpes (herpes simplex virus).

Hand-to-hand transmission is the mode of direct contact seen with the spread of the common cold due to rhinovirus. This route is also involved in the transmission of various GI infections when the hands are not properly washed and are fecally contaminated.

Infectious respiratory secretion or droplet infection serves as a route for several respiratory viruses, as well as bacterial pathogens, including *Streptococcus pyogenes* (the agent in strep throat) and *N. meningitidis.* Infectious secretions include coughing, sneezing, kissing, and nasal drainage. Respiratory secretions can become dried on clothing, bedding, or floors and converted to dust, which may serve as a route of indirect transmission.

Indirect routes of infection include fomites, ingestion of contaminated food and water, airborne routes, and animal or arthropod vectors.

Fomites are inanimate objects such as eating utensils, hospital instruments, clothing, money, doorknobs, and tampons. Frequently, these inanimate objects may serve as a route of **nosocomial** (hospital acquired) infection.

Water may be contaminated as a result of improper sanitary measures or after it has been treated. Microorganisms that may be associated with contaminated water include *Shigella, Salmonella,* enteropathogenic *E. coli,* and hepatitis A virus (HAV). Improperly prepared, processed, preserved, or stored **food** may become contaminated with various microorganisms, including *Salmonella* and *S. aureus.* Milk and milk products may be contaminated through improper or lack of pasteurization, while undercooked meats may serve as sources of contamination. Ingestion of the microorganisms or of preformed toxins plays a role in infections acquired through contaminated foods.

Infections may be incidentally transmitted to humans through infected **animals** or **insect** or **arthropod vectors.** Rabies, pasteurellosis *(Pasteurella multo- cida)*, and tularemia *(Francisella tularensis)* are examples of infections that can be acquired through the bite or scratch of an infected animal. Arthropod vectors such as flies, mites, lice, ticks, and mosquitoes may transmit microorganisms from an infected animal to a human host. Malaria *(Plasmodium)* is transmitted by mosquitoes, whereas Lyme disease *(Borrelia burgdorferi)* is transmitted by the bite of an infected tick.

Airborne routes of infection include the **inhalation** of infectious particles that may be suspended in the air. **Infectious aerosols** can be formed in the laboratory that can serve as a route for laboratory-acquired infection. *Mycobacterium tuberculosis,* the agent in tuberculosis, can remain suspended in droplets that serve as infectious aerosols. Dimorphic fungi causing systemic infections, such as *Coccidioides immitis,* can cause airborne infections through the inhalation of infectious spores.

Once established in a particular area, the microorganism may multiply and spread from its original site of entry to contiguous tissue or disseminate through the blood to other, distant sites. Microorganisms spread and multiply when host defense mechanisms are overcome.

HOST DEFENSE MECHANISMS

Host defense mechanisms include **innate** or **natural immunity, acquired immunity,** and **phagocytosis. Immunity** refers to host properties that confer resistance of the host to foreign substances. It is the sum of all mechanisms used by the body as protection against environmental agents that are not normally present in the body.

Innate or **natural immunity** is inborn, mainly genetically determined, and nonspecific. It is not acquired through previous contact with an infectious agent. The **skin** acts as a protective barrier, and a limited number of microorganisms can penetrate the intact skin barrier. Many microorganisms, however, can enter the body through breaks in the skin resulting from bites, wounds, cuts, or needles. In addition, microorganisms can enter through the sweat and fat glands. The normal flora bacteria of the skin produce free fatty acids from oil, which will produce low pH on the skin, preventing the establishment of infection.

Mucus covers the surfaces of the **respiratory tract.** The mucus can trap bacteria and, with the assistance of **cilia** that are also present in the nasal cavity, can trap many microorganisms. The bacteria are either swallowed, entering the stomach where they are destroyed by the acidic environment, or are removed through external openings such as the nose and mouth by sneezing or coughing. **Lysozyme,** an enzyme that lyses bacterial cell walls, is also present in respiratory secretions. Some types of immunoglobulin A (IgA) have a secretory component that can prevent attachment of the microorganisms to the mucous membranes of the respiratory tract. Those bacteria that are phagocytized are transported through the lymphatic system and eventually removed from the body.

The respiratory tract is a common portal of entry for several microorganisms, including *Streptococcus pneumoniae, M. tuberculosis, Mycoplasma pneumoniae,* and several respiratory viruses. Those microorganisms possessing **pili,** appendages for attachment, are able to attach to the mucous membranes.

Saliva in the oral cavity possesses various hydrolytic enzymes that can break down bacteria. The low pH of the **stomach** and the presence of gastric enzymes result in a limited amount of microorganisms that can sustain life in the stomach. The rapid peristalsis in the **small intestine** together with the presence of enzymes and bile keep the microbial population in this site at very low levels. The **large intestine** has a large amount of normal flora that competes with pathogens, thus decreasing the chance for establishment of infection. The anaerobic normal flora of the large intestine produces fatty acids, while facultative anaerobes produce bacteriocins, which also hinder the multiplication of pathogens.

The constant flushing action and low pH of **urine** prevent pathogens from establishing in the urinary system. Females, who have shorter urethras, are more prone to UTIs than males, who have longer urethras. Bacteria have easier access to the female bladder from the GI and vaginal tracts.

Lactobacilli, a major normal flora in the female vaginal tract, produce large amounts of lactic acid, which results in a low pH. This acidic environment decreases the amount of other microorganisms that can cause infection in this area.

The **eyes** are protected through the constant flushing provided by tears as well as the presence of lysozyme in tears.

Other elements of innate immunity include fever, interferon, phagocytosis, and various serum proteins. These components are described with the inflammatory response.

Natural immunity can be affected by a number of factors. For example, very young and very old persons are more susceptible to infection then other age groups. Hormonal changes, such as those occurring during pregnancy, diabetes mellitus, and Addison's and Cushing's diseases can alter the metabolism and immune response, which results in increased susceptibility to infection. The use of broad-spectrum antibiotics, which alter the host's normal flora, can also promote the growth of pathogens. The normal flora is no longer present in large amounts to compete with the pathogenic organisms. Such infections are termed **secondary infections** or **superinfections** because the infection results from use of an antibiotic.

The **inflammatory response** can be activated by trauma or tissue injury. **Inflammation** is the total of the changes occurring in tissue factors upon injury. Hemodynamic changes, such as increased vascular permeability, dilation of arterioles and capillaries, and increased blood flow to the injured area, occur. Plasma proteins, such as complement, interferon, and antibodies, are also released. Edema may occur as a result of vasodilation, while there is also an influx of red blood cells to the area.

TABLE 1–1
Chemical Mediators of Inflammation

COMPOUND	EFFECT
Histamine	Dilates blood vessels, increases permeability of blood vessels
Kinins	Increase vascular permeability and initiate or enhance release of other mediators from white blood cells; derived in the clotting cascade from activation of the precursor **kininogen** by **kallikrein**
Leukotrienes	Affect white blood cell mobility and metabolism
Prostaglandins	Formed in the hypothalamus in the thermoregulation center; induce fever
C-reactive protein, serum amyloid A, antitrypsin	Liver proteins playing a role in the acute response
Interleukin-1	Stimulates cells of immune response, increases fever by interaction with prostaglandins, increases adhesion of neutrophils to endothelium, promotes T cell proliferation
Interleukin-2	Causes proliferation of activated T and B cells
Cytokines	Stimulate white blood cells, promoting their growth and differentiation
Gamma interferon	Promotes growth of T and B cells

Phagocytic cells—neutrophils (PMNs) and macrophages—have four functions: **migration, chemotaxis, ingestion,** and **killing.** The cells may **adhere** to the vascular endothelium or **migrate** from the blood to the affected tissues in a process known as **diapedesis. Chemotaxis** refers to the attraction of the phagocytes to the affected area by the microorganisms or its products from the blood to the injured site. Neutrophils and monocytes are attracted by bacterial products, such as endotoxin and enzymes. **Attachment** initiates the phagocytic process. The microorganism must be coated with opsonins (such as IgG or complement units) for facilitation of the process. Those organisms that have a capsule are resistant to the effects of phagocytosis. The next step is **ingestion,** which involves the formation of a **phagosome,** which undergoes a respiratory burst. The respiratory burst results in the release of superoxide anion and peroxide, both of which are toxic to microorganisms. Lysosomes within the cell combine with phagosomes to form phagolysosomes, which eventually release hydrolytic enzymes.

Neutrophils are formed in the bone marrow and enter the blood and tissue. Monocytes, also formed in the bone marrow, are known as macrophages once the cells have entered the tissue. Macrophages are present in tissues but are also fixed to the blood vessels of the liver, spleen, and lymph nodes. Macrophages can become activated by microorganisms, endotoxins, and antigen-antibody complexes. Once activated, macrophages produce an increased number of lysosomes, which produce interleukin-1. Interleukin-1 is associated with the stimulation of fever and activation of phagocytosis.

Inflammation caused by microorganisms may be initiated through activation of the complement system or the blood coagulation cascade. These systems initiate the release of several chemical mediators of inflammation, which are summarized in Table 1-1.

Acquired immunity can be either passive or active. **Passively acquired immunity** refers to the temporary resistance to infectious agents by administration of antibodies preformed in another host. Common examples include gamma globulin and antitoxin to *Clostridium botulinum* toxin. Passive acquisition is also seen in the fetus, who acquires antibodies from the mother's blood during pregnancy. These antibodies remain active in the newborn until 4 to 6 months of age. Newborns may also acquire immunity passively from their mother through antibodies carried in breast milk.

Actively acquired immunity is a state of resistance built in an individual following contact with foreign antigens, such as microorganisms. The immunity may result from clinical or subclinical infection, through injection of live killed microorganisms or their antigens, or through the absorption of bacterial products, such as toxins or toxoids. In active immunity the host actively produces antibody in reaction to a foreign antigen.

TABLE 1–2

Summary of Human Immunoglobulins

	IgG	IgM	IgA	IgD	IgE
Percentage in normal serum	75%-85%	5%-10%	5%-15%	0.001%	0.0003%
Molecular weight (approximate)	150,000	900,000	160,000 (serum) 400,000 (secretory)	180,000	190,000
Heavy chain class	gamma (γ)	mu (μ)	alpha (α)	delta (δ)	epsilon (ϵ)
Heavy chain subclasses	$\gamma_1\gamma_2\gamma_3\gamma_4$	$\mu_1\mu_2$	$\alpha_1\alpha_2$	None	None
Cross placenta	yes	no	no	no	no
Activate complement	yes for IgG-1, -2, -3	Yes	No	No	No

Acquired immunity involves contact with a foreign agent or **antigen.** This process is known as **immunization,** and it initiates a series of reactions that leads to the activation of **lymphocytes** and the synthesis of specialized serum proteins known as **antibodies.** Thus antigens are substances foreign to the body that initiate the production of antibodies.

Three major cell types are involved in the immune response: T cells, B cells, and macrophages. **T** and **B cells** arise from a common lymphoid precursor cell but mature in different areas of the body. T cells mature in the thymus while B cells, named for the bursa of Fabricius (the area in the chicken where the cells were first isolated), mature in the bone marrow. Although B and T cells have different functions, both play a role in the recognition of antigen and reaction toward it. The third type of cell, **macrophages,** are phagocytic cells that ingest, process, and present antigens to T cells.

Humoral immunity is mediated by serum antibodies secreted by B cells. These antibodies are known as **immunoglobulins.** There are five major classes of immunoglobulins: IgG, IgM, IgA, IgD, and IgE. Each immunoglobulin class has unique biological abilities.

IgG is able to cross the placenta and is most active at 37°C. It is the major immunoglobulin in normal serum. IgG is primarily involved in the secondary or anamnestic immune response.

IgM is involved mainly in the primary immune response and appears in the serum following initial exposure to an antigen. IgM has its greatest activity at 20°C to 25°C.

IgA is unique in that it is the only immunoglobulin found in secretions, such as tears, saliva, and secretions of the respiratory tract.

Important characteristics of the immunoglobulins are summarized in Table 1-2, and a summary of their primary functions is found in the box at right.

Primary Functions of Human Immunoglobulins

IgG Passive immunity for newborns, neutralization of viruses and exotoxin; responds best to protein antigens, mainly involved in secondary (anamnestic) immune response

IgM Endotoxin neutralization, bacterial agglutination, complement-mediated bacteriolysis, strong opsonization ability; responds best to polysaccharide antigens, mainly involved in primary immune response

IgA Prevention of bacterial and viral invasion of mucous membranes through interference with adherence of microorganism to site; found in tears, milk, saliva, and respiratory and GI secretions

IgD Little is known; may serve as a B cell receptor or play a role in autoallergic diseases

IgE Major role in allergic response

The **complement system** is another important aspect of humoral immunity. The complement system involves more than 20 different serum proteins and enzymes that can be activated by immune (antigen-antibody) complexes or nonimmune routes, such as lipopolysaccharide. If the complement cascade is activated, the target cell may be lysed or phagocytic cells may be stimulated.

Cell-mediated immunity (CMI) involves the T lymphocytes, which circulate to the antigen to perform their function. There are several populations of T cells, including:

- **T helper (inducer) cells**
  Enhance proliferation and differentiation of B cells and precursors to cytotoxic T cells
  Increase ability of macrophages to ingest and destroy pathogens
  Enhance the production of antibody by B cells
  Release lymphokines, including interleukin-1 (IL-1) and interleukin-2 (IL-2), and B cell–stimulating factor, which helps to activate B cells
- **Cytotoxic T cells**—destroy targets on direct contact through the recognition and destruction of antigen-bearing cells
- **T suppressor cells**—suppress or regulate the response of T and B cells
- **Null cells (natural killer [NK] and killer [K] cells)**—kill tumor or viral-infected cells, although not with the specificity of cytotoxic T cells

Although presented as separate functions, the humoral and cell-mediated immune systems interact in the immune response.

EXOTOXINS AND ENDOTOXINS

Bacteria produce systemic effects of infection through the production of **toxins.** **Exotoxins** are associated with gram-positive organisms and are secreted by the living bacterial cell. Exotoxins are usually found in high concentration in fluid media and are not associated with the production of fever. Examples include leukocidin produced by *S. aureus,* which inhibits white blood cells (WBCs); the toxic shock syndrome toxin of *S. aureus;* diphtheria toxin of *Corynebacterium diphtheriae;* and theta toxin, a necrotizing toxin produced by *Clostridium perfringens.* Other exotoxins are extracellular enzymes such as DNAse, which inhibits the host deoxyribonucleic acid (DNA); coagulase, which converts fibrinogen into fibrin; hemolysins, which lyse red blood cells (RBCs); proteases; which break down protein, and fibrinolysins, which lyse fibrin clots. **Endotoxins** are usually associated with gram-negative bacteria and consist of **lipopolysaccharide (LPS),** the component of the cell wall. Endotoxins are released at cell lysis or death and are capable of inducing fever in the host.

Signs of Infection

The entire process for clinical microbiology begins with a patient who is exhibiting one or more signs of infection. Some common general or systemic signs of acute infection include a high-grade, spiking fever; chills; vasodilation with flushing; and an increased pulse rate. Chronic or subacute infections may be accompanied by the following systemic signs: intermittent, low-grade fever; weight loss; and fatigue. Local signs of infection include pain, heat, redness, and swelling.

In the laboratory, specific procedures are used to diagnose infection. These include the **leukocyte count,** which is elevated for most infectious processes, and the **differential white blood cell count,** which enables the clinician to determine the type of infection. In general, but not always, bacterial infections are associated with an elevated WBC count and an increased percentage of **neutrophils.** By contrast, **lymphocytes** are the predominant WBC in most viral infections. The **erythrocyte sedimentation rate (ESR)** is a nonspecific indicator of inflammation and is frequently increased in infectious disease and in numerous other inflammatory states. **C-reactive protein** is another plasma protein that is present during infectious disease. Finally, the presence of **type-specific antibodies** in a patient's serum can be used to identify the presence of a particular pathogen. On exposure to a bacterial or viral pathogen, the patient produces antibodies against the antigens of the organism. The antibodies can then be detected through use of antigenic markers.

Radiographic signs of infectious disease that a clinician would note include pulmonary infiltrates, gas and swelling in the tissues, and the accumulation of fluid in a body cavity.

Gastrointestinal signs, such as nausea, vomiting, and diarrhea as well as various neuromuscular and cardiopulmonary signs, are also noted by the clinician.

NOSOCOMIAL INFECTIONS

A **nosocomial infection** is acquired in the hospital or other health care setting. The organism is not present and not incubating in the patient on entry or admission into the health care facility. A **community-acquired infection** is present or incubating at the time of admission into the health care facility. As with other infections, nosocomial and community-acquired infections can be categorized as endogenous or exogenous. **Endogenous infections** result from organisms that are a part of the patient's normal flora, whereas **exogenous infections** result from organisms from external sources. These sources may include contaminated medical instruments or equipment, inanimate objects in the health care setting, or from contact with health care personnel. Individuals, including health care providers, may be **colonized** with an organism. **Colonization** is defined as the presence and multiplication of a microorganism in a host, with no clinical signs of infection. Such individuals may serve as a reservoir of infection and transmit the organism to susceptible individuals.

The most common types of nosocomial infections are urinary tract infections (35% to 40%), surgical wound infections (20%), lower respiratory tract infections (15%), and bacteremia (5%). These percentages may vary with each health care setting. Those bacteria most often associated with nosocomial infections include *S. aureus, E. coli, Enterococcus,* and *Pseudomonas aeruginosa.* Many nosocomialpathogens are resistant to multiple antimicrobial agents.

Nosocomial UTIs may follow catheterization, the presence of indwelling catheters, or other urological techniques, such as cystoscopy. The organism is frequently of endogenous origin, as with *E. coli,* which is a member of the normal flora of the large intestine. Exogenous sources include the contaminated hands of health care providers or contaminated equipment or solutions.

Nosocomial surgical wound infections usually involve *S. aureus* or gram-negative bacilli. These infections may be endogenous or exogenous.

Nosocomial pneumonia may result from aspiration of the organisms from the stomach or upper respiratory tract. The airways or stomach may become colonized with bacteria, including *S. aureus, P. aeruginosa,* and *Klebsiella pneumoniae.* Respiratory care procedures, such as endotracheal suctioning and inhalation therapy, also present a greater risk for nosocomial pneumonia. A high mortality rate is associated with nosocomial infections of the lower respiratory tract.

Bacteremia may result from the patient's own flora as well as that of the health care provider. In addition, IV devices or solutions may be contaminated.

Host factors that lead to increased susceptibility to nosocomial infections include a compromised immune system, underlying medical disease or diseases, age, trauma, burns, poor nutritional status, anatomical abnormalities, use of medical instrumentation, and diagnostic procedures.

Some, but not all, nosocomial infections can be prevented. The universal use of gloves and practice of aseptic techniques, including thorough handwashing, can decrease the incidence of nosocomial infections. The routine disinfection of inanimate surfaces and prevention of aerosols are also important factors.

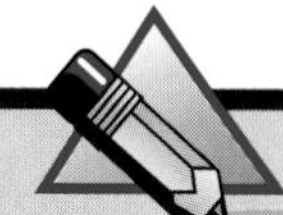

REVIEW QUESTIONS

MATCHING

Match the following terms with the correct definition:

____ **1. Infection**
____ **2. Infectious disease**
____ **3. Opportunistic infection**
____ **4. Nosocoimal infection**
____ **5. Colonization**

a. Condition associated with functional and structural harm to the host, accompanied by signs and symptoms
b. Infection in an immunocompromised host that does not cause infection in an immunocompetent individual
c. Infection acquired in the health care setting
d. Presence and multiplication of a microorganism in a host with no clinical signs of infection
e. Entrance and multiplication of a microorganism in a host

MULTIPLE CHOICE

6. All the following sites contain normal flora *except:*
   a. Oral cavity
   b. Skin
   c. Colon
   d. Cerebrospinal fluid

7. Which of the following is *not* classified as a direct route of infection?
   a. Ingestion of contaminated food or water
   b. Sexual
   c. Hand to hand
   d. Congenital

8. Droplet infection through contact with infectious respiratory secretions may be described as:
   a. Inhalation of infectious aerosols during laboratory procedures
   b. Transmission of rhinovirus through failing to wash hands
   c. Spread of respiratory viruses and *Streptococcus pyogenes* through coughing or sneezing
   d. Inhalation of bacteria or viruses that have dried on bedding or clothing

REVIEW QUESTIONS

(Continued)

9. Which of the following organisms are typically spread through the ingestion of contaminated food or water?
   a. *Neisseria meningitidis* and *S. pyogenes*
   b. *Salmonella* and *Shigella*
   c. Herpes simplex virus and *Treponema pallidum*
   d. *Plasmodium* and *Borrelia*

10. Which of the following organisms are spread through arthropod vectors?
   a. *N. meningitidis* and *S. pyogenes*
   b. *Salmonella* and *Shigella*
   c. Herpes simplex virus and *T. pallidum*
   d. *Plasmodium* and *Borrelia*

11. Innate or natural immunity involves which of the following mechanisms?
   a. Mucus and cilia in the respiratory tract that help to trap and clear microorganisms
   b. Humoral immunity
   c. Cell-mediated immunity
   d. Immunity resulting from vaccination

12. The movement of neutrophils and monocytes from the blood to injured tissue is known as:
   a. Diapedesis
   b. Chemotaxis
   c. Ingestion
   d. Hematopoiesis

13. Antibody-producing white blood cells are:
   a. Macrophages
   b. Neutrophils
   c. T lymphocytes
   d. B lymphocytes

14. Which of the following cells play a major role in cell-mediated immunity?
   a. Macrophages
   b. Neutrophils
   c. T lymphocytes
   d. B lymphocytes

15. The immunoglobulin found in the highest concentration in normal serum is:
   a. IgA
   b. IgD
   c. IgE
   d. IgG
   e. IgM

16. Which of the following immunoglobulins is involved mainly in the primary immune response?
   a. IgA
   b. IgD
   c. IgE
   d. IgG
   e. IgM

BIBLIOGRAPHY

Bartlett RC, Mazens-Sullivan M, Tetreault JZ: Evolving approaches to management of quality in clinical microbiology, *Clin Microbiol Rev* 7:55, 1994.

Benjamini E, Leskowitz S: *Immunology, a short course,* ed 2, New York, 1991, Wiley-Liss.

Berkowitz FE: Bacterial exotoxins: how they work, *Pediatr Infect Dis J* 8:42, 1989.

Finlay BB, Falkow S: Common themes in microbial pathogenicity, *Microbiol Rev* 53:210, 1989.

Haley RW, Culver DH, White JW, et al: The efficacy of infection surveillance and control programs in preventing nosocomial infections in US hospitals, *Am J Epidemiol* 121:182, 1985.

Lubran MM: Bacterial toxins, *Ann Clin Lab Sci* 18:58, 1988.

Mackowiak PA: The normal microbial flora, *N Engl J Med* 307:83, 1982.

Schaechter M, Eisenstein BI: Establishment of infectious diseases. In Schaechter M, Medoff G, Schlessinger D: *Mechanisms of microbial disease,* Baltimore, 1993, Williams & Wilkins.

Schwab JH: Suppression of the immune response by microorganisms, *Bacteriol Rev* 39:121, 1975.

Smith H: The bacterial challenge of microbial pathogenicity, *J Appl Bacteriol* 57:395, 1984.

Soule BM, LaRocco MT: Nosocomial infections: an overview. In Howard BJ et al, editors: *Clinical and pathogenic microbiology,* ed 2, St Louis, 1993, Mosby.

Stansfield WD: *Serology and immunology: a clinical approach,* New York, 1981, Macmillan.

Walter JB: *An introduction to the principles of disease,* ed 3, Philadelphia, 1992, Saunders.

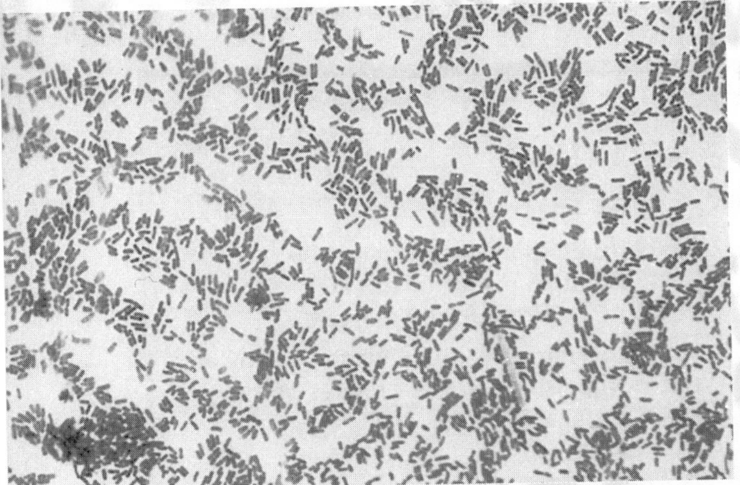

BACTEROIDES FRAGILIS

CHAPTER OUTLINE

KEY TERMS

ANTIBIOTIC MEDIA
ASYMPTOMATIC CARRIER
BACTEREMIA
BARTLETT'S CLASSIFICATION
CAPNOPHILIC
COLONY COUNT
DIFFERENTIAL MEDIA
ENRICHMENT BROTH
FACULTATIVE ANAEROBE
FASTIDIOUS
GENERAL ISOLATION MEDIA
MENINGITIS
MESOPHILIC
NONSELECTIVE MEDIA
NORMAL FLORA
OBLIGATE AEROBE
OBLIGATE ANAEROBE
SELECTIVE MEDIA
SEPTICEMIA

Specimen Collection, Transport, and Processing

LEARNING OBJECTIVES

1. List and discuss the basic concepts for proper specimen collection in diagnostic microbiology. Recognize samples that are not suitable and suggest appropriate corrective action.
2. For each of the following specific sites, describe specific collection requirements:
   a. Throat
   b. Nasopharyngeal
   c. Sputum
   d. Urine (clean catch, catheterized, suprapubic)
   e. Wound
   f. Stool
   g. Cerebrospinal fluid
   h. Genital (male urethral, female vaginal and cervical)
   i. Blood
3. Discuss proper specimen transport and processing methods. Name the typically used transport media.
4. Describe the gross examination of specimens for microbiology.
5. Using Bartlett's classification, determine if a sputum sample is a "good" specimen or contaminated.
6. List and discuss important quality control measures used in the microbiology laboratory.
7. For each of the following media, state the purpose and describe the important components:
   a. Sheep blood agar
   b. Colistin–nalidixic acid
   c. Chocolate agar
   d. Modified Thayer-Martin, Martin-Lewis, New York City

Continued.

e. MacConkey
f. Eosin–methylene blue
g. Gram-negative broth, selenite broth, tetrathionate broth
h. Thioglycollate
i. Hektoen enteric, *Salmonella-Shigella,* xylose-lysine-deoxycholate

8. List and describe the types of hemolysis observed on sheep blood agar.
9. Streak an agar plate correctly to obtain isolated colonies.
10. Define and differentiate the following terms:
    a. Aerobe and anaerobe
    b. Facultative anaerobe and obligate anaerobe
    c. Mesophile and thermophile

The time-honored adage in laboratory medicine, "Your results are only as good as your specimen," holds very true in the clinical microbiology laboratory. Specimens collected improperly provide the physician with misleading and erroneous results that may lead to overtreatment, undertreatment, or mistreatment of a suspected infection. Guidelines for proper specimen collection must be established and enforced by the microbiology laboratory to gain valid, consistent results. Failure to properly collect specimens for culture may result in the failure to isolate the organism that is actually causing the infection. The recovery of contaminants or normal flora may lead to inappropriate or unnecessary antibiotic therapy.

This chapter discusses general guidelines for specimen collection, then specific guidelines for some common collection sites.

GENERAL SPECIMEN GUIDELINES

When possible, the specimen should be collected from the actual site of infection. Contamination from adjacent tissue and the **normal flora** should be avoided in specimen collection. Normal flora may overgrow the pathogen and lead to an erroneous result.

For example, the area adjacent to a wound infection should not be cultured. Instead, a needle aspiration of the wound is recommended. A swab of the adjacent area may simply lead to the isolation of *Staphylococcus epidermidis,* a normal flora of the skin. Similarly, in the collection of a specimen for the diagnosis of bronchitis or pneumonia, the specimen collected should be representative of the lower respiratory tract. A sputum sample is representative of this area; however, saliva from the oral cavity would simply yield normal oropharyngeal flora.

When possible, one should culture for a specific pathogen and culture the site where a particular pathogen is most likely found.

When possible, one should obtain cultures before the initiation of antibiotic therapy. Antibiotics may inhibit the growth of pathogens, which may result in a negative culture, even if the patient has a bacterial infection. When this is not possible, it is important for the physician or nurse to note any antibiotics prescribed for the patient.

One must also consider the history and physiology of the disease when considering the time of specimen collection. The causative organism may be recovered from different sources at different times during the course of the illness. Also, a higher yield of the organism may be obtained at different stages of the illness. For example, the enteric pathogens associated with gastroenteritis are most efficiently cultured when the patient is in the acute, diarrheal stage. When one considers viral meningitis, the optimal collection time for highest viral yield is shortly after the onset of the illness.

Probably the best example of optimal collection time is the physiology of *Salmonella typhi,* the agent of typhoid fever. The organism first attacks the blood and can therefore be isolated from the blood during the first week of illness. During weeks 2 and 3, the highest yield is found in the urine or feces. Finally, antibody titers become positive in the fifth week. Culturing the correct site will initiate the process for proper specimen identification.

The specimen should also be in a sufficient quantity to perform all procedures requested. Inadequate specimens should be marked "QNS" (quantity not sufficient) and held until the physician determines which tests, if any, should be performed. Specimens should always be held and not discarded until this information is obtained. If a recollection is necessary, the physician or nurse should be notified. Although some samples are easily collected, others (such as cerebrospinal fluid and catheterized urine) are more difficult to obtain. For this reason, it is important to note that no guarantee exists that a repeat specimen can be collected.

Specimens must be collected with sterile collection methods. Contaminated containers may lead to an incorrect identification. Also, when possible, swabs are not recommended for collection because organisms have a tendency to dry out. Swabs are never appropriate for anaerobic culture, since the atmospheric oxygen is toxic to these organisms. Culturettes, which contain swabs and a transport media, are recommended for many cultures of bacterial specimens. Figure 3-1 illustrates examples of various specimen collection devices.

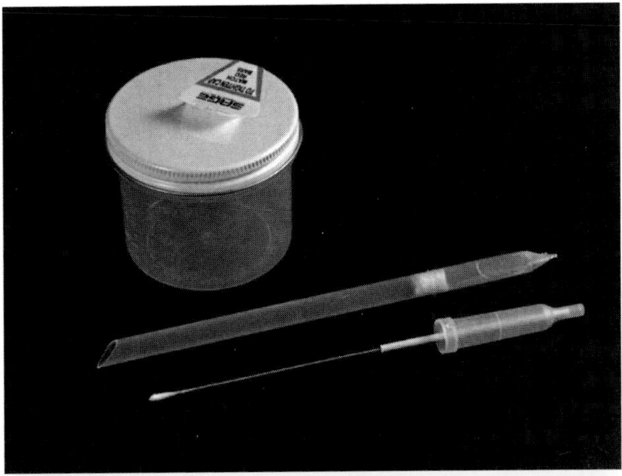

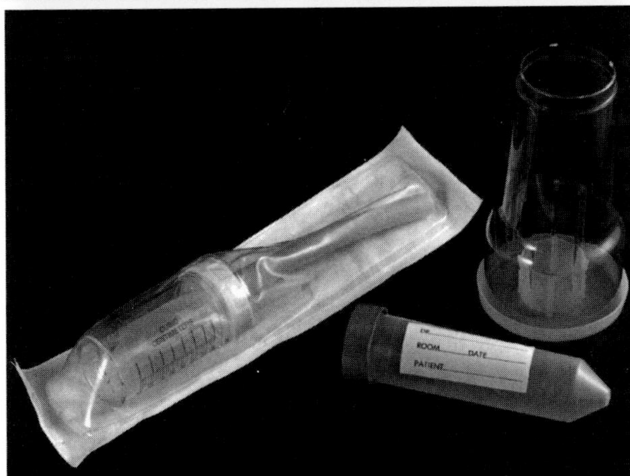

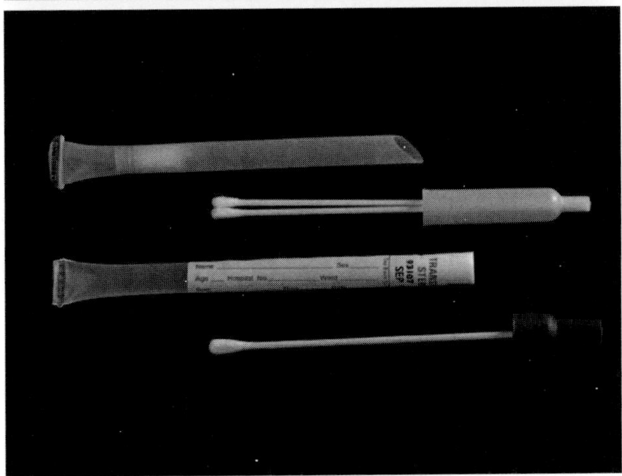

FIGURE 3–1
Specimen collection and transport devices.

The actual time between specimen collection and plating to media should be kept to a minimum. Any delay may lead to the decline of the pathogen and the multiplication of the normal flora. Certain bacteria, such as the pathogenic *Neisseria* and *Haemophilus*, are very susceptible to changes in temperature and to drying out. Thus it is important to culture immediately samples suspected of harboring any fastidious organism. **Fastidious** bacteria are those organisms that require special cultivation measures, such as enriched media, or special atmospheric conditions, such as increased carbon dioxide (CO_2). In general, a 2-hour limit between collection and receipt of the specimen in the laboratory is established for those specimens not preserved in a transport medium. Cerebrospinal fluids should be transported immediately to the laboratory and examined. It is crucial to avoid any delay in the workup of cerebrospinal fluid when one considers the morbidity and mortality of the infection and the fastidious nature of those bacteria associated with meningitis.

Finally, a complete and accurate label is essential. The label should include the patient's full name, identification number, date and time of collection, room number, and source of collection. The physician's name should be available so that the laboratory knows who to contact if a problem arises.

Specimen quality assurance means that the collection of suitable specimens for the microbiology laboratory depends on proper communication among the director of the microbiology laboratory, medical staff, laboratory personnel, and nursing staff. Procedure manuals and thorough instructions for specimen collection are helpful, as is direct verbal communication between the laboratory and medical and nursing personnel. When a specimen is not suitable for culture, the physician should be informed of the reason(s) so that the error does not continue to occur. In addition to improving the quality of patient care, proper specimen collection also is an important cost containment measure for the laboratory.

SPECIMEN COLLECTION REQUIREMENTS FOR SPECIFIC SITES

Respiratory Tract

Specimens collected from the upper respiratory tract include throat cultures, nasopharyngeal cultures, and specimens from the oral cavity. The normal flora of the upper respiratory tract includes alpha-hemolytic streptococci (viridans streptococci), *S. epidermidis*, diphtheroids, nonpathogenic *Neisseria* species, some anaerobes, *Haemophilus* species, and a few *Candida albicans.*

Throat cultures are primarily requested to diagnose **group A streptococcal** *(Streptococcus pyogenes)* infection. The most important consideration in the collection of a throat culture is to avoid the normal oropharyngeal flora. The posterior pharynx between the tonsillar pillars should be swabbed while the roof and sides of the mouth and the tongue should be avoided.

Throat cultures may also be requested for the following suspected infections:

Whooping cough: *Bordetella pertussis*
Epiglottitis: *Haemophilus influenzae*
Oral thrush in infants and immunosuppressed patients: *Candida albicans*
Oral gonorrhea: *Neisseria gonorrhoeae*

The **nasopharynx** is cultured by guiding a swab through the nasal septum until the posterior pharynx is reached. A nasopharyngeal specimen is preferred for the diagnosis of pertussis and may rarely be used to diagnose middle ear infections. Also, the specimen may be used to identify the carrier state of *Staphylococcus aureus* or *Neisseria meningitidis.* If an individual is an **asymptomatic carrier,** the bacterium is present but does not cause infection. However, the carrier can serve as a source of infection to susceptible individuals.

Cultures of the **lower respiratory tract** are requested to diagnose bronchitis or pneumonia. Although usually viral, bacterial types and *Mycoplasma pneumoniae* are also associated with bronchitis. Specific bacterial species typically associated with pneumonia include *Streptococcus pneumoniae, Klebsiella pneumoniae, Serratia* species, *Pseudomonas aeruginosa, Escherichia coli, S. aureus,* anaerobes, and fungi.

Sputum samples are frequently collected to diagnose infections of the lower respiratory tract. Sputum samples are difficult to collect without contamination from saliva. It is important to obtain deep cough secretions that will yield productive results. A saline gargle may enhance the collection.

Several classification schemes are available to assess the quality of sputum samples. In **Bartlett's classification** (see the box at left) the number of neutrophils and epithelial cells per low-power field (LPF) are enumerated. Based on these findings, the sputum is given a score. Scores of 0 or less indicate a lack of inflammation or the presence of saliva.

Other methods of determining the suitability of a sputum sample include simply scanning the slide for the presence of squamous epithelial cells (SECs), polymorphonuclear neutrophils (PMNs), alveolar macrophages (AMs), and columnar cells (CCs). The relative number of each is quantitated as follows:

Few: less than 10/LPF
Moderate: 10 to 25/LPF
Abundant: greater than 25/LPF

In general, PMNs are associated with acute bacterial pneumonia, whereas AMs and CCs are found in the lower respiratory tract and indicate that the specimen was collected properly. Their presence may or may not indicate infection. SECs that line the mucous membranes of the oral cavity usually indicate oral flora contamination. **Purulent secretions** contain more than 25 PMNs and less than 10 SECs/LPF, whereas a predominance of AMs or CCs (greater than 25/LPF) indicate respiratory secretions. Oral secretions are indicated by more than 25 SECs/LPF and less than 10 PMNs/LPF. Other combinations are considered borderline samples. It is recommended that all specimens containing purulent secretions should be cultured, whereas those containing oral secretions should be recollected.

Bartlett's Classification

Number of neutrophils per low-power field	Grade
Less than 10	0
10-25	+1
Greater than 25	+2
Mucus	+1
Number of epithelial cells per low-power field	
10-25	−1
Greater than 25	−2
TOTAL SCORE	____

Scores of 0 or less indicate lack of inflammation or presence of saliva.

Gastrointestinal Tract

Specimens from the gastrointestinal tract may be cultured to diagnose the cause of gastroenteritis. Bacterial infections of the stomach are rare because of its acidic pH; thus most infections involve the intestines. The clinical symptoms of gastroenteritis include nausea, vomiting, and diarrhea. The nausea and vomiting usually result from the ingestion of preformed toxins instead of bacterial invasion.

The patient's history is of particular significance in determining the type of infection. The type and quality of food or water ingested, travel to areas with poor sanitation, recent antibiotic use, and knowledge of similar problems with family members are all important points to consider.

Stool specimens are preferred over rectal swabs. When examining for ova and parasites, the specimen should be analyzed as soon as possible. A direct examination of the stool for fecal white blood cells, parasites, and yeast can be performed. The presence of many leukocytes is often an indication of a bacterial infection. When a delay is anticipated, the specimen should be preserved in polyvinyl alcohol for the examination of ova and parasites.

When analysis of bacterial pathogens is required, an enrichment media such as selenite broth or gram-negative broth should be inoculated to enhance the isolation of the pathogen by inhibiting the growth of the normal flora enteric bacteria.

Urine

A urine culture may be requested to diagnose a urinary tract infection (UTI) of the upper or lower tract. Lower UTIs may involve the bladder (**cystitis**) or the urethra (**urethritis**). Such infections frequently ascend through the urethra and consist of normal flora coliforms that may be present in the periurethral flora. Other sources of infection include urinary catheters or other types of instrumentation, which may also involve the normal flora coliforms, or contaminating bacteria from health care personnel.

Upper UTIs include infections of the kidney, such as **pyelonephritis** and **glomerulonephritis.** In addition, the renal pelvis can be involved **(pyelitis)** as well as the ureters.

The specimen of choice for bacterial culture of urine is the **clean-catch midstream specimen.** A **routine** or **randomly voided specimen** is not acceptable due to the presence of contaminating bacteria from the periurethral and vaginal areas. In collection of the clean-catch midstream specimen, the periurethral area is cleansed with soap, sterile water, and sterile gauze using a front-to-back motion. The first few milliliters of the specimen is discarded to flush bacteria from the urethra. The "midstream" portion is collected into a sterile container.

A **catheterized specimen** may be used for bacterial culture only if the patient cannot void or if the catheter has been inserted for another medical reason. Urine is normally sterile in the bladder, and therefore a catheterized specimen should contain no bacteria. A catheter should never be inserted for the single purpose of bacterial culture, due to the risk of infection to the patient.

A **suprapubic aspiration** may be performed on infants and young children. Because this is an invasive technique, it is only performed when absolutely necessary. The skin is disinfected over the urinary bladder, and the area is locally anesthetized. A small incision with a surgical blade is made, and a needle is inserted into the bladder to withdraw the specimen. This procedure is reserved for patients who cannot be catheterized when a urine sample is urgently needed.

Uncultured urine should be refrigerated to minimize bacterial multiplication. Routine or randomly voided samples should be examined for contamination.

A **colony count** is performed on all urine samples submitted for bacterial culture. A 1 μl calibrated inoculating loop is used to deliver 1 μl (0.001 ml) of urine. The plate is incubated overnight and the number of colonies counted. The number is multiplied by 1000 to convert microliters to milliliters. The value obtained indicates the number of colonies per milliliter of urine. For example, if a 1 μl calibrated loop yields 145 colonies, the colony count is 145,000 or 1.45×10^5 colonies/ml urine. Values greater than 1.0×10^5 indicate infection. Values between 1.0×10^3 and 1.0×10^5 colonies/ml are considered to be contaminated or may represent cultures taken during the period of recovery from a UTI after antibiotics have been initiated.

Those organisms most frequently causing UTIs include the Enterobacteriaceae. The most common cause of UTIs is *E. coli,* which is associated with approximately 90% of all UTIs in ambulatory persons and also a large percentage of those occurring in hospitalized patients. Other members of the Enterobacteriaceae, including *Klebsiella, Proteus,* and *Enterobacter,* as well as *Enterococcus faecalis* and *P. aeruginosa,* are also associated with UTIs. *Staphylococcus saprophyticus* is known to cause UTIs with colony counts in a lower range of less than 1×10^5 colonies/ml.

Blood

Bacteremia refers to the presence of bacteria in blood, which is considered a sterile site. In **transient bacteremia,** normal flora bacteria may be introduced into the blood. For example, after brushing or cleaning the teeth, the viridans streptococci may be introduced into the blood. In **intermittent bacteremia,** bacteria are sporadically discharged from extravascular abscesses or infections into the blood. In **continuous bacteremia,** there is a constant release of bacteria into the blood from subacute bacterial endocarditis, contaminated indwelling catheters, or intravascular infections. Bacteremia is frequently accompanied by fever, chills, increased pulse rate, and decreased blood pressure.

The normal immune system clears bacteria from the blood within 30 to 45 minutes. This does not occur as readily in patients who are immunosuppressed or have overwhelming infections. In **septicemia** the circulating bacteria multiply faster than phagocytosis can occur, and multiple organs and body systems may be infected.

Even when bacteremia is significant, organisms in the blood are usually not of great enough numbers to be grown from a single specimen. As few as 1 to 10 bacteria per milliliter of blood can be associated with bacteremia. Also, the highest concentration of bacteria in the blood occurs *before* the fever spikes. Since this cannot be predicted, it is recommended to collect blood at two to three different venipuncture sites at least 1 hour apart. This serves to maximize the chances of isolating the organism.It is imperative to prepare the patient's skin properly before phlebotomy to ensure that no skin contaminants are collected. Typical methods include a 70% to 95% alcohol rinse to remove dirt, lipids, and fatty acids. A circular motion moving in to out is needed. This is followed by either a 2% iodine or iodophor scrub, which is left on for 1 minute. Next, a second alcohol rinse is applied. A second method uses a wash with green soap followed by a sterile water rinse. Tincture of iodine is applied and allowed to dry. The final step is the application of 70% alcohol.

Typically, 10 ml of blood is collected from adults during each phlebotomy, and approximately 1 to 5 ml is collected from children.

Cerebrospinal Fluid

Cerebrospinal fluid (CSF) is collected by lumbar puncture in the third or fourth lumbar vertebra by a physician. A local anesthetic is used, and a needle is inserted into the spinal canal. In most adults the collection consists of three tubes. Because the first two tubes may contain skin contaminants, it is usually recommended that the third tube be used for microbiology.

A normal CSF is clear and colorless, and on receipt in the laboratory the volume, color, and appearance should be recorded. The specimen should be screened immediately for the presence of bacteria or fungi by using a methylene blue or Gram stain. The presence of any microorganisms should be reported to the physician immediately.

There should be no delay in the processing or workup of CSF, since some of the organisms associated with **meningitis** are fastidious and prone to chilling or drying. These include *N. meningitidis* and *H. influenzae.* Delays must also be avoided because of the high mortality rate and rapid proliferation associated with the infection.

Genital Tract

Microorganisms associated with genital tract infections include Neisseria gonorrhoeae, herpes simplex virus type 2, Chlamydia trachomatis, and the parasite *Trichomonas vaginalis.* Some of these pathogens represent new syndromes and require new methods for identification. For example, kits specific for sexually transmitted diseases for gonorrhea and chlamydia are available. *Trichomonas* may be identified by a standard wet mount procedure. *N. gonorrhoeae* requires chocolate agar to grow. It is imperative to inoculate the media and incubate the plates in increased CO_2 soon after specimen collection to enhance the chances of recovery. Transport media, such as Gono-Pak or JEM-BEC,* may alternatively be used to provide proper nutrient and atmospheric requirements.

For the diagnosis of male urogenital infections, the urethral discharge is usually collected. In female patients, specimens of the uterine cervix, urethra, or cervix may be collected. Because of the abundance of normal flora in the female genital tract, it is important to use a plate selective for *N. gonorrhoeae,* such as Martin-Lewis or modified Thayer-Martin. Such media inhibit the normal flora and allow a better recovery of the pathogen.

Wound Cultures and Abscesses

It is generally preferred to collect specimens for wound culture using a needle and syringe to aspirate the drainage. This avoids the collection of normal flora and also enhances the recovery of anaerobes, which are often associated with wound infections and abscesses. The isolation of normal flora may hinder the recovery of both aerobic and anaerobic bacteria in such infections. **Exogenous** wound infections result from animal and human bites, burns, ulcers, and traumatic wounds (gunshot or stabbing). **Endogenous** wound infections may be attributed to bacterial sources within the patient and include cellulitis, dental infections, and septic arthritis. Many endogenous infections are nosocomial and occur as a result of contamination during an invasive procedure.

Specific guidelines related to the processing and culturing of each specimen type are addressed in more detail in Chapter 22.

SPECIMEN TRANSPORT AND PROCESSING

It is important to maintain the specimen as close to its original state as possible. Exposure to heat, cold, and drying should be avoided. In general, a 2-hour limit between collection and reception into the laboratory is required. If a delay is anticipated, a transport medium such as Stuart's should be used to increase the viability of the pathogen. The Stuart's system consists of swabs in a test tube with transport media that can be activated by crushing an ampule. The buffered semisolid agar, which contains sodium thioglycollate, can maintain bacteria for up to 72 hours. Amies is a modified Stuart's medium that can be used in its place. Cary-Blair medium is designed for the transport of stool speci-

---

**Gono-Pak, Becton Dickinson Microbiological Systems; JEM-BEC, James E. Martin Biological Environmental Chamber.*

mens and is recommended for the transport of enteric pathogens.

Because cotton swabs may release toxic fatty acids, calcium anginate or Dacron swabs are usually preferred for collection. Specimen collection devices are often incorporated into a transport medium. The medium is released by crushing an ampule after the swab has been inserted into the collection tube. Systems for both aerobes and anaerobics are commercially available.

The specimen should be examined for adherence to collection guidelines on receipt in the laboratory. If any violations exist, the physician or nurse should be notified. When possible, the specimen should be recollected. However, it is the physician's right to request analysis even when collections may not be correct. The laboratory should note any problems with collection on the requisition and report to ensure proper communication of results.

A **gross examination** of the specimen is performed. This includes examination of the color, volume, and appearance of the specimen. The gross examination may provide initial clues. For example, a cloudy CSF may indicate infection, and a rust-tinged sputum may indicate *Streptococcus pneumoniae.*

The ultimate identification of bacteria and its designation as normal flora or pathogen depend on proper specimen collection. Guidelines must be established and followed for proper specimen workup to provide the clinician with accurate results.

SELECTION AND INOCULATION OF PRIMARY MEDIA

Culture medium is a mixture of the nutrients needed by microorganisms. Most media contain an energy source, such as carbon, nitrogen, sulfur, phosphorus, hydrogen, oxygen, and buffers. In addition, various agents, such as dyes or antibiotics, may be added to either increase or decrease the viability of a particular organism or group of organisms.

Media in the liquid form are known as **broth.** When the medium is in a gel or semisolid form, it is known as **agar.** Most agar is solidified by using the red algae polysaccharide **agar agar.** Bacterial growth can be observed as discrete colonies on agar, which is essential to obtain isolated colonies or to enumerate colonies.

Several different classification methods for media exist. Table 3-1 summarizes some of the frequently used media and their purpose.

General isolation media, also known as **supportive media,** support the growth of most nonfastidious bacteria. Examples include nutrient agar, trypticase soy agar, and nutrient broth. No advantage is given to any group of bacteria.

Nonselective isolation media, also known as **enriched media,** contain a nutrient supplement. Examples include **sheep blood agar (SBA)** and **chocolate agar.** SBA has a trypticase soy agar base to which has been added 5% defibrinated sheep red blood cells. Other agar bases that can be used include Columbia agar and brain-heart infusion agar. Sheep blood is the preferred blood to use because other sources, such as horse blood, may give erratic results for hemolysis (see the box at left and Figure 3-2 [Color Plate 1]). For example, the enterococci of group D streptococci are nonhemolytic on sheep blood agar but beta hemolytic on rabbit, horse, or human blood agar. Sheep blood agar does not support the growth of *Haemophilus influenzae* or *Haemophilus haemolyticus.* The former requires NAD (nicotinamide dinucleotide, coenzyme I), which is destroyed by NADase in the sheep blood agar. The latter is considered normal flora of the oropharynx, and its beta-hemolytic properties may be misinterpreted as *Streptococcus pyogenes,* a pathogen.

Chocolate agar is prepared in a similar manner as blood agar, except the agar is either heated or enzyme treated to hemolyze the red blood cells. By doing so, the red blood cells are destroyed and NAD is released

Hemolytic Patterns

Alpha: incomplete; greening or browning of the medium

Beta: complete; total clearing of the medium

Gamma: nonhemolytic; no change in the color of the medium

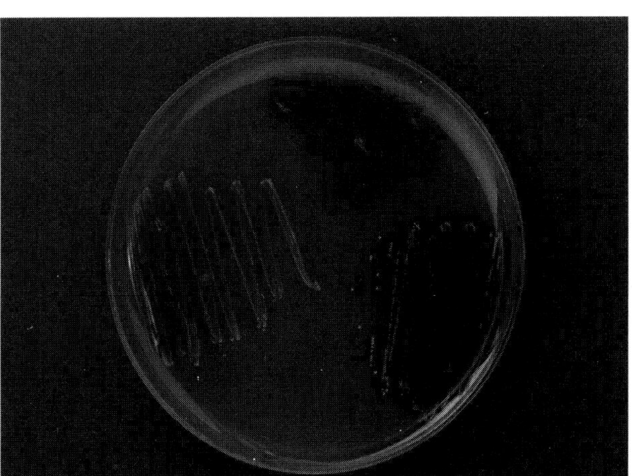

FIGURE 3–2
Hemolytic patterns on sheep blood agar (also see the box at left).

TABLE 3–1

Frequently Used Isolation Media

MEDIUM	PURPOSE
Sheep blood agar	Enriched, nonselective medium
Chocolate agar	Enriched, nonselective medium to isolate fastidious organisms, such as *Neisseria* and *Haemophilus*
Colistin–nalidixic acid	Isolation of gram-positive bacteria
Modified Thayer-Martin	Isolation of *Neisseria gonorrhoeae*
Martin-Lewis	Isolation of *N. gonorrhoeae*
MacConkey	Differential: isolation of gram-negative bacilli and differentiation of lactose fermenters from nonlactose fermenters
Eosin–methylene blue	Differential: isolation of gram-negative bacilli and differentiation of lactose fermenters from nonlactose fermenters
Hektoen enteric	Selective: isolation of stool pathogens through inhibition of normal flora coliforms
Salmonella-Shigella	Selective: isolation of stool pathogens through inhibition of normal flora coliforms
Xylose-lysine-deoxycholate	Selective: isolation of stool pathogens through inhibition of normal flora coliforms
Selenite broth	Enrichment broth to enhance recovery of stool pathogens and inhibit normal flora coliforms
Tetrathionate	Enrichment broth to enhance recovery of stool pathogens and inhibit normal flora coliforms
Gram-negative broth	Enrichment broth to enhance recovery of stool pathogens and inhibit normal flora coliforms
Anaerobic phenylethyl alcohol	Isolation of gram-positive and gram-negative anaerobes
Anaerobic kanamycin-vancomycin	Isolation of gram-negative anaerobes
Thioglycollate	Enriched broth that permits growth at various oxygen levels
Löwenstein-Jensen	Primary isolation medium for *Mycobacterium*
Petragnani	Primary isolation medium for *Mycobacterium*
Middlebrook	Primary isolation medium for *Mycobacterium*

from the cells. In addition, chocolate agar is enriched with IsoVitaleX, which contains dextrose, cysteine, vitamin B_{12}, thiamine, and ferric nitrate.

Chocolate agar supports the growth of fastidious bacteria, such as *N. gonorrhoeae* and *H. influenzae.*

Differential media provide distinct colonial appearances of microorganisms to aid in their identification. Most differential media are used to isolate gram-negative bacteria through the addition of (a) compound(s) that is (are) inhibitory for gram-positive bacteria. **MacConkey agar** contains lactose, bile salt, neutral red indicator, and crystal violet. The bile salt and crystal violet inhibit the growth of the gram-positive bacteria. If the organism can ferment lactose, the colonies appear pink to red in color. If the organism is unable to ferment lactose, the colonies appear clear. Another example is **eosin–methylene blue (EMB),** which contains lactose and the dyes eosin and methylene blue. The dyes are toxic to gram-positive bacteria and allow one to isolate gram-negative bacteria. In addition, bacteria that can ferment lactose cause the pH of the medium to decrease, which decreases the solubility of the methylene blue-eosin complex. This results in a purple color. Gram-negative bacteria that cannot ferment lactose appear clear on the medium. *E. coli* produces colonies with a unique green metallic sheen.

Some authors prefer to categorize MacConkey agar and EMB agar as **selective-differential,** since they "select" for gram-negative bacteria and "differentiate" lactose fermenters from lactose nonfermenters. These media are used interchangeably based on the laboratory's preference.

Enrichment broths are used to inhibit the growth of one organism while enhancing that of another organism. These broths are used most frequently for stool cultures to inhibit the normal flora bacteria, such as *E. coli,* so that pathogens, such as *Salmonella* and *Shigella,* can be isolated. Examples of such broths include gram-negative, selenite, and tetrathionate. **Gram-negative broth** contains bile salt in the form of sodium deoxycholate, which is toxic to gram-positive bacteria and inhibitory to the normal flora coliforms. **Selenite broth** contains sodium hydrogen selenite, which allows for the isolation of *Salmonella* and *Shigella.* **Tetrathionate broth** contains bile salts and sodium thiosulfate, which enhance the isolation of *Salmonella* and *Shigella.* All three media can be used interchangeably at the laboratory's preference.

Thioglycollate broth, another type of enrichment broth, contains thioglycolic acid as a reducing agent, a small percentage of agar to prevent oxygen from reaching all areas of the broth, and numerous nutrients, such as yeast and beef extracts, vitamins, and hemin. The medium allows for the differentiation of aerobes and anaerobes. For example, strict aerobes grow at the surface of the broth while facultative bacteria grow throughout the media. Anaerobes usually grow in the deeper portion of the tube, where the oxygen level is lowest.

Selective media allow one to select for pathogens through the inhibition of normal flora. Examples include **Hektoen enteric (HE) agar, *Salmonella-Shigella* (SS) agar,** and **xylose-lysine-deoxycholate (XLD) agar.** All these media selectively inhibit gram-positive bacteria and gram-negative coliform bacteria and permit the isolation of stool pathogens. HE medium contains lactose, sucrose, salicin, sodium thiosulfate, ferric ammonium citrate, and bromthymol blue indicator. Organisms that ferment one or more of the carbohydrates will appear as yellow-orange colonies while nonfermenters appear green or blue in color. The medium also permits the differentiation of hydrogen sulfide-producing bacteria (black precipitate) from those that cannot produce hydrogen sulfide. SS medium contains lactose, bile salts, sodium thiosulfate, neutral red indicator, and ferric citrate. It allows for the differentiation of lactose fermenters from nonfermenters, as well as the detection of hydrogen sulfide producers. XLD contains xylose, lysine, lactose, sucrose, phenol red indicator, sodium deoxycholate, sodium thiosulfate, and ferric ammonium citrate. The medium is selective for gram-negative enteric pathogens and allows for the detection of xylose fermentation, lysine decarboxylation, and hydrogen sulfide production.

Antibiotic media are selective for a certain group of bacteria through the addition of specific antibiotics. Examples include **colistin–nalidixic acid (CNA)** and **modified Thayer-Martin (MTM).** CNA contains sheep blood agar base with the antibiotics colistin and naladixic acid added. Colistin (polymyxin E) disrupts the cell membrane of gram-negative organisms while nalidixic acid blocks DNA replication in gram-negative bacteria. Thus CNA allows for the selection of gram-positive bacteria.

MTM is a chocolate agar base with the antibiotics vancomycin, colistin, nystatin, and trimethoprim lactate added. The medium selectively isolates *N. gonorrhoeae.* Vancomycin inhibits gram-positive bacteria through interference with cell wall synthesis, colistin inhibits gram-negative bacteria by interfering with synthesis of the cell wall, and nystatin is inhibitory to yeast. Trimethoprim inhibits the swarming of *Proteus.* **Martin-Lewis medium,** also selective for *N. gonorrhoeae,* contains similar components to MTM, except anisomycin replaces nystatin as the yeast inhibitor.

Primary plating media are usually selected on the basis of specimen type. The growth requirements of those bacteria most often isolated from a particular site must be met. For example, since most UTIs are caused by gram-negative bacilli, such as *E. coli,* it is imperative that a differential plate be inoculated. Since most throat cultures are performed to determine the presence of *S. pyogenes,* it is essential to inoculate a blood agar plate.

In addition, it is essential to obtain isolated colonies for biochemical and serological testing. Streaking an agar plate for isolation can be accomplished using several different methods. For all methods, when using sheep blood agar, it is important to "stab" the medium and force some of the growth into the medium to observe for subsurface hemolysis (see the Procedure box on pp. 32-33).

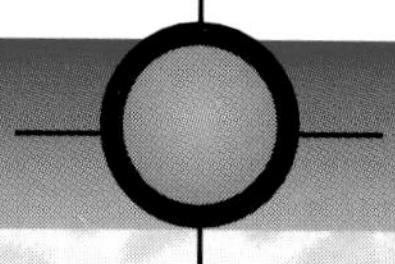

PROCEDURE

STREAKING FOR ISOLATION

Method A can be used on either liquid specimens (such as urine) or swabs.

1. Transfer a drop of the liquid specimen using a sterile pipette to a corner of the agar plate. Swabs are plated directly by rolling over an area in the corner of the plate.
2. Sterilize the wire loop and pass it through the initial inoculum several times, streaking the top quarter of the plate into the second quadrant. This is streak area 1.
3. Rotate the plate 90 degrees and repeat the streaking from the second quadrant into the third quadrant. This is streak area 2.
4. Rotate the plate again 90 degrees and continue the streaking from the third quadrant into the fourth quadrant. This is streak area 3. Flame between quadrants unless inoculum is light.

This method can be semiquantitated by using the following scale:

GROWTH RATING	QUADRANT 2	3	4
1+	*Less than 10*		
2+	*More than 10*	*Less than 5*	
3+	*More than 10*	*More than 5*	*Less than 5*
4+	*More than 10*	*More than 5*	*More than 5*

1 2 3 4

Method B can be used for cultures in heavy broth or solid media.

1. Streak specimen or inoculum in top quarter of plate.
2. With sterile loop, make a light sweep through inoculated area and streak entire top quarter of plate with parallel strokes. Sterilize loop.
3. Turn plate 90 degrees and make a light sweep into lower portion of area streaked in step 2. Streak as in step 2, covering approximately one half of remaining plate.
4. Turn plate 180 degrees and streak remaining plate with sterilized loop. Avoid any previously streaked areas.

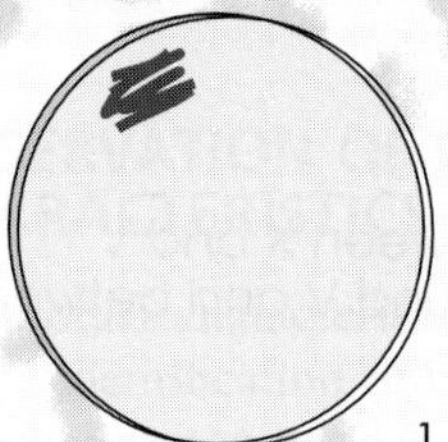
1

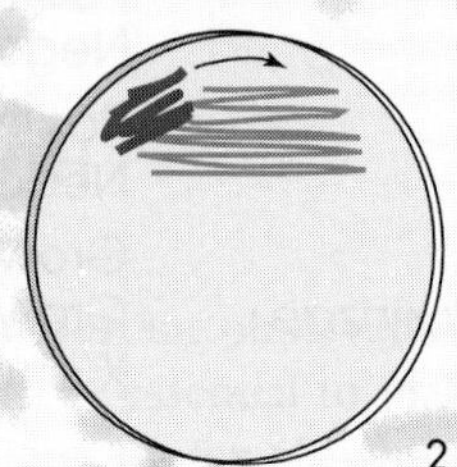
2

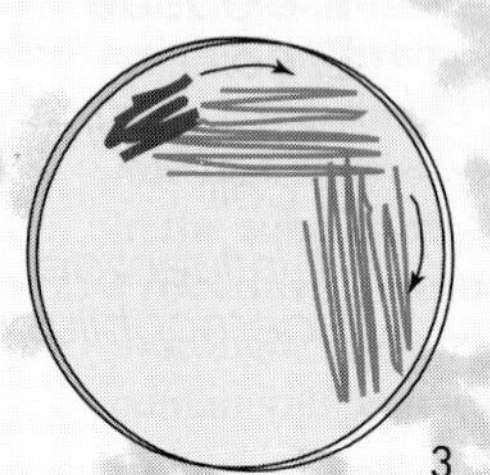
3

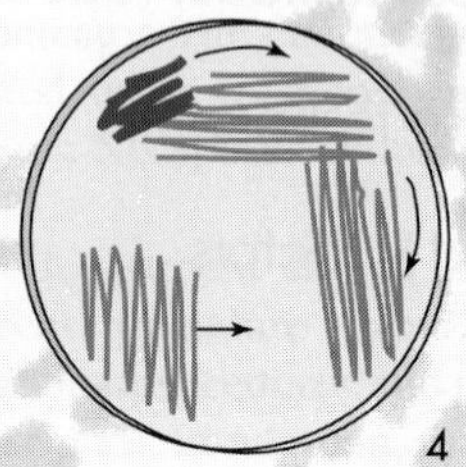
4

PROCEDURE
STREAKING FOR ISOLATION
(Continued)

Method C is a method preferred by some microbiologists for broth cultures.

1. Apply a loopful of inoculum near periphery of plate. Cover approximately one fourth of the plate with close parallel streaks. Sterilize loop.
2. Make one light sweep through lower portion of streaked area. Turn plate 90 degrees and streak approximately one half of remaining plate.
3. Turn plate 180 degrees and streak remainder of plate. Avoid any previously streaked areas.

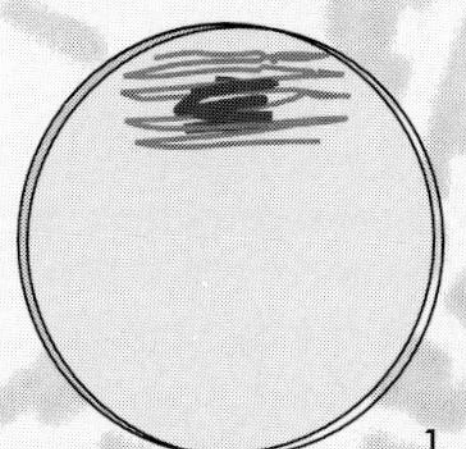

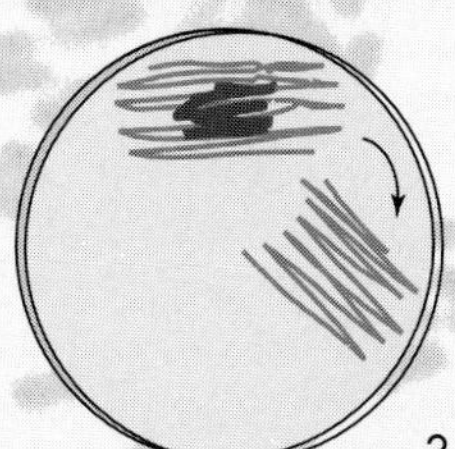

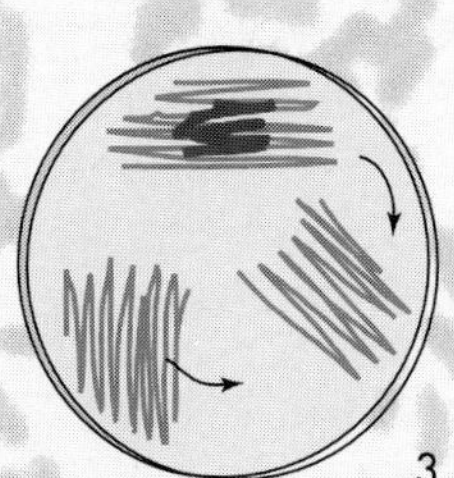

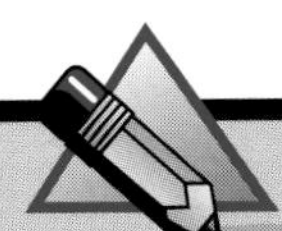

REVIEW QUESTIONS

MATCHING

Match the medium with its classification (some responses may be used more than once):

_____ **1. Modified Thayer-Martin agar**
_____ **2. Colistin–nalidixic acid agar**
_____ **3. MacConkey agar**
_____ **4. Hektoen enteric agar**
_____ **5. Blood agar**
_____ **6. Eosin–methylene blue agar**
_____ **7. Chocolate agar**

a. Enriched, nonselective
b. Differential recovery of gram-negative bacilli
c. Selective for fecal pathogens
d. Antibiotic, selects for gram-positive bacteria
e. Antibiotic, selects for pathogenic *Neisseria*

MULTIPLE CHOICE

8. Complete hemolysis of blood is known as:
a. Alpha hemolysis
b. Beta hemolysis
c. Gamma hemolysis
d. Synergistic hemolysis

9. The specimen of choice for bacterial culture of urine is a:
a. Clean-catch midstream
b. Catheterized sample
c. Suprapubic
d. Routine void

Continued.

REVIEW QUESTIONS
(Continued)

10. The optimal wound specimen for culture of anaerobic organisms should be:
a. A swab of lesion obtained before administration of antibiotics
b. A swab of lesion obtained after administration of antibiotics
c. A syringe filled with pus obtained before administration of antibiotics
d. A syringe filled with pus obtained after administration of antibiotics

11. A throat swab is submitted for anaerobic culture. This specimen should be:
a. Set up immediately
b. Rejected
c. Inoculated into thioglycollate broth
d. Sent to a reference laboratory

12. A spinal fluid specimen is submitted for Gram stain and culture during an afternoon shift. The physician also requests that an aliquot be saved for possible serological studies, which are only performed on day shift. The most correct action is:
a. Inoculate culture, perform a Gram stain, and refrigerate remaining spinal fluid.
b. Inoculate culture, perform a Gram stain, and incubate remaining spinal fluid at 35° to 37°C.
c. Incubate entire specimen at 35° to 37°C and perform culture and Gram stain the next day.
d. Refrigerate entire specimen and perform culture and Gram stain the next day.

13. The general guidelines for collection of blood cultures state:
a. Disinfect skin with an alcohol swab only.
b. Large amounts of bacteria are required to cause bacteremia.
c. Two to three sets per 24 hours are usually sufficient to diagnose bacteremia.
d. One specimen per 24 hours is sufficient to diagnose bacteremia.

14. Prompt delivery of specimens for microbiology is essential for accurate culture workup. Which of the following is *not* a consequence of delay in specimen delivery?
a. Normal flora may overgrow pathogen.
b. Fastidious organisms may no longer be viable.
c. Swabs may dry out, resulting in loss of pathogens.
d. Normal flora may no longer be isolated.

15. Optimal collection time to diagnose gastrointestinal infection caused by bacterial or viral pathogens is:
a. Any time during the course of the illness
b. During the acute stage of the illness
c. During the convalescent stage of the illness
d. Through collection of serum to identify type-specific antibodies

16. Which of the following is *not* considered to be a sterile site?
a. Blood
b. Urinary bladder
c. Spinal fluid
d. Oral cavity

17. An abdominal abscess specimen received in the laboratory produced abundant growth when grown anaerobically but produced no growth when the culture plates were incubated aerobically. This culture contains:
a. An obligate aerobe
b. An obligate anaerobe
c. A facultative anaerobe
d. None of the above

18. The optimal time to collect blood cultures is:
a. Shortly before the fever spikes
b. While the fever spikes
c. Shortly after the fever spikes
d. No more than one set daily

19. Most pathogenic bacteria prefer an incubation temperature of:
a. 30° to 32°C
b. 33° to 35°C
c. 35° to 37°C
d. 42° to 45°C

20. Those bacteria that prefer growth under increased CO_2 are known as
a. Mesophiles
b. Microaerophiles
c. Capnophilic
d. Facultative anaerobes

21. Which of the following should be monitored as part of the quality control program in the microbiology laboratory?
a. Temperature of incubators and refrigerators
b. Plating media with known positive and negative controls
c. Oxygen content and CO_2 content of incubators
d. All the above

BIBLIOGRAPHY

Baron EJ, Peterson LR, and Finegold SM: Selection, collection, and transport of specimens for microbiologic examination. In *Bailey and Scott's diagnostic microbiology,* ed 9, St Louis, 1994, Mosby.

Bartlett RC: Making optimum use of the microbiology laboratory. II. Urine, respiratory, wound and cervicovaginal exudate, *JAMA* 247:1336, 1982.

Campos JM, McNamara AM, Howard BJ: Specimen collection and processing. In Howard BJ et al, editors: *Clinical and pathogenic microbiology,* ed 2, St Louis, 1993, Mosby.

Collingnon P, Munro R: Limitations of semiquantitative methods for catheter culture, *J Clin Microbiol* 26:1074, 1988.

Difco Laboratories: Difco Manual, ed 10, Detroit, 1984, Difco.

Estevez EG: Bacteriologic plate media: review of mechanisms of action, *Lab Med* 15:4, 1984.

Gray LD, Fedorko DP: Laboratory diagnosis of bacterial meningitis, *Clin Microbiol Rev* 5:130, 1992.

Gross PA, Flower M, Barden G: Polymicrobic bactinuria: significance associated with bacteremia, *J Clin Microbiol* 3:246, 1976.

Johnson C: Definitions, classification, and clinical presentation of urinary tract infections, *Med Clin North Am* 75:241, 1991.

Lauer BA, Reller LB, Mirrett S: Comparison of acridine orange and Gram stains for detection of microorganisms in cerebrospinal fluid and other clinical specimens, *J Clin Microbiol* 14:201, 1981.

Lipsky B, Ireton RC, Fihn SC et al: Diagnosis of bacteriuria in men: specimen collection and culture interpretation, *J Infect Dis* 155:847, 1987.

Merrick TA: Specimen quality assurance for the microbiology laboratory, *Lab Med* 13:498, 1982.

Miller JM: *Handbook of specimen collection and handling in microbiology,* Atlanta, 1987, US Dept of Health and Human Services, Centers for Disease Control.

National Committee for Clinical Laboratory Standards: *Standard procedures for the handling and transport of diagnostic specimens and etiologic agents,* H5-A2, Villanova, Pa, 1985, NCCLS.

Tenney JH, Reller LB, Mirrett S, et al: Controlled evaluation of the volume of blood cultured in the detection of bacteremia and fungemia, *J Clin Microbiol* 15:558, 1982.

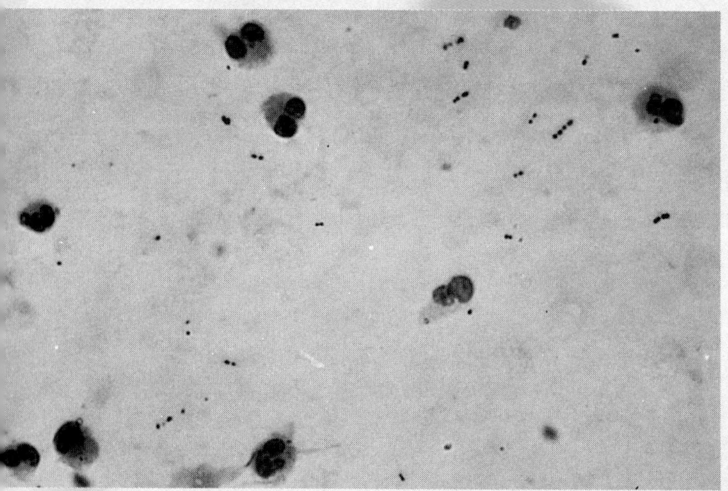

STREPTOCOCCUS PNEUMONIAE

CHAPTER OUTLINE

DIRECT EXAMINATION METHODS

STAINING METHODS

- Acid-Fast Stains
- Fluorescent Stains
- Fungal Stains
- Antibody-Conjugated Stains

KEY TERMS

BRIGHTFIELD MICROSCOPY

DARKFIELD MICROSCOPY

FLUORESCENT MICROSCOPY

GRAM STAIN

PHASE-CONTRAST MICROSCOPY

Microscopic Methods of Examination

LEARNING OBJECTIVES

1. Recognize and state the function of the following parts of the compound microscope:
   a. Ocular
   b. Objectives
   c. Condenser
   d. Iris diaphragm
2. Describe the use of darkfield microscopy in clinical microbiology.
3. Explain the principle of fluorescent microscopy.
4. State the purpose of each of the following direct methods of examination:
   a. Saline mount
   b. Hanging drop
   c. Iodine mount
   d. Potassium hydroxide preparation
   e. Nigrosin
   f. Neufeld (Quellung) reaction
5. Prepare smears from stock cultures or clinical specimens without error.
6. State the reagents used in the Gram stain and the function of each.
   a. Perform Gram stains on stock cultures or clinical specimens without error.
   b. Interpret Gram stains to include the shape, morphology, and Gram stain reaction.
7. Name the stains used to stain *Mycobacterium* and explain why these bacteria are termed *acid-fast bacilli.*
8. Name two fluorescent stains and state the purpose of each.
9. Describe the use of antibody-conjugated stains in clinical microbiology.

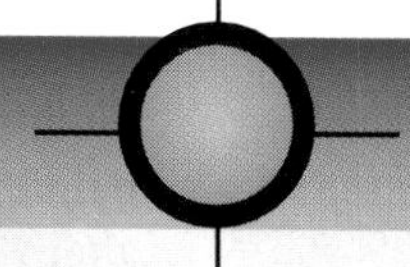

PROCEDURE
GRAM STAIN

PURPOSE

To categorize bacteria as gram positive or gram negative and to observe the cellular morphology. The Gram stain is also a valuable tool in the direct observation of clinical material.

PRINCIPLE

Bacteria will differentially retain the primary stain based on the characteristics of the cell wall. Gram-positive bacteria, with a high content of peptidoglycan and teichoic acid, retain the primary stain and appear blue to purple. Gram-negative bacteria, with a high content of lipopolysaccharide in the cell wall, lose the primary stain during decolorization. Gram-negative bacteria take up the counterstain and appear pink to red.

MATERIALS

Crystal violet
Gram's iodine
Acetone or ethyl alcohol
Safranin O
95% methanol

PROCEDURE

1. Prepare a thin smear of the culture or specimen to be observed. Allow the smear to air dry and heat fix. Alternatively fix the smear by flooding with 95% methanol and allowing to air dry
2. Overlay smear with crystal violet for 30 seconds to 1 minute
3. Rinse with distilled water, tapping off excess
4. Flood smear with Gram's iodine for 1 minute
5. Rinse with distilled water, tapping off excess
6. Add acetone or ethyl alcohol to decolorize drop by drop until no violet color appears in rinse. This requires less than 10 seconds
7. Rinse with distilled water immediately
8. Flood smear with safranin O for 30 seconds
9. Rinse with distilled water and allow slide to drain
10. Blot dry with paper towel (bulbous paper) or air dry for delicate smears
11. Examine each slide under oil immersion objective for characteristic Gram stain reaction, morphology, white blood cells, and other important structures.

INTERPRETATION

Gram-positive organisms stain blue-purple.
Gram-negative organisms stain pink-red.

PROCEDURE
GRAM STAIN
(Continued)

QUALITY CONTROL
Prepare a mixed suspension of *Staphylococcus* and *Escherichia coli* in saline. Place a drop on the surface of the slide and allow to air-dry. Fix and stain smear as in above method.

Results
Staphylococcus appear as purple cocci in clusters.
E. coli appears as pink bacilli.

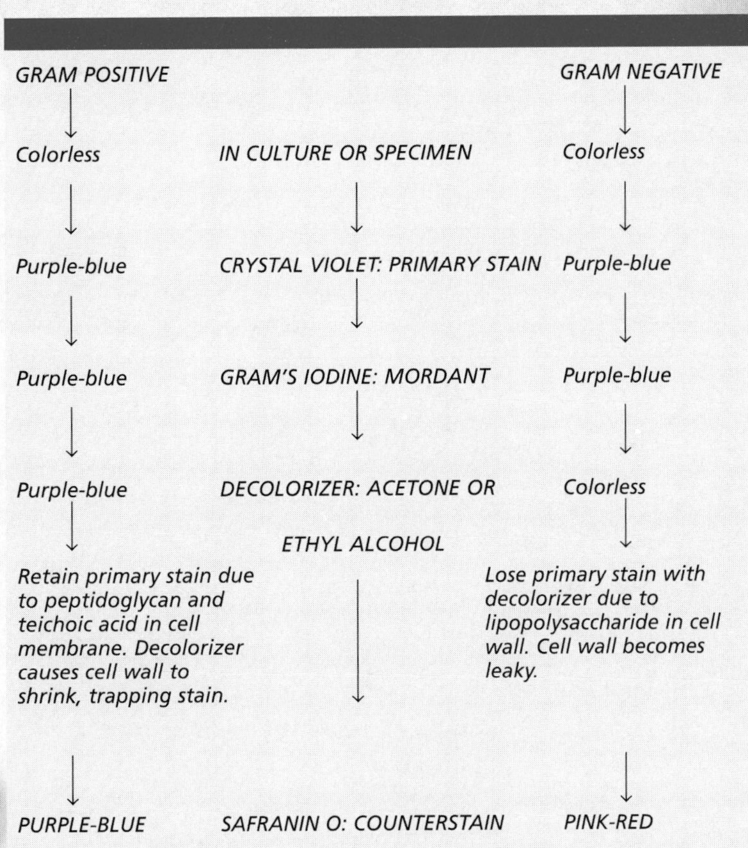

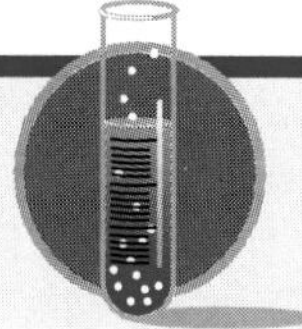

LABORATORY EXERCISES

1

Prepare one smear of each of the following specimens. Perform a Gram stain on each. Observe your stains under the oil immersion lens. Record your results.

a. *Staphylococcus epidermidis* ______

b. *Streptococcus pneumoniae* ______

c. *Enterococcus faecalis* ______

d. *Escherichia coli* ______

e. *Moraxella catarrhalis* ______

f. *Bacillus subtilis* ______

2

Observe prepared acid-fast smears. Record your results. ______

3

Observe the following prepared smears and describe your findings.

a. Sputum ______

b. Stool ______

c. Wound ______

d. Blood ______

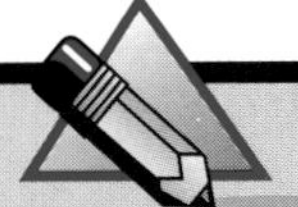

REVIEW QUESTIONS

MATCHING

Match the direct method of examination with its purpose:

____ 1. Iodine mount
____ 2. Nigrosin
____ 3. Potassium hydroxide preparation
____ 4. Hanging drop

a. Motility
b. Fungal elements
c. Parasitic nuclei
d. Capsules
e. *Trichomonas vaginalis*

MULTIPLE CHOICE

5. The oil immersion objective provides a *total* specimen magnification of:
a. 10×
b. 100×
c. 450×
d. 1000×

6. The higher the numerical aperture, the lower the resolving power of the microscope.
a. True
b. False

7. The function of the ____ is to gather and focus light rays on the specimen.
a. Objective
b. Iris diaphram
c. Condenser
d. Ocular

8. Darkfield microscopy is most often used to study:
a. Fungi
b. Mycobacteria
c. Parasitic nuclei
d. Spirochetes

9. The typical morphology of *Staphylococcus* is:
a. Cocci in chains
b. Cocci in clusters
c. Filamentous bacilli
d. Coccibacilli

10. In the Gram stain technique, Gram's iodine functions as the:
a. Primary stain
b. Mordant
c. Decolorizer
d. Counterstain

11. Gram-positive bacteria stain blue to purple.
a. True
b. False

12. The dye used to stain *Mycobacterium* is:
a. Methylene blue
b. Crystal violet
c. Carbolfuchsin
d. Iodine

13. Which of the following is *not* used to stain fungal mycelium?
a. Calcofluor white
b. Lactophenol cotton blue
c. Carbolfuchsin
d. Periodic acid–Schiff

BIBLIOGRAPHY

American Optical: AO series 150 reference manual, Buffalo, NY, Scientific Instrument Division, American Optical.

Barenfanger JE, Dick BW, Rabinovich S: Significance of visualization of bacteria in blood smears, *Lab Med* 21:579, 1990.

Baron EJ, Peterson LR, and Finegold SM: Optical methods for laboratory diagnosis of infectious diseases. In *Bailey and Scott's diagnostic microbiology,* ed 9, St Louis, 1994, Mosby.

Douglas SD: Microscopy. In Lenette EH, editor: *Manual of clinical microbiology,* ed 4, Washington, DC, 1985, American Society for Microbiology.

Glossary of optical terms, Buffalo, NY, Microscopy and Scientific Instruments Division, Leica.

Phase contrast equipment according to Zernike. In Leitz reference manual, Midland, Ontario, Canada, Leitz.

Rice-Spearman L: The Gram stain: still a diagnostic tool? *Clin Lab Sci* 6:16, 1993.

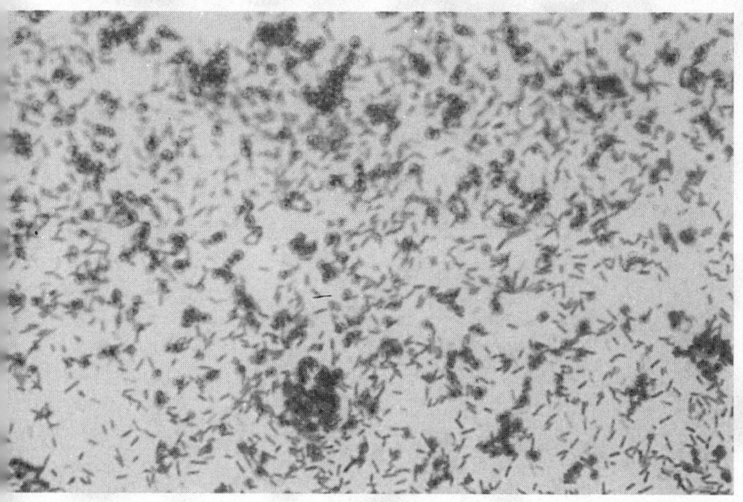

BACTINURIA

CHAPTER OUTLINE

MULTITEST SYSTEMS

AUTOMATION
- Fully Automated Systems
- Blood Culture Systems
- Automated Urine Screening Methods

IMMUNOSEROLOGICAL METHODS
- Agglutination
- Enzyme-Linked Immunosorbent Assay (ELISA)
- Immunofluorescence

INTRODUCTION TO MOLECULAR TECHNIQUES

KEY TERMS

ACUTE PHASE SPECIMEN
AGGLUTINATION
ANTIBODY TITER
COLORIMETRY
CONVALESCENT PHASE SPECIMEN
COUNTERIMMUNOELECTROPHORESIS
DIRECT AGGLUTINATION
DIRECT IMMUNOFLUORESCENCE
ENZYME-LINKED IMMUNOSORBENT ASSAY (ELISA)
FLUOROMETRIC
GENETIC PROBE
IMMUNOSEROLOGICAL METHODS
INDIRECT AGGLUTINATION
INDIRECT IMMUNOFLUORESCENCE
MONOCLONAL ANTIBODY
MULTITEST SYSTEMS
NEPHELOMETRY
NEUTRALIZATION
NUCLEIC ACID HYBRIDIZATION
POLYMERASE CHAIN REACTION (PCR)

Miscellaneous Methods in Identification

AUTOMATION AND IMMUNOSEROLOGY

CHAPTER FIVE

LEARNING OBJECTIVES

1. Discuss the use of miniaturized, multitest systems in the microbiology laboratory.
2. State the principle of colorimetry, and explain how it is used in semi-automated and automated identification systems.
3. State the principle of nephelometry, and explain how it is used in semi-automated and automated identification systems.
4. List at least two semi-automated identification systems.
5. For each of the following automated identification systems, state the principle(s) of operation and capabilities:
   a. Vitek
   b. AutoSCAN W/A
   c. Aladin
6. Describe and compare the Bactec and BacT/Alert with respect to principle and capabilities.
7. List two automated urine screening methods.
8. Discuss the significance of collecting both an acute phase and a convalescent phase specimen for serological testing.
   a. Define titer.
   b. Indicate the rise in titer that is necessary to diagnose a current infection.
9. For each of the following immunoserological methods, state the principle and discuss the application of the test to clinical microbiology:
   a. Agglutination
   b. Coagglutination
   c. Enzyme-linked immunosorbent assay
   d. Immunofluorescence: direct and indirect
10. Briefly describe molecular methods that are available in clinical microbiology.

Conventional methods to identify microorganisms have been the mainstay in clinical microbiology for several years. These methods rely on the use of several organic substrates, their reaction with microbial enzymes, and the determination of metabolic end products. These systems may incorporate a pH indicator whose color changes in a positive reaction. Numerous biochemical tests are available, but because these tests are cumbersome to inoculate and often require incubation periods of 24 to 48 hours, alternative testing methods have evolved.

Several conventional methods have been adapted into a rapid format. These methods often involve paper disks or strips that are impregnated with reagent or substrate. Such methods may utilize a large concentration of substrate or a heavy inoculum. Examples include the spot oxidase test, which can detect the enzyme cytochrome oxidase, and the spot indole test, which uses filter paper impregnated with paradimethylaminobenzaldehyde (Kovac's reagent). A loopful of the organism is rubbed onto the filter paper, and a red color indicating a positive reaction results within 20 to 30 seconds.

MULTITEST SYSTEMS

Several miniaturized, **multitest systems** have been developed that have converted multistep procedures into single-step procedures. These include the Minitek system (BBL of Becton Dickinson Microbiology Systems), which utilizes a multiwell plate with filter paper disks impregnated with various substrates. Minitek systems (Figure 5-1 [Color Plate 8]) are available for the identification of Enterobacteriaceae, anaerobes, and *Neisseria.* The specific reactions can be chosen by the user; when used with a heavy inoculum, the results can be read within 4 hours. The API systems (bioMérieux Vitek), including the API 20E for Enterobacteriaceae and nonfermentative gram-negative bacilli, API 20S for streptococci, API 20C for yeast identification, and API 20A for anaerobe identification, as well as the Rapid NFT for nonfermentative gram-negative bacilli, utilize dried reagents that are inoculated with a heavy suspension. Results may be read in 4 to 6 hours for rapidly metabolizing bacteria while other results can be read in 18 hours. After interpretation of reactions, a profile number is determined that can be matched with that in a profile index from a data base. Some of these systems are illustrated in Figure 5-2 (Color Plate 9).

Other multitest systems include the Enterotube II for identification of Enterobacteriaceae and the Oxi-Ferm tube for nonfermenters. These systems (Becton Dickinson Microbiology Systems) contain several small pieces of agar substrates in a long plastic tube (Figure 5-3 [Color Plate 10]). The entire tube is inoculated with a long wire that is enclosed in the system. After incubation and interpretation of results, a profile number is determined that can be matched to a data base.

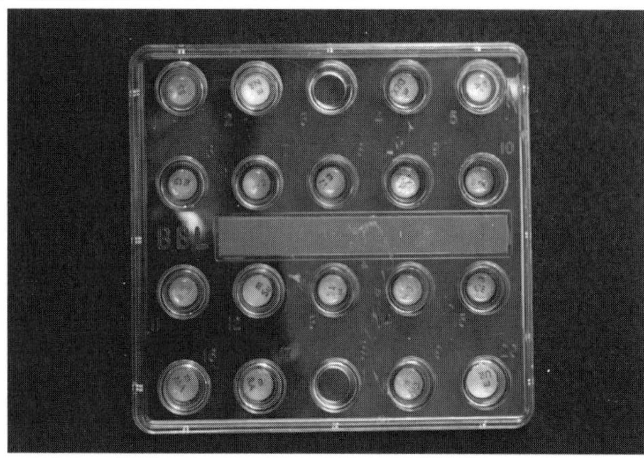

FIGURE 5-1
Minitek system is a miniaturized, multitest system for the identification of Enterobacteriaceae, anaerobes, and *Neisseria.* The system uses filter paper disks impregnated with various substrates. (Becton Dickinson Microbiology Systems.)

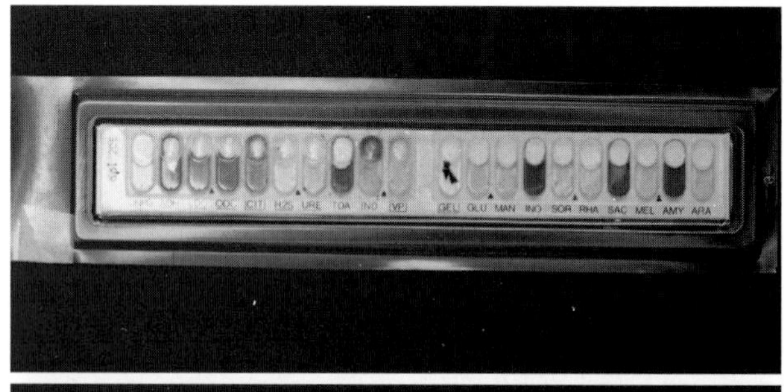

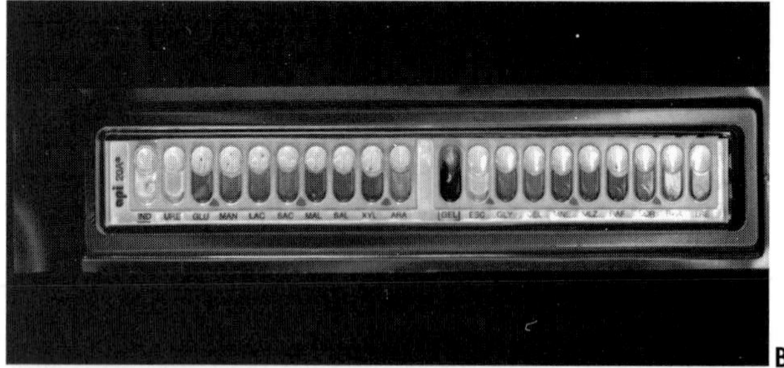

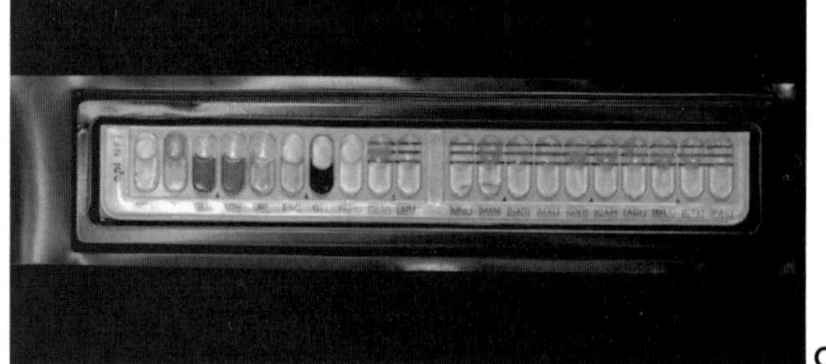

FIGURE 5-2
A, API 20E for identification of Enterobacteriaceae, **B,** API 20A for identification of anaerobes, and **C,** NFT for identification of nonfermentative gram-negative bacilli. Miniaturized, multitest systems use dehydrated reagents; a profile number is determined after interpretation of reactions and compared with profile numbers in extensive data bases. (bioMérieux Vitek.)

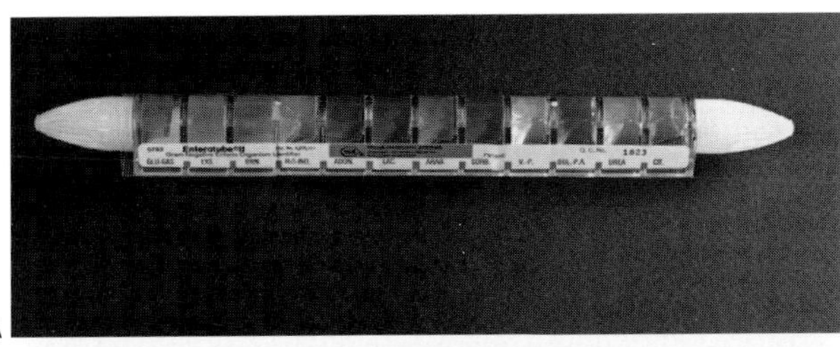

A

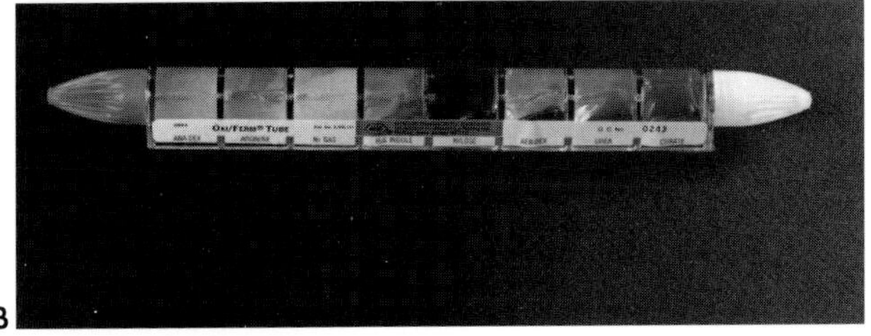

B

FIGURE 5–3

Enterotube **(A)** and Oxi-Ferm **(B)** multitest systems, which feature small pieces of agar substrates and an inoculation wire that is contained within the system. (Becton Dickinson Microbiology Systems.)

Other agar-based multitest identification systems include the Enteric-Tek for identification of Enterobacteriaceae, Uni-N/F-Tek for identification of nonfermentative gram-negative bacilli, Uni-Yeast-Tek for yeast, and Anaerobe-Tek for anaerobes. These systems are manufactured by Remel.

Several of these systems have been adapted as a part of semi-automated procedures that may aid in inoculation, incubation, interpretation, and reporting of results. These systems provide for shorter incubation and reaction times and for more reliable, reproducible results with the identification of a greater number of organisms.

AUTOMATION

Semi-automated systems usually involve a plastic tray with various substrates contained in multiple wells. These systems are available both for the identification of microorganisms and for antibiotic susceptibility testing, including qualitative results and determination of the minimal inhibitory concentration (MIC). Many of these systems have a computer module with software available from the manufacturer to aid in the reporting of results. The panels can be either inoculated manually or automatically. Often, a multipronged inoculator is used.

Semi-automated systems usually rely on the principles of **colorimetry** or **nephelometry.** Colorimetry uses a spectrophotometer to measure a color change in the pH indicator as an organism metabolizes a particular substrate. Nephelometry is based on the principle of light scattering. It is usually used for antibiotic susceptibility testing. As an organism grows, the well becomes turbid. Photometers are placed at angles to the turbid suspension, and the scattering of light is measured. Alternatively, the absorbance of the solution can be measured. The percentage of light transmitted through the solution is compared with that transmitted through a clear control well. Substrates are either dehydrated or freeze-dried and are inoculated with a standard concentration of inoculum. Incubation times may vary from 4 to 24 hours, and results are read either manually or automatically. The identification is made through comparison with a data base.

An example of a semi-automated system is the Pasco MIC/ID (Difco Laboratories). The principle of the system is colorimetry, and results can be read in 16 to 20 hours. Frozen microtiter panels are used for the identification and antibiotic susceptibility testing of gram-negative and gram-positive bacteria. The panels are manually inoculated using a multipronged disposable inoculator. Trays typically have 20 to 30 different substrates to determine fermentation, hydrolysis, and other biochemical reactions. The MicroMedia system (MSI/MicroMedia Systems) is very similar to the Pasco system.

The Sceptor system (Becton Dickinson Microbiology Systems) resembles the Pasco system except it utilizes dehydrated panels. It uses the principles of colorimetry and turbidity. The Sceptor system provides for the identification of gram-positive and gram-negative bacteria, as well as anaerobes. Susceptibility testing for gram-negative and gram-positive bacteria are also a part of the system. Inoculation is facilitated through an automated, multitip pipette.

The Sensititre system (Radiometer America) uses the principle of fluorometry to identify and determine antibiotic susceptibility of both gram-negative and gram-positive bacteria. Because of the **fluorometric** procedure, results can be read as quickly as 5 hours. Twenty-four biochemical tests are provided; all substrates have a fluorescent component. If the organism has the enzyme to metabolize a substrate, fluorescence results. In some reactions, fluorescence is used to detect a change in pH. For example, the pH increases a positive decarboxylase reaction that causes the production of fluorescence. Alternatively, in other reactions, an acidic pH would be noted by the lack of fluorescence.

Fully Automated Systems

Currently, three fully automated microbiology systems are available: the Vitek (bioMérieux Vitek), the AutoSCAN W/A (Walkaway 40 and Walkaway 96) available from the MicroScan Division of Baxter Health Care Corporation, and the Aladin (Automated Laboratory Diagnostic Instrument), also manufactured by bioMérieux Vitek.

The Vitek (Figure 5-4) identifies most clinically significant bacteria and yeast and also performs qualitative and quantitative antibiotic susceptibility tests. Plastic cards containing 30 wells with various substrates to

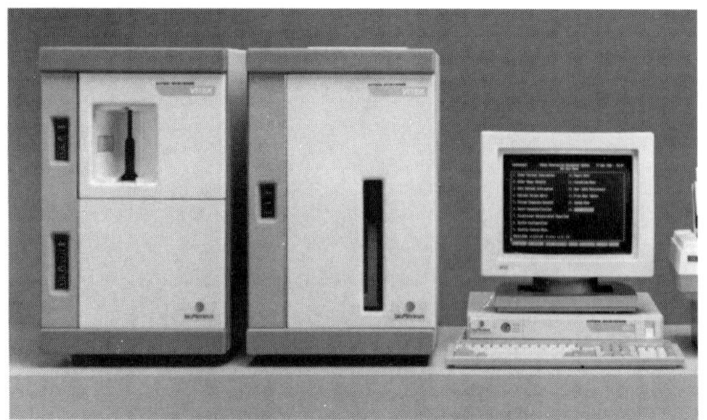

FIGURE 5–4
Fully automated Vitek identification system. (bioMérieux Vitek.)

identify and perform antibiotic susceptibility tests on the microorganisms are used. Plastic identification test cards are available for the following microorganisms: gram-negative bacteria, gram-positive bacteria, *Neisseria* and *Haemophilus,* yeast, and anaerobes. There is also a test card for the enumeration and identification of urine pathogens and an enteric pathogen screen card.

The Vitek has several modules, including a reader/incubator module, which has a capacity of 30, 60, 120, or 240 cards depending on the specific Vitek model. The card-filling unit inoculates test cards in a vacuumized, repressurization procedure. The sealer module seals the test cards after the inoculation procedure. The card-filling and card-sealing modules can hold one to eight trays, each capable of holding 30 test cards. The reader/incubator processes and incubates the cards at 35°C and monitors each card optically once an hour for data collection. The computer module stores, analyzes, and interprets test data and also controls reader/incubator functions. The data terminal and printer module allow the visual examination of results and provide an automatic printed copy of results.

The inoculum is prepared from a growing isolate, and the cards are inoculated automatically. The card is placed in the reader/incubator module, where it is scanned by a series of emitted diodes. The light source directs light through the wells to the reader. The data are sent to a computer, which records and interprets the readings. Changes in absorbance resulting from changes in turbidity as the organism grows or from color changes that occur as the pH changes are measured. Readings are taken from each well once per hour, and the change in percent transmittance of light is determined. The change in transmission of light is compared with a preset threshold value for each well. Values greater than or equal to the threshold value are considered to be positive reactions, whereas values less than the threshold are considered to be negative until the next reading.

The Vitek also can be used for antibiotic susceptibility testing for gram-positive and gram-negative organisms. A gram-positive or gram-negative susceptibility card is inoculated, and the reader measures the amount of light passing through each well hourly for 15 hours. As the organism grows, the amount of light transmitted decreases. Increased turbidity and resulting decreased transmission of light usually indicate the organism is resistant to the antibiotic. A growth curve is developed based on the decline of percent transmission. MICs can be determined based on the growth curve and slope of the curve.

The AutoSCAN W/A is a fully automated, computer-controlled system that uses both colorimetric and fluorometric principles for the identification and susceptibility testing of microorganisms. Currently, identification systems are available for gram-positive bacteria, gram-negative bacteria, yeast, anaerobes, *Haemophilus,* and *Neisseria.* Susceptibility testing is available for gram-negative and gram-positive bacteria. The fluorometric system allows for rapid identification results within 2 hours for certain bacteria. The rapid colorimetric system can identify other microorganisms within 4 hours, and susceptibility results are available in 4 to 7 hours. The system uses microtiter trays that contain fluorescent-labeled substrates containing a synthetic and metabolic component. A halogen quartz incandescent lamp is focused on the trays. If the organism produces the enzyme to act on a substrate, the synthetic moiety is released, which enables it to fluoresce. The degree of fluorescence is measured using a fluorometer. Some of the substrates contain fluorescent pH indicators that emit or fail to emit fluorescence when the pH changes. The colorimetric tests are read spectrophotometrically for a color change. For antibiotic susceptibility testing, the microtiter wells contain a growth medium, a fluorogenic substrate, and various concentrations of antibiotics. The wells are inoculated and incubated, and the amount of fluorescence in each test well is compared with that in a control well with no antibiotic present. If growth is inhibited, less fluorescence occurs, indicating susceptibility. If more fluorescence occurs, indicating the presence of bacterial growth, resistance may be indicated.

The Aladin can be used to test several panels, including the UniScept 20E (Enterobacteriaceae and antibiotics), 20GP (*Staphylococcus* and *Streptococcus*), the AN-IDENT (anaerobes), and the UniScept MIC (minimal inhibitory concentrations). The system also provides for the identification of fastidious *Neisseria* and *Moraxella.* The user inoculates the identification or susceptibility panel and places it in the instrument's incubator. The instrument automatically incubates, adds reagents, processes the panels, and reads the results.

The Aladin uses the unique principle of video capture for interpretation of results. The entire system is computer controlled. A video camera reads the entire area where the reaction occurs, not simply at one detection point. The metabolic reaction to various substrates is determined by focusing the camera in each well of the test panel to capture any color change or change in turbidity. Images are captured and manipulated for viewing enhancement. Picture elements known as pixels are formed and then interpreted by the image processor. Readings are converted into positive or negative results. A digital profile number is obtained that can be compared to a data base for identification.

For susceptibility testing, a suspension of the organism is placed in wells with different antibiotic concentrations. The image processor reads each well by passing light through the cupules. The amount of light passing through each well is compared with that passing through a sterile well where no growth is present. The panel is interpreted, and the video image obtained is transferred to the image processor, which analyzes the data and interprets and records the results.

Blood Culture Systems

Automation in the detection of bacteria in the blood has significantly improved the quality of blood-culturing systems. The Bactec (Becton Dickinson Diagnostic Instrument Systems) was the first automated blood culture system. The early models, such as the Bactec 460, used a radiometric principle and relied on the release of $^{14}CO_2$ from ^{14}C radioactively labeled substrates. These models have been replaced by newer versions, such as the Bactec 660 and Bactec NR 860, which detect the release of CO_2 directly with an infrared spectrophotometer. The newer models alleviate the disadvantages associated with radioactivity, including safety hazards and strict disposal guidelines.

In the nonradiometric Bactec models (Figure 5-5), blood culture vials are injected with the patient's blood sample. Media are available for aerobic and anaerobic bacteria, as well as for fungi and some species of *Mycobacterium*. Trays with the vials are incubated in the appropriate atmosphere: 2.5% CO_2 with air for aerobes and 5% CO_2 with nitrogen for anaerobes. The vials are agitated periodically by a rotary shaker that is part of the system. Periodically, the vials enter the monitoring module, where they are moved by a detector. The detector penetrates the rubber stopper at the top of the vial with two needles, removing any gas that has accumulated above the liquid medium. This gas is known as the "headspace gas." The headspace gas is replaced with a fresh mixture of the appropriate aerobic or anaerobic gaseous mixture. The amount of CO_2 in each vial is measured with an infrared spectrophotometer. Any level of CO_2 above a preset threshold is monitored and processed by the microbiologist. A computer handles the data and interprets and records the results.

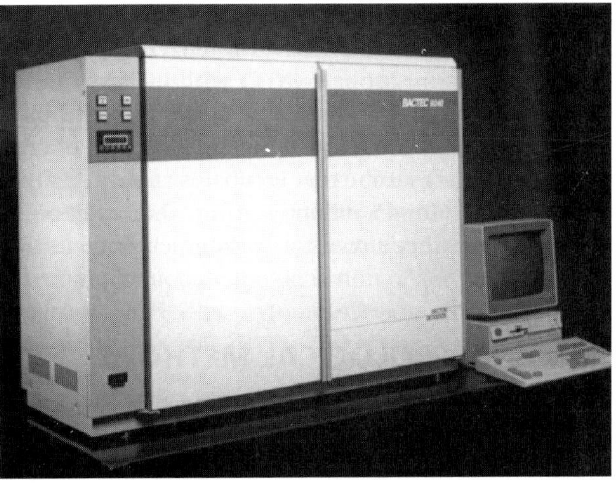

FIGURE 5–5
Bactec model blood culture system. (Becton Dickinson Microbiology Systems.)

The BacT/Alert (Organon Teknika) also measures microbial-produced CO_2 photometrically. The system is automated and noninvasive and utilizes a colorimetric CO_2 sensor that is placed at the bottom of each blood culture bottle. A CO_2 permeable membrane separates the sensor from microbial growth. CO_2 generated from microbial metabolism diffuses across the membrane into the sensor and dissolves in a pH-sensitive water solution. This results in the production of hydrogen ions, which lowers the pH, changing the color of the sensor from dark green to yellow. Light reflected from the sensor is detected and measured photometrically. Changes in reflectance are determined, and a voltage signal proportional to the intensity of the reflected light is generated. The voltage signal is analyzed by a computer, which determines if growth is present based on changes in absorbance, rate of change, and the color threshold produced. A significant advantage of the BacT/Alert is continuous monitoring of each vial, since the vials remain in one place during incubation, decreasing the time necessary to detect a positive result.

Automated Urine Screening Methods

Automated instruments are also available for the rapid detection of bacteriuria, the presence of significant bacteria in the urine. The Bac-T-Screen (bioMérieux Vitek) method is based on the principle of colorimetric filtration. Bacteria and white blood cells are trapped on a filter, and safranin O stain is used to dye the trapped cells. One milliliter of urine is added to a filter in one well of the instrument. The instrument automatically adds acetic acid and dye. The acetic acid functions as both a diluent and a decolorizer, removing unbound dye. The filter card is removed and placed in the spectrophotometric reader. Results are compared against a negative control and are available in 1 to 2 minutes.

REVIEW QUESTIONS

(Continued)

13. Indirect fluorescent antibody techniques:
   a. Can only detect antigen
   b. Use both an unlabeled antibody and labeled antibody
   c. Are not very sensitive detection methods
   d. Cannot be quantitated

14. The interaction between single-stranded nucleic acid molecules to form a double-stranded molecule is known as:
   a. Blotting
   b. Hybridization
   c. Denaturation
   d. A DNA probe

15. The molecular method that involves the synthetic amplification of a known DNA sequence using several denaturation and polymerization cycles is known as:
   a. Southern blot
   b. DNA hybridization
   c. Polymerase chain reaction
   d. DNA cloning

BIBLIOGRAPHY

Barry AL: Simple and rapid methods for bacterial identifications, *Clin Lab Med* 5:3, 1985.

Birkenmeyer LG, Mushahwar IK: DNA probe amplification methods, *J Virol Methods* 35:117, 1991.

Burdash NM et al: A comparison of four commercial systems for the identification of nonfermentative gram-negative bacilli, *Am J Clin Pathol* 73:564, 1980.

Carter JH: Enzyme immunoassays: practical aspects of their methodology, *J Clin Immunol* 7:64, 1984.

Coovadia YM, Naidu KK: Evaluation of a latex particle Bactigen latex agglutination and Phadebact coagglutination for detection of bacteria antigens in cerebrospinal fluid, *J Clin Pathol* 38:561, 1985.

D'Amato RF, Isenberg HD, McKinley GA et al: Novel application of video image processing to biochemical and antimicrobial susceptibility testing, *J Clin Microbiol* 26:1492, 1988.

Drow DL, Manning DD: Comparison of coagglutination, latex agglutination, and enzyme linked immunosorbent assay for detection of *Haemophilus influenzae* type b infection, *Diagn Microbiol Infect Dis* 1:317, 1983.

Enns RK: DNA probes: an overview and comparison with current methods, *Lab Med* 19:295, 1988.

James K: Immunoserology of infectious diseases, *Clin Microbiol Rev* 3:132, 1990.

Klosinski DD, Mattson JC: The growth of DNA technology in the clinical laboratory. Part I, *Lab Med* 24:553, 1993.

Morello JA, Matushek SM, Dunne MC et al: Performance of a BACTEC non-radiometric method for pediatric blood cultures, *J Clin Microbiol* 29:359, 1991.

Murray PR, Smith TB, McKinney TC: Clinical evaluations of three urine screening tests, *J Clin Microbiol* 25:467, 1987.

National Committee for Clinical Laboratory Standards: *Glossary and guidelines for immunodiagnostic procedures, reagents, and reference materials,* Document D11-A1, vol 6, no 16, Approved guideline, 1986.

Persing DH: Polymerase chain reaction: trenches to benches, *J Clin Microbiol* 29:1281, 1991.

Pezzlo MT: Detection of bacteriuria by automated methods, *Lab Med* 15:539, 1984.

Polymerase chain reaction, International Conference Series, vol 1, 1992, Roche.

Rhoden DL, Smith PB, Schable B et al: Evaluation of PASCO MIC/ID system for identifying gram negative bacilli, *J Clin Microbiol* 22:915, 1985.

Rosebrock JA: Labeled-antibody techniques: fluorescent, radioisotopic, immunochemical. In Balows A, editor: *Manual of clinical microbiology*, ed 5, Washington, DC, 1991, American Society for Microbiology.

Stager CE, Davis JR: Automated systems for identification of microorganisms, *Clin Microbiol Rev* 5:302, 1992.

Tenover FC: Diagnostic deoxyribonucleic acid probes for infectious diseases, *Clin Microbiol Rev* 1:82, 1988.

Thorpe TC et al: BacT/Alert: an automated colorimetric microbial detection system, *J Clin Microbiol* 28:1608, 1990.

Tinghitella TJ, Edberg SC: Agglutination tests and *Limulus* assay for the diagnosis of infectious disease. In Balows A, editor: *Manual of clinical microbiology,* ed 5, Washington, DC, 1991, American Society for Microbiology.

Ward KM, Lehmann CA, Leiken AM: *Clinical laboratory instrumentation and automation: principles, applications, and selection,* Philadelphia, 1994, Saunders.

Wilson AJ et al: Enzyme based methods for IgM serology: standard indirect ELISA versus antibody capture ELISA, *Lab Med* 23:259, 1992.

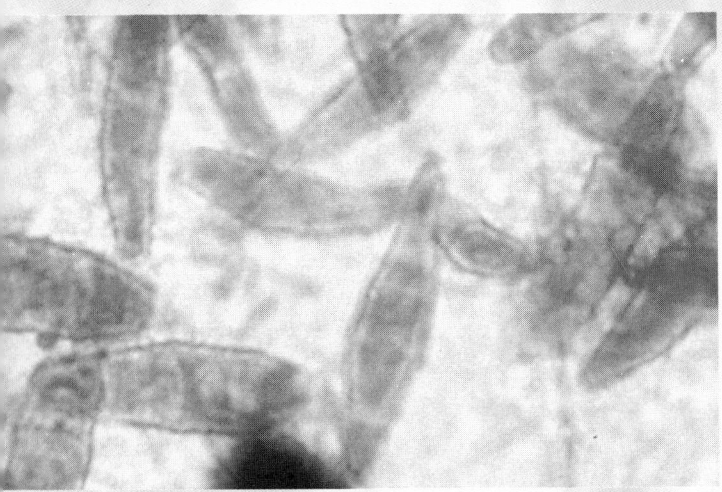

MICROSPORUM CANIS

CHAPTER OUTLINE

OVERVIEW OF ANTIBIOTIC SUSCEPTIBILITY TESTING

BACTERIAL RESISTANCE TO ANTIMICROBIAL AGENTS

LABORATORY METHODS FOR SUSCEPTIBILITY TESTING

- Disk Diffusion Susceptibility Testing
- Quantitative Dilution Susceptibility Testing

BETA LACTAMASE

MACRODILUTION BROTH SUSCEPTIBILITY TEST

KIRBY-BAUER DISK DIFFUSION TEST

MICRODILUTION BROTH SUSCEPTIBILITY TEST

KEY TERMS

ACQUIRED RESISTANCE
ADDITIVE
ANTAGONISTIC
ANTIBACTERIAL
ANTIBIOGRAM
ANTIBIOTIC
ANTIFUNGAL
ANTIMICROBIAL
ANTIVIRAL
AUTONOMOUS
BACTERIOCIDAL
BACTERIOSTATIC
BETA LACTAMASE
BROAD-SPECTRUM ANTIBIOTIC
INTRINSIC RESISTANCE
MINIMAL BACTERIOCIDAL CONCENTRATION
MINIMAL INHIBITORY CONCENTRATION
NARROW-SPECTRUM ANTIBIOTIC
PEAK AND TROUGH SPECIMENS
PLASMID
RESISTANT
SERUM BACTERIOCIDAL TEST
SUPERINFECTION
SUSCEPTIBLE
SYNERGISTIC
TRANSPOSONS

Antimicrobial Susceptibility Testing

LEARNING OBJECTIVES

1. Define the following terms:
   a. Antibiotic
   b. Antimicrobial agent
   c. Bacteriocidal
   d. Bacteriostatic
2. Differentiate narrow-spectrum from broad-spectrum antibiotics.
3. Describe the factors that are considered in the selection of an antimicrobial agent.
4. State the mode of activity and describe the indications for use for the major antibiotics.
5. List at least five antiviral agents.
6. List at least five antifungal agents.
7. Describe acquired resistance.
8. List and describe at least three mechanisms of resistance.
9. Define the following terms:
   a. Susceptible
   b. Resistant
   c. Synergistic
   d. Antagonistic
10. Describe the important test characteristics in Kirby-Bauer susceptibility testing that must be met to obtain consistent results.
11. Explain how the results of disk diffusion testing are affected when:
    a. Inoculum is too dense.
    b. Inoculum is too light.
    c. pH is too acidic.
    d. Disks are placed too close together.
    e. Plates are incubated in increased carbon dioxide.
12. Describe how the following situations are handled in disk diffusion testing:
    a. Colonies within zone of inhibition
    b. Zone overlapping
    c. Zone within a zone
    d. *Proteus* swarming into a zone of inhibition
13. Perform a minimum of 5 Kirby-Bauer susceptibility tests, using the correct quality control strains. Interpret all results without error.
14. State the principle and purpose of quantitative dilution susceptibility testing.
    a. Define minimal inhibitory concentration (MIC).
    b. Define minimal bacteriocidal concentration (MBC).

Continued.

15. When given the volumes of broth, concentration and volume of antibiotic, and concentration and volume of inoculum, determine the antibiotic concentration in each dilution of a macrotube dilution susceptibility test.
16. Perform one macrobroth dilution susceptibility test, determining the MIC and MBC.
17. Perform and interpret at least four microbroth dilution susceptibility tests.
18. List the three types of procedures available for detection of beta-lactamase.
19. Perform and interpret at least three procedures to detect beta-lactamase.
20. Describe the serum bacteriocidal test (SBT).
21. Define *peak* and *trough* and relate these terms to drug assays.

OVERVIEW OF ANTIBIOTIC SUSCEPTIBILITY TESTING

Proper selection of antimicrobial agents to treat an infection first requires the isolation and identification of the causative agent. Next, the susceptibility and resistance of the organism to several antimicrobial agents are determined. Based on these results and other important factors, the physician can determine appropriate therapy for the patient.

Antibiotics are chemicals produced by microorganisms that inhibit the growth of other microorganisms. Some antibiotics are chemically modified. **Antimicrobial agents** are agents that destroy microorganisms through inhibiting their development or action. Such agents may be obtained either from microorganisms or synthetically in the laboratory. More specifically, **antibacterial agents** inhibit the action of bacteria; **antiviral agents** inhibit the action of viruses; and **antifungal agents** inhibit the action of fungi.

Antimicrobial agents may be classified as bacteriocidal or bacteriostatic. **Bacteriocidal agents** kill the microbe, and cell lysis results. Most often these agents are used for life-threatening infections and infections in immunosuppressed hosts. Examples of bacteriocidal antibiotics include the penicillins, cephalosporins, and vancomycin. **Bacteriostatic agents** inhibit the growth of the microorganism but rely on the host immune system to follow through to destroy the organism. Some examples of bacteriostatic agents include tetracycline, the sulfonamides, and erythromycin. The categories may overlap, and classification of an agent as bacteriostatic or bacteriocidal also depends on the dosage, route of administration, and site of infection.

Those antimicrobial agents with a limited spectrum of action are known as **narrow-spectrum antibiotics.** For example, penicillin G is effective only against gram-positive bacteria. **Broad-spectrum antibiotics** have action against both gram-positive and gram-negative bacteria. An example of a broad-spectrum antibiotic is tetracycline. A disadvantage of broad-spectrum antibiotics is the inhibition or destruction of the normal flora of the patient. A new infection, or **superinfection,** may appear as a result of treatment of the primary infection. Superinfections frequently involve the mouth, respiratory tract, and genitourinary tract and are often difficult to treat. Examples of organisms typically associated with superinfections include *Pseudomonas aeruginosa, Candida albicans,* and *Staphylcoccus aureus.*

Selection of the appropriate agent depends on several factors. The box on p. 65 summarizes some of these important considerations.

The mode of activity of the antibiotic must be considered. For example, the beta-lactam antibiotics function by inhibition of cell wall synthesis. When treated with an antibiotic that inhibits cell wall synthesis, nucleotide intermediates accumulate in the cell wall, which results in cell lysis and death. Other examples of cell wall–inhibiting antibiotics include vancomycin and the cephalosporins.

Other antibiotics function by inhibition of protein synthesis. The aminoglycosides, such as tobramycin and gentamicin, interfere with the protein synthesis at the 30S ribosomal subunit. This is also the mechanism for tetracycline. Clindamycin and erythromycin inhibit protein synthesis by binding to the 50S ribosomal subunit. The sulfonamides function by competitive inhibition of folic acid formation, whereas the quinolones inhibit deoxyribonucleic acid (DNA) gyrase activity.

The box on pp. 66-68 summarizes some of the frequently used antibacterial agents, antimycobacterial agents, antifungal agents, and antiviral agents and their mode of action and use.

In general, the cephalosporins, erythromycin, penicillins, and vancomycin can be used for infections involving gram-positive bacilli and *Staphylococcus.* Increasing numbers of strains of *Staphylcoccus aureus* are resistant to penicillin, including the penicillinase-resistant

Selection of Antimicrobial Agents

- Antimicrobial agent has strong activity against microorganism
- Agent has low toxicity toward the host
- Agent is least toxic toward normal flora of host; narrow-spectrum antibiotics should be used when possible
- Appropriate pharmacological properties of antibiotic
- Host immune status: use of steroids, prolonged antibiotic therapy, chemotherapy
- Host organ function: consideration toward renal function for drug elimination and hepatic function for biotransformation
- Underlying medical disease in host, including circulatory problems
- Age of patient: certain agents are toxic to very young patients and may affect geriatric patients in an atypical manner
- Site of infection
- Route of administration
- Does the antibiotic cross the placenta, which may be toxic to the fetus?
- Does the antibiotic penetrate the blood-brain barrier?
- Is surgical intervention a part of the treatment, such as drainage or débridement for anaerobic infections?
- Can effective blood or tissue levels be achieved?
- Is the host allergic or hypersensitive to the agent?

penicillins. An increased resistance to methicillin has been identified. Methicillin-resistant *S. aureus* (MRSA) has become a serious problem, particularly with nosocomial infections. Serious *Enterococcus* infections (endocarditis) are treated with a combination therapy of penicillin and an aminoglycoside or vancomycin. Less serious enterococcal infections usually respond to penicillin or ampicillin. Nonenterococcal streptococci generally respond well to the penicillins. Group A *Streptococcus* is universally susceptible to penicillin, and there is usually no need for susceptibility testing in most patients. Groups B, C, F, and G are likewise generally susceptible to penicillin. Erythromycin can be substituted in individuals who are hypersensitive or allergic to penicillin. The viridans streptococci have recently shown an increased resistance to penicillin, and infections are usually treated with a combination therapy of a penicillin with an aminoglycoside. *Streptococcus pneumoniae,* once universally susceptible to penicillin, has recently shown a resistance to this agent.

Gram-negative bacteria other than *P. aeruginosa* can be treated with aminoglycosides, extended-spectrum penicillins, cephalosporins, quinolones, and imipenem. *P. aeruginosa* can be treated with the aminoglycosides, extended-spectrum penicillins, third-generation cephalosporins, and imipenem. *Haemophilus influenzae* is generally resistant to the first-generation cephalosporins; some strains are also resistant to ampicillin. Third-generation cephalosporins are recommended for treatment. *Neisseria gonorrhoeae* was susceptible to penicillin until the 1970s, when penicillinase-producing *N. gonorrhoeae* (PPNG) was detected. An increase in resistance to tetracycline has also occurred. Today the recommended therapy for this pathogen is ceftriaxone with doxycycline (a tetracycline). *Neisseria meningitidis* has remained susceptible to penicillin but has developed some resistance to the sulfonamides and rifampin, used for prophylactic contacts.

Most anaerobic infections can be treated with extended-spectrum penicillins, beta-lactam drugs that are resistant to beta-lactamase, cefoxitin, chloramphenicol, imipenem, or metronidazole.

The box on p. 69 summarizes the interactions that can occur when two or more antibiotics are given together.

BACTERIAL RESISTANCE TO ANTIMICROBIAL AGENTS

Consideration of bacterial resistance to an antibiotic or group of antibiotics is another important factor in antimicrobial susceptibility testing. **Intrinsic resistance** refers a characteristic of the organism before antibiotic use. Examples include the intrinsic resistance of *Staphylococcus saprophyticus* to novobiocin. An example in the Enterobacteriaceae includes the resistance of *Proteus, Providencia, Morganella,* and *Edwardsiella* to the polymyxins. Most other members of the Enterobacteriaceae are susceptible to these agents. Intrinsic resistance may be useful for identification of the organism.

Acquired resistance is necessitated by prior exposure to the antimicrobial agent. Organisms that were once susceptible are now resistant. Acquired resistance may result from chromosomal mutations or from plasmids. In chromosomal mutations the antibiotic

ANTIBACTERIAL AGENTS: MODE OF ACTIVITY AND INDICATIONS

BETA-LACTAM ANTIBIOTICS

Mode of activity: inhibition of cell wall synthesis

PENICILLINS

Natural penicillins

Penicillin G, penicillin V

Source is the mold *Penicillium notatum;* primarily a gram-positive spectrum with major indications for *Streptococcus* infections, other than *Enterococcus;* most *Staphylococcus* species are resistant.

Penicillinase-resistant penicillins

Methicillin, nafcillin, oxacillin, cloxacillin, dicloxacillin

Various side chains added to the penicillin molecule confer resistance to penicillinase; gram-positive spectrum; active against penicillinase-producing *Staphylococcus,* although these organisms are becoming increasingly resistant to these agents.

Extended-spectrum penicillins: aminopenicillins

Ampicillin, amoxicillin, bacampicillin, ticarcillin

Extended spectrum of gram-positive and gram-negative bacteria, including *Escherichia coli, Proteus mirabilis, Haemophilus influenzae, Salmonella,* and *Shigella;* they are slightly less active than penicillin G against *Streptococcus pneumoniae* and *Streptococcus pyogenes.*

Extended-spectrum penicillins: carboxypenicillins

Carbenicillin

Primarily a gram-negative spectrum; treatment of serious gram-negative enteric infections and *Pseudomonas aeruginosa;* may be used in combination with an aminoglycoside; *Klebsiella* species are resistant.

Extended-spectrum penicillins: acyclaminopenicillins

Azlocillin, mezlocillin, piperacillin

Primarily a gram-negative spectrum; greater activity against enteric bacteria and *P. aeruginosa;* also active against *H. influenzae, Serratia,* and *Bacteroides fragilis;* synergistic activity occurs with the aminoglycosides.

Penicillin co-drugs (beta-lactam with beta-lactamase inhibitor)

Augmentin (amoxicillin with clavulanate potassium (clavulanic acid))

Timetin (ticarcillin with clavulanate potassium (clavulanic acid))

Gram-negative and gram-positive spectrum; they also exhibit activity against beta-lactamase-producing *Staphylococcus, H. influenzae, Bacteroides,* and some enteric bacteria.

CEPHALOSPORINS

The cephalosporins are structurally similar to penicillin, but better withstand the action of beta-lactamase and are more modifiable. Original cephalosporin was cephalosporin C, which was modified to aminocephalosporanic acid, which has been modified into first-, second-, and third-generation cephalosporins.

First-generation cephalosporins

Cephalothin, cephapirin, cefazolin, cephalexin, cefadroxil, cephradine

Active against gram-positive cocci, other than *Enterococcus* and methicillin-resistant *Staphylococcus aureus* (MRSA), active against enteric bacteria (*E. coli, P. mirabilis, Klebsiella*), and anaerobes other than *Bacteroides fragilis;* they may be inactivated by beta-lactamase.

Second-generation cephalosporins

Cefamandole, cefoxitin, cefuroxime, cefonicid, ceforanide, cefotetan

Slightly more active than first-generation cephalosporins against Enterobacteriaceae, but less active against *Staphylococcus,* also active against *H. influenzae,* and *Moraxella;* cefaclor is active against anaerobes.

Third-generation cephalosporins

Cefoperazone, cefotaxime, ceftriaxone, moxalactam, ceftizoxime, ceftazidime

Greatly increased activity against gram-negative bacilli, with increased stability against beta-lactamase and less active against gram-positive cocci when compared with other cephalosporins; useful in nosocomial and multidrug-resistant gram-negative infections; cefotaxime is useful for *E coli, Serratia,* and *Klebsiella* infections, whereas ceftriaxone has activity against *Neisseria gonorrhoeae;* several

ANTIBACTERIAL AGENTS: MODE OF ACTIVITY AND INDICATIONS (Continued)

are active against *P. aeruginosa* and most anaerobes.

MISCELLANEOUS BETA-LACTAM DRUG

Imipenem: activity similar to third-generation cephalosporins, with slightly greater activity toward Enterobacteriacea; they are also active against gram-positive cocci, including *Enterococcus*

AMINOGLYCOSIDES

Mode of activity: interference with protein synthesis at 30S ribosomal subunit; gram-positive and gram-negative spectrum; dosage should be monitored using peak and trough values.

Gentamicin: bacteriocidal; used to treat nosocomial infections caused by gram-negative bacilli; often used synergistically with beta-lactam drugs to treat severe systemicinfections

Tobramycin: similar to gentamicin with increased activity against *P. aeruginosa*

Amikacin: similar to gentamicin and tobramycin; used to treat gram-negative bacilli that are resistant to these agents; also has activity against *Nocardia asteroides* and *Mycobacterium avium-intracellulare* complex

Netilmicin: similar to gentamicin and tobramycin; slightly less active against *P. aeruginosa* and *Serratia*

Neomycin: oral and topical antibacterial agent

Spectinomycin: used only for treatment of gonorrhea, although the organism has shown resistance

Streptomycin: may be used in combination therapy for tuberculosis and with a beta-lactam for enterococcal infections

TETRACYCLINE

Mode of activity: interference with protein synthesis at 30S ribosomal subunit; broad-spectrum with activity against gram-positive and gram-negative bacteria; also useful for mycoplasma and chlamydial infections; bacteriostatic; growing resistance is noted.

CHLORAMPHENICOL

Mode of activity: interference with protein synthesis by binding to 50S ribosomal subunit

Used for serious gram-negative infections, such as typhoid fever and salmonellosis; should be limited because of serious side effect of bone marrow aplasia.

SULFONAMIDES

Mode of activity: competitive inhibition of folic acid synthesis; all have para-amino sulfonamide group, which acts as an antimetabolite of para-aminobenzoic acid, forming a nonfunctional analog of folic acid.

Sulfamethoxazole: primarily for acute urinary tract infections (UTIs).

Trimethoprim-sulfamethoxazole: treatment of chronic UTIs, Enterobacteriaceae, *H. influenzae, Moraxella catarrhalis, Pseudomonas cepacia;* anaerobes are resistant.

MACROLIDES

Mode of activity: inhibition of protein synthesis by binding to 50S ribosomal subunit

Erythromycin: gram-positive spectrum; respiratory infections from *S. pyogenes* and *S. pneumoniae* in penicillin-allergic patients; it is also effective for *Mycoplasma pneumoniae* and *Legionella* infections.

Clindamycin: gram-positive spectrum; it is active against most aerobic gram-positive cocci other than MRSA and *Enterococcus,* as well as most anaerobes, including *B. fragilis,* although resistance has been noted.

GLYCOPEPTIDE

Mode of activity: inhibition of cell wall formation through inhibition of peptidoglycan synthesis

Vancomycin: gram-positive spectrum; used for MRSA and nosocomial infections from coagulase-negative *Staphylococcus;* it is also used for *Clostridium difficile* colitis and as a penicillin alternative to treat endocarditis from viridans streptococcus and with a penicillin for enterococcal endocarditis.

Continued.

ANTIBACTERIAL AGENTS: MODE OF ACTIVITY AND INDICATIONS (Continued)

QUINOLONES

Mode of activity: inhibition of DNA gyrase activity

Nalidixic acid: first quinolone; used to treat UTIs

Fluoroquinolones: broader spectrum; used to treat serious infections (complicated UTIs, invasive ear infections) from Enterobacteriaceae, *N. gonorrhoeae, Neisseria meningitidis, M. catarrhalis, H. influenzae;* They have decreased activity against *Streptococcus* and *Enterococcus;* effective against *Staphylococcus* other than MRSA.

MISCELLANEOUS AGENTS

Polymyxins
Mode of activity: disruption of cell membrane. Gram negative-spectrum; used as topical agents in combination with other antibiotics to treat wound infections

Nitrofurantoin
Mode of activity: inhibition of bacterial enzymes
Treatment of UTIs; not effective against *P. aeruginosa, Serratia,* or *Proteus*

Rifampin
Mode of activity: inhibition of DNA-dependent ribonucleic acid (RNA) polymerase
Treatment of tuberculosis and prophylaxis for contacts of those with meningococcal disease

Metronidazole
Mode of activity: reduction products of metronidazole are toxic when taken in by the organism.
Treatment of *Gardnerella* vaginosis and *Trichomonas;* active against most anaerobes, including *C. difficile*; parasitic infection; no activity against most aerobes

ANTIMYCOBACTERIAL AGENTS

Multiple drugs are used to prevent resistance of organism to agents. Some of these agents function by inhibiting mycolic acid formation in the cell wall while others inhibit DNA-dependent RNA protein.

First-line drugs

Isoniazid

Rifampin

Pyrazinamide

Second-line drugs

Ethambutol

Streptomycin

ANTIFUNGAL AGENTS

Amphotericin B: treatment of systemic fungal infections

5-Fluorocytosine (5-FC): inhibition of RNA and DNA synthesis in yeasts; *Cryptococcus* and *Candida* infections; given with amphotericin B for cryptococcal meningitis

Imidazoles

Clotrimazole: dermatophytic, yeast, and superficial fungal infections

Ketoconazole: fungistatic, non-life-threatening histoplasmosis, and blastomycosis

Fluconazole: severe or disseminated candidiasis and cryptococcis; can penetrate into cerebrospinal fluid

Miconazole: topical agent for cutaneous and subcutaneous candidiasis

Itraconazole: aspergillosis and *Sporothrix* infections

Griseofulvin: dermatophytic infections

Nystatin: superficial skin and mucous membrane infections caused by yeast and dermatophytes

ANTIVIRAL AGENTS

Amantadine: influenza A

Vidarabine: herpes simplex virus (HSV) 1 and 2

Idoxuridine, trifluridine, acyclovir: HSV 1 and 2

Ribavirin: respiratory syncytial virus

Azidothymidine, Zidovudine (AZT): inhibits replication of retroviruses; used in HIV infections

Ganciclovir: herpes viruses

Foscarnet: CMV retinitis, varicella, and acyclovir-resistant HSV infections exerts selective pressure on the susceptible strain of the organism. The resistant mutant strain overgrows the susceptible cells, and the new population consists of resistant cells. **Plasmids** are extrachromosomal elements of DNA that are associated with virulence and antibiotic resistance. Plasmids act independently from the chromosome, and the resistance genes may be transferred from chromosome to plasmid, or vice versa.

Transposons, commonly known as "jumping genes," can insert pieces of DNA in areas even if no homology exists. Thus the host range is much broader when compared with plasmids. Transposons can carry part of plasmids or pieces of chromosomes to other bacteria.

The specific mechanisms of resistance include modification of the target site. The antibiotic's ability to bind to the cell wall or ribosome is altered. The binding affinity of the antibiotic is decreased or nonexistent. This mechanism is seen in the beta-lactams, macrolides, tetracyclines, aminoglycosides, vancomycin, and trimethoprim. Beta-lactams bind to penicillin-binding proteins in the cell wall. Resistance to these agents usually involves interference with the penicillin-binding proteins.

A second mechanism for resistance is inactivation of the antimicrobial agent. In this case, bacterial enzymes convert the active drug into an inactive form. The **beta lactamases (penicillinases)** are a group of enzymes that convert the beta-lactams into inactive forms. This resistance may be plasmin mediated or chromosomally mediated. Beta-lactamase production was first directed against the natural penicillins, but this enzyme group is now directed against broad-spectrum penicillins and some cephalosporins.

Other mechanisms for resistance include decreased permeability of the cell wall, which results in poor entry of the antibiotic into the bacterial cell. This is seen in gram-negative bacteria whose outer membrane renders them impermeable to certain antibiotics. Other bacteria can prevent the accumulation of the antibiotic through a pumping mechanism. This is known as active transport from the cell; the efflux of tetracycline is an example. Another mechanism is an alteration of the binding of ribosomes, which is illustrated by the resistance of *Pseudomonas* to certain aminoglycosides.

Antibiotic Interactions

Autonomous: **Indifferent**

Result obtained with two drugs is equal to result with most effective drug by itself.

Antagonistic

Result with two drugs is significantly less than the autonomous result.

Additive

Result with two drugs is equal to combined action of each of the drugs used separately.

Synergistic

Result with two drugs is significantly greater than additive response. The antibiotics may have different modes of action or function at different sites. One member of the combination may be resistant to beta-lactamase. The uptake of aminoglycosides into the bacterial cell is enhanced by beta-lactam drugs. For example, a penicillin derivative with an aminoglycoside shows synergistic action and is used to treat enterococcal endocarditis.

LABORATORY METHODS FOR SUSCEPTIBILITY TESTING

Selection of the specific type of susceptibility test to be performed and selection of specific antibiotics to be tested should be determined jointly by the director of microbiology, the infectious disease department, and the medical staff. The pharmacy department may also have input into the selection of specific antibiotics, since this department may be responsible for the delivery and supply of the antimicrobial agents.

Various susceptibility testing methods are currently available, and each has both advantages and disadvantages.

Disk Diffusion Susceptibility Testing

The **Kirby-Bauer disk diffusion test** is performed by inoculating a standardized suspension of bacteria onto Mueller-Hinton agar. Paper disks impregnated with specific antibiotics are placed on the agar and incubated under well-defined conditions. The antibiotics diffuse into the surrounding medium. After overnight incubation, the zones of inhibition around each are measured and compared with established interpretative values. The diameter of the zone of inhibition is an indicator of relative susceptibility of the organism to the antibiotic. Results are reported as **susceptible, resistant, intermediate,** or **moderately susceptible.**

Susceptible results indicate that the antibiotic appears to be effective against the bacteria because growth is inhibited in vitro. Resistant results indicate the antibiotic appears to be ineffective against the bacteria tested. In vivo activity of the antibiotic against the microbe also depends on host factors, the site of infection, the specific antibiotic used, and specific properties of the microorganism.

The principle of the disk diffusion test is based on the inverse linear relationship between the diameter of the zone of inhibited growth around the antibiotic disk

for a routine microbiology laboratory. Its routine use has been in anaerobic susceptibility testing and in research facilities.

The macrobroth dilution (or macrodilution broth) test uses Mueller-Hinton broth with calcium and magnesium ions (Ca^{2+} and Mg^{2+}) added. The medium supports the growth of most bacteria. When testing *Staphylococcus* with methicillin, oxacillin, or nafcillin, the medium should be supplemented with 2% sodium chloride (NaCl). In this method, 13 tubes are labeled and 1.0 ml of Mueller-Hinton broth is pipetted into tubes 2 through 10, 11, and 13. Next, 2.0 ml of broth is pipetted into tube 12. Tubes 1, 2, and 13 receive 1.0 ml of the working antibiotic solution. Twofold serial dilutions in 1.0 ml amounts in tubes 2 through 10 are performed. Then 1.0 ml of the standardized inoculum is pipetted to tubes 1 through 11. The tubes are mixed and incubated at 35°C for 18 to 24 hours. After incubation the first tube showing no visible growth is considered to be the MIC. One should subculture all tubes showing no growth to media, incubate, and note the lowest antibiotic concentration that has resulted in 99.9% killing. This is the MBC. The MBC should be performed on immunosuppressed patients or those with diminished immunity and serious infections, such as endocarditis. Agents that are bacteriocidal usually produce MBCs within one or two dilutions of the MIC. Figure 6-6 depicts a typical broth dilution test, showing determination of the MIC and MBC.

The macrobroth dilution test is useful for laboratories testing a few antibiotics with a few organisms. It is cumbersome to perform in laboratories where large volumes of organisms and large numbers of antibiotics must be tested. The microbroth dilution (or microdilution broth) test is more practical in such cases. In this technique, plastic trays with approximately 80 wells are filled with minute volumes (50 to 100 μl) of serial twofold dilutions of several antibiotics that have been diluted in Mueller-Hinton Broth. A standardized inoculum of the organism is inoculated into each well through use of a multipronged dilutor. The system includes a growth control and purity control. The plastic trays are commercially available from a number of manufacturers, and the user may also select the battery of antimicrobial agents to be included. The antibiotics are either frozen or lyophilized when obtained from the manufacturer. With the advent of automation, the plates can be automatically inoculated and read with an instrument (see Chapter 5). The method for the microdilution broth susceptibility test is described later in this chapter. Figure 6-7 shows a typical microtiter dilution tray; Table 6-3 provides typical values to interpret MIC values for antimicrobial agents for this technique.

Bacterial isolates can also be tested for the production of a specific enzyme that may result in the resistance of the organism to an antibiotic or a group of antibiotics. The beta-lactamase enzymes cleave the beta-lactam ring of penicillins and cephalosporins. Both gram-negative and gram-positive organisms are known to produce beta lactamase. Bacteria that most often produce beta lactamase are *Staphylococcus* species, *H. influenzae, N. gonorrhoeae, Moraxella catarrhalis,* and *Enterococcus* species. The substrate to detect beta-lactamase may be a penicillin or a cephalosporin, and the principles that may be used include iodometric, acidometric, and chromogenic techniques. In iodometric methods, the end products of the activity of beta lactamase on the penicillin substrate reduce iodine, which is bound to starch. A positive reaction is indicated by the disappearance in color as the starch-iodine complex is degraded. In acidometric methods, penicillin is hydrolyzed into acidic end products in the presence of beta lactamase. An indicator that changes color in the presence of acid is used to visualize the reaction. The most sensitive method and the method that has been effective in detecting many types of beta-lactamase is that using the chromogenic cephalosporin Nitrocefin. In the presence of beta lactamase the amide bond in the beta-lactam ring is hydrolyzed. This results in a color change of the chromogen from yellow to red. The test can be commercially obtained as the Cefinase procedure (BBL Microbiology Systems), which uses filter paper disks impregnated with Nitrocefin. The Cefinase procedure is described later in this chapter and is illustrated in Figure 6-8 (Color Plate 12).

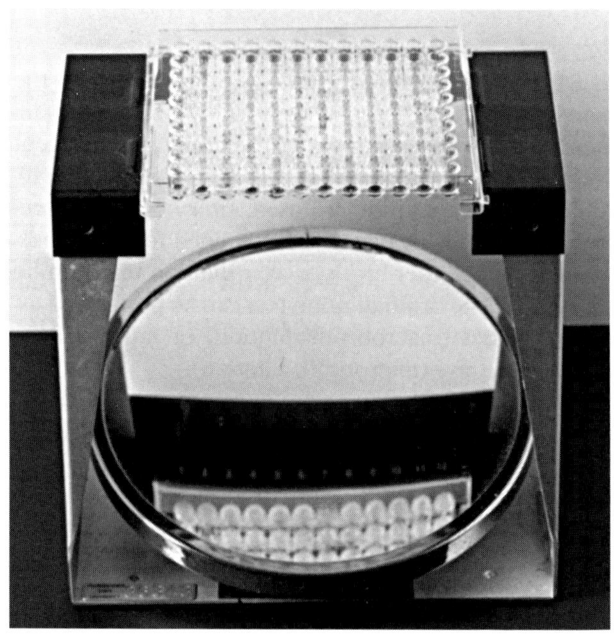

FIGURE 6–7
Microdilution tray with viewing mirror used to observe for the presence or absence of growth in each well.

TABLE 6–3

Interpretation of Breakpoints: Minimal Inhibitory Concentration (MIC) Interpretative Guidelines*

ANTIMICROBIAL AGENT	S	I	R
Amikacin	16	32	64
Amoxicillin/clavulanate/potassium			
Staphylococcus	4/2	—	8/4
Other organisms	8/4	16/8	32/16
Ampicillin			
Enterobacteriaceae	8	16	32
Staphylococcus	0.25	—	0.5
Enterococcus	8	—	16
Nonenterococcal *Streptococcus*	0.12	0.25-2	4
Ampicillin/sulbactam	8/4	16/8	32/16
Carbenicillin			
Pseudomonas	128	256	512
Other gram-negative bacteria	16	32	64
Cefaclor	8	16	32
Cefamandole	8	16	32
Cefazolin	8	16	32
Cefixime	1	2	4
Cefmetazole	16	32	64
Cefonicid	8	16	32
Cefoperazone	16	32	64
Cefotaxime	8	16	32
Cefoxitin	8	16	32
Ceftriaxone	8	16-32	64
Cephalothin	8	16	32
Chloramphenicol	8	16	32
Ciprofloxacin	1	2	4
Clindamycin	0.5	1-2	4
Erythromycin	0.5	1-4	8
Gentamicin	4	8	16
Methicillin	8	—	16
Mezlocillin			
Pseudomonas	64	—	128
Other gram-negative bacteria	16	32-64	128
Nafcillin			
Staphylococcus	2	—	4
Nitrofurantoin	32	64	128
Norfloxacin	4	8	16
Ofloxacin	2	4	8
Oxacillin			
Staphylococcus	2	—	4
Penicillin G			
Staphylococcus	0.12	—	0.25
Enterococcus	8	—	16
Nonenterococcal *Streptococcus*	0.12	0.25-2.0	4
Pneumococcus	0.06	0.12-1.0	2
Piperacillin			
Pseudomonas	64	—	128
Other gram-negative bacteria	16	32-64	128
Ticarcillin			
Pseudomonas	64	—	128
Other gram-negative bacteria	16	32-64	128

Continued.

TABLE 6-3

Interpretation of Breakpoints: Minimal Inhibitory Concentration (MIC) Interpretative Guidelines* (Continued)

ANTIMICROBIAL AGENT	S	I	R
Ticarcillin-clavulanate potassium			
Pseudomonas	64/2	—	128/2
Other gram-negative bacteria	16/2	32/2-64/2	128/2
Sulfonamides	256	—	512
Tetracycline	4	8	16
Trimethoprim	8	—	16
Trimethoprim/sulfamethoxazole	2/38	—	4/76
Tobramycin	4	8	16
Vancomycin	4	8-16	32

*These values are intended for student use in interpretation of Macrodilution and Microdilution MIC procedures. The values have been adapted from NCCLS Document M100-S4 (vol 12, no 20, December 1992) and are not intended for use in the clinical microbiology laboratory with patient specimens.

S, Susceptible; I, intermediate; R, resistant.

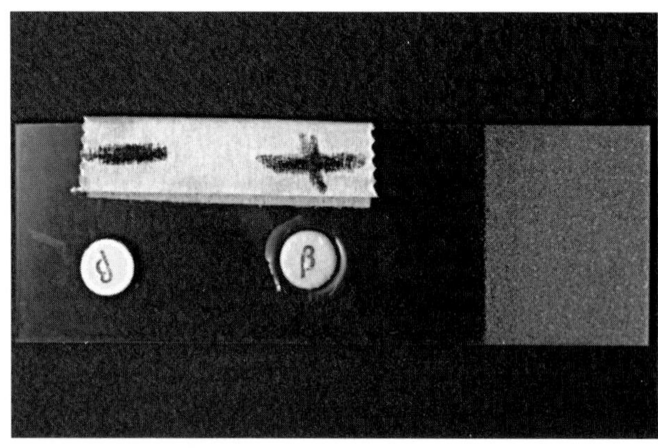

FIGURE 6-8

Cefinase procedure for determination of beta lactamase activity. (Becton Dickinson Microbiology Systems.)

The **serum bacteriocidal test (SBT)**, or **Schlichter test,** is a measure of the activity of the antibiotic in the patient's own serum against the pathogen. It is used as a guideline to determine if the patient is receiving effective therapy for a serious infection, such as meningitis, endocarditis, or osteomyelitis. The SBT is defined as the lowest dilution of the patient's serum that kills a standardized inoculum of bacteria. A trough specimen is collected within 15 minutes before the next antibiotic dose, and a peak specimen is collected approximately 30 to 60 minutes after the antibiotic is given. Twofold serial dilutions of the patient's serum samples are then tested against the standardized inoculum. The highest dilution (or lowest amount of antibiotic) that inhibits the organism (MIC for SBT) is determined. An MBC, or serum bacteriocidal titer for the procedure, can also be determined by following the macrobroth dilution susceptibility procedure.

Assays of specific antimicrobial agents may be indicated for those drugs that have a low therapeutic index. Such drugs have a small window between a level that is therapeutic and a level that is toxic to the host. Agents that may require assays include the aminoglycosides (tobramycin, gentamicin), vancomycin, and choramphenicol. Often the assays are requested to determine the amount of antibiotic that is in the circulation or that has reached a particular body fluid, such as cerebrospinal fluid. This level may be affected by the biotransformation of the agent (hepatic function), elimination of the agent (renal function), and other host factors. The assays require the collection and analysis of a peak and a trough specimen. The **peak specimen** is collected 30 minutes after the agent is administered through the intravenous route and approximately 60 minutes when given intramuscularly. The peak specimen represents the highest level of antibiotic that has reached the blood. The **trough specimen** should be collected 15 minutes before the next dose. At least one dose of the antibiotic must have been given to collect a valid trough specimen.

Antibiograms can be used to compare the susceptibility of a particular bacterial isolate to several antibiotics with the standard predictable pattern of that microorganism. In doing so, the development of resistance to a certain agent can be detected. In addition, an antibiogram can alert the clinician to verify and investigate any "unusual" resistant patterns.

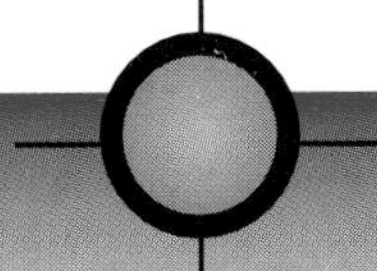

PROCEDURE
BETA LACTAMASE (CEFINASE)

PURPOSE
Cefinase disks are used to detect beta lactamase production by testing isolated colonies of *Staphylococcus* species, *Haemophilus influenzae, Neisseria gonorrhoeae,* and anaerobic bacteria. Isolates containing these organisms should be routinely tested for beta lactamase activity.

PRINCIPLE
The Cefinase disk is impregnated with the chromogenic cephalosporin Nitrocefin. A rapid color change from yellow to red results when the amide bond in the beta-lactam ring is hydrolyzed by beta lactamase.

MATERIALS
Cefinase disks (available through Becton Dickinson Microbiology Systems)
Microscope slides or Petri plates
Sterile loop or application sticks

PROCEDURE
1. Dispense a Cefinase disk from the dispenser or remove one disk from the vial using sterile forceps and place on a microscope slide or empty Petri plate.
2. Moisten each disk with one drop of purified water.
3. Using a sterile loop or applicator stick, select several well-isolated colonies and smear onto the moistened disk surface.
4. Observe disk for color change.
5. Alternatively, using forceps, moisten disk with one drop of purified water and wipe across surface of colony.

RESULTS
Positive: color change from yellow to red; color change usually does not occur over entire disk. Most bacterial strains develop a positive result within 5 minutes. Positive reactions for some strains of *Staphylococcus* may take up to 1 hour to develop.
Negative: color change does not occur on the disk.

QUALITY CONTROL
Positive: *Staphylococcus aureus* ATCC 29213: color change from yellow to red
Negative: *Haemophilus influenzae* ATCC 10211: no color change

LIMITATIONS
The efficacy of the test in predicting the beta-lactam resistance of microorganisms not listed in the Purpose is not proved.

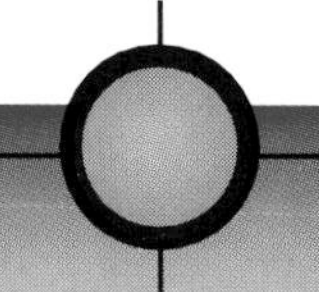

PROCEDURE

MACRODILUTION BROTH SUSCEPTIBILITY TEST

PURPOSE

The minimal inhibitory concentration (MIC) and minimal bacteriocidal concentration (MBC) of a particular antibiotic are determined through serially diluting an antibiotic.

PRINCIPLE

Dilutions of an antibiotic are added to Mueller-Hinton broth and a standard concentration of the inocolum. The tubes are incubated overnight and read visually for turbidity. The lowest concentration showing no visible growth or macroscopic inhibition is the MIC. Broth cultures showing no visible growth are subcultured onto appropriate agar and incubated to determine if the organism has been killed. The lowest concentration of antibiotic that exhibits at least 99.9% killing on subculture is the MBC.

MATERIALS

Antibiotic standard—for penicillin use a working solution of 20 U of activity/ml; for other antibiotics, use a 200 mg/ml working solution.
Subculture of organism to be tested; an overnight culture grown at 35° C on blood agar is recommended. Inoculate a trypticase soy broth with the overnight culture.
Mueller-Hinton broth
Sterile 13 × 100 mm test tubes with screw caps

PROCEDURE

1. Set up 13 sterile 13 × 100 mm test tubes with caps and label 1 through 13.
   Tube 11 will be the inoculum control.
   Tube 12 will be the broth control.
   Tube 13 will be the antibiotic control.
2. Pipet 1.0 ml of Mueller-Hinton broth into tubes 2 through 10, tube 11, and tube 13. Pipet 2.0 ml of MH broth into tube 12.
3. Pipet 1.0 ml of the working antibiotic solution into tubes 1, 2, and 13.
4. Make two-fold dilutions in 1.0 ml amounts in tubes 2 through 10. Mix and change pipettes at each dilution. This is done by mixing tube 2 and transferring 1.0 ml of its contents to tube 3. The process is continued to tube 10. Discard 1.0 ml from tube 10.
5. Standardize the inoculum to a 0.5 McFarland standard. Then further adjust the inoculum by adding 0.1 ml of the inoculum to 19.9 ml of MH broth. This is a 1:200 dilution. The final concentration of bacteria is approximately 1×10^5 to 1×10^6 CFU/ml.
6. Pipet 1.0 ml of the standardized inoculum into tubes 1 through 11. Mix each tube well and incubate at 35° C for 18 to 24 hours. Do not incubate under increased CO_2 unless this is required for growth.

PROCEDURE
MACRODILUTION BROTH SUSCEPTIBILITY TEST
(Continued)

7. Prepare plate for colony count. This is done by preparing a 1:100 dilution of the inoculum and plating 0.01 ml of the dilution onto a blood agar plate. Incubate at 35° C for 18 to 24 hours. Do not incubate under increased CO_2 unless this is required for growth.

INTERPRETATION

Determination of MIC: The tube with the lowest antibiotic concentration showing no visible growth is considered to be the MIC.
Inoculum Control (Tube 11): Must show visible growth for test to be valid.
Broth Control (Tube 12): Must show no visible growth for test to be valid.
Antibiotic Control (Tube 13): Must show no visible growth for test to be valid.

DETERMINATION OF MBC

1. Subculture 0.01 ml from each tube showing no visible growth and the first tube with visible growth onto a blood agar plate. Streak the inoculum in several directions to maximally dilute the antibiotic.
2. Incubate the plates for 18 to 24 hours at 35° C. Do not incubate under increased CO_2 unless required for growth.
3. The MBC is the lowest antibiotic concentration that results in 99.9% killing. This is illustrated by the lowest antibiotic concentration permitting no survival of the organism.

14. State the principle and purpose of the following techniques to identify *S. aureus:*
   a. Latex agglutination
   b. Hemagglutination

15. List medically significant species classified as coagulase-negative staphylococci (CoNS) and describe infections attributed to these organisms.

16. Describe the identification of *Staphylococcus epidermidis.* Identify *Staphylococcus epidermidis* from an unknown culture without error.

17. Name infections attributed to *Staphylococcus epidermidis* and describe the patient population typically infected.

18. State the purpose and principle of the novobiocin test. Perform and interpret this test without error.

19. Discuss the clinical significance of isolating *Staphylococcus saprophyticus.*

20. Identify *Staphylococcus saprophyticus* from an unknown culture without error.

21. Explain the identification of *Stomatococcus* and discuss its role as a pathogen.

GRAM-POSITIVE COCCI

The medically significant gram-positive cocci can be generally classified as either *Staphylococcus* or *Streptococcus.* The gram-positive cocci all contain a high content of peptidoglycan and a low level of lipid in the cell wall. This accounts for the fact that alcohols and other solvents do not penetrate the gram-positive cell wall but instead cause the cell wall to crenate. This is why gram-positive organisms retain the primary stain, crystal violet, in the Gram stain procedure. The decolorizer, acetone/alcohol, causes the gram-positive cell wall to seal tightly, trapping the crystal violet within.

The gram-positive cocci are natural habitants of skin and mucous membranes in humans and can be found throughout the environment in dust and inanimate objects. Gram-positive infections are spread through direct contact with infected individuals or contaminated objects. Such infections are termed **pyogenic** due to the accumulation of neutrophils, bacterial cells, and fluids at the infection site.

The bacterial family Micrococcaceae comprises four genera: *Micrococcus, Staphylococcus, Planococcus,* and *Stomatococcus.* Members of the Micrococcaceae are gram-positive cocci, which are catalase positive. The *Micrococcus* organisms may colonize human skin but are rarely infectious, and thus they are identified to the genus level by most microbiology laboratories. The *Planococcus* organisms, from the marine environment, are likewise rarely associated with human infection. The *Stomatococcus* organisms are emerging as rare opportunistic pathogens.

Staphylococcus is the genus of Micrococcaceae most frequently associated with human infection. Staphylococci are facultative anaerobes and ferment glucose anaerobically, whereas micrococci are strict aerobes, which utilize glucose oxidatively or are nonsaccharolytic. Micrococci are resistant to 200 μg/ml of lysostaphin and are modified oxidase positive, whereas staphylococci are susceptible to lysostaphin and are modified oxidase negative. Lysostaphin is a peptidase that breaks the glycine peptide linkages in the cell wall of the staphylococci. In addition, *Staphylococcus* is resistant to 0.04 units of bacitracin while *Micrococcus* is susceptible. Table 7-1 lists characteristics for the differentiation of *Micrococcus* from *Staphylococcus.*

STAPHYLOCOCCUS

The genus *Staphylococcus* is composed of approximately 24 species, several of which are associated with human colonization or infection. The list of species found in humans or animals includes *S. aureus, S. epidermidis, S. saprophyticus, S. hominis, S. hemolyticus, and S. warneri.* All listed species except *S. aureus* are classified as coagulase-negative staphylococci (CoNS) due to the lack of production of this enzyme.

Important characteristics of the genus *Staphylococcus* are as follows:

Gram-positive cocci arranged in tetrads or clusters
Facultative anaerobes
Medium-sized, raised, creamy colonies on blood agar or colistin–nalidixic acid with white, cream, or golden pigmentation
Catalase positive
Modified oxidase negative
Nonmotile
Non–spore forming
Reduces nitrates to nitrites
Grows in 7.5%–10% NaCl
Lysostaphin susceptible
Bacitracin resistant

TABLE 7–1

Differentiation of *Staphylococcus* from *Micrococcus*

	STAPHYLOCOCCUS	***MICROCOCCUS***
Catalase	+	+
Aerobic growth	+	+
Anaerobic growth	+	−
Glucose utilization (of media)	Fermentative	Oxidative or nonsaccharolytic
Modified oxidase	−	+
Benzidine	−	+
Resistant to lysostaphin (200 μg/ml)	−	+
Resistant to bacitracin (0.04 U)	+	−

These criteria are very important in differentiating *Staphylococcus* from *Streptococcus* species, which are typically arranged in pairs or chains and are pinpoint, flat, colorless colonies with wide zones of hemolysis. Streptococci are typically catalase negative. Figure 7-1 illustrates positive and negative catalase reactions.

FIGURE 7–1
Positive catalase reaction is indicated by the presence of bubbles.

Staphylococci are easily isolated on blood agar, colistin-nalidixic acid (CNA), or mannitol salt agar (MSA). On blood agar, colonies are medium convex, creamy, and dome shaped. The pigment varies from white to golden yellow. Figures 7-2 (Color Plate 13), 7-3 (Color Plate 14), and 7-4 (Color Plate 15) illustrate staphylococcal species on sheep blood agar. CNA is a selective medium with a blood agar base that contains the antibiotics colistin and nalidixic acid. The medium is selective for gram-positive cocci, inhibiting the growth of gram-negative bacilli. MSA contains 7.5% to 10% sodium chloride (NaCl), the carbohydrate-alcohol mannitol, and phenol red indicator. The medium is typically used for the selective isolation of *Staphylococcus,* since most other bacteria cannot sustain this high salt concentration. The plate is first read for growth and then read for fermentation of mannitol, which is characterized by a yellowing of the medium as the phenol red indicator takes on its acidic color of yellow. Positive fermentation of MSA is illustrated in Figure 7-5 (Color Plate 16), and negative fermentation is illustrated in Figure 7-6 (Color Plate 17).

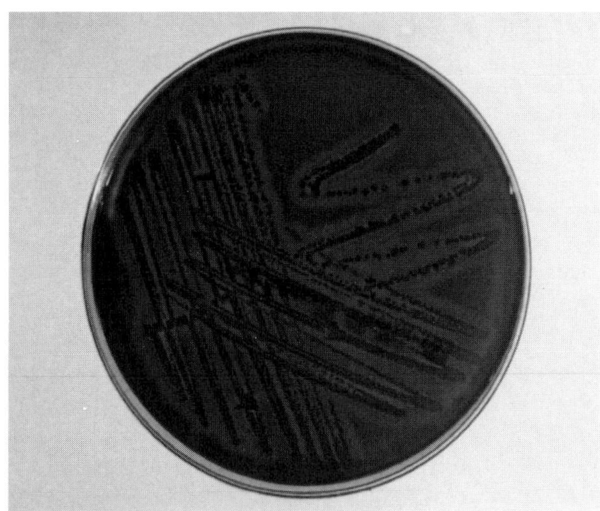

FIGURE 7–2
Staphylococcus aureus on sheep blood agar. Large, convex, creamy colonies of *S. aureus* may be pigmented white to golden yellow with a narrow zone of beta hemolysis.

Staphylococcus aureus

Most strains of *Staphylococcus aureus* appear as medium to large colonies, 2 to 3 mm in diameter with a convex, creamy appearance. The edge is entire, and the colonies may be pigmented white to golden yellow. Most strains of *S. aureus* exhibit a narrow zone of beta

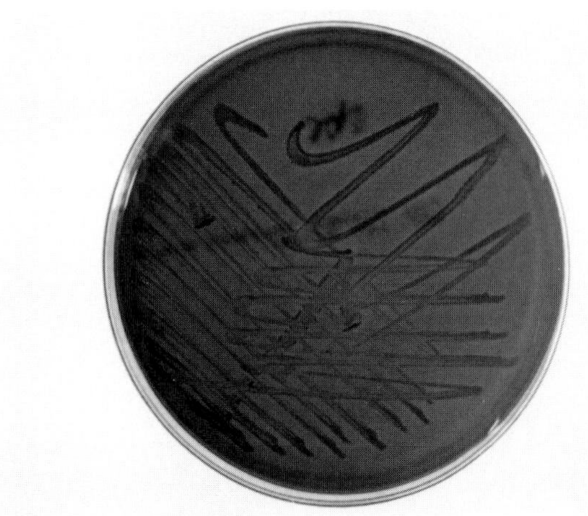

FIGURE 7-3
Staphylococcus epidermidis on sheep blood agar shows medium, white, creamy, nonhemolytic colonies.

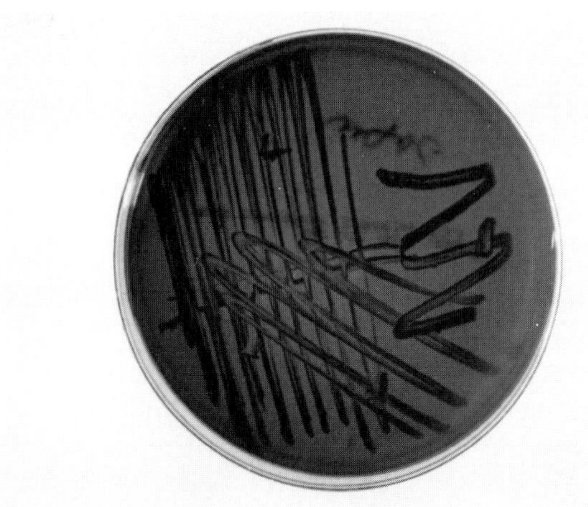

FIGURE 7-4
Staphylococcus saprophyticus on sheep blood agar shows medium, white, creamy, nonhemolytic colonies.

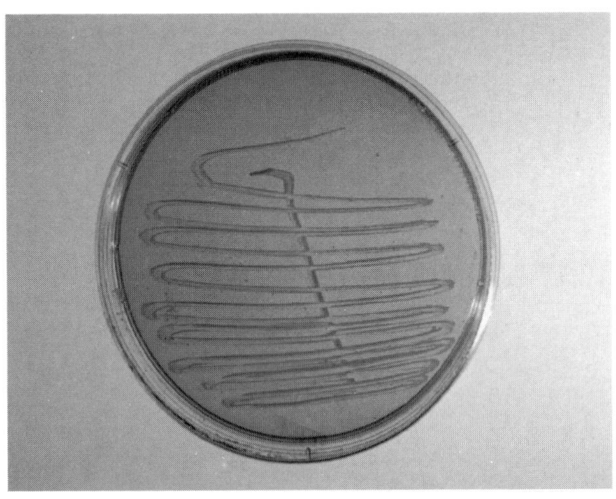

FIGURE 7-5
Mannitol salt agar showing positive fermentation of mannitol, as indicated by a yellow color. Reaction is typical of *Staphylococcus aureus.*

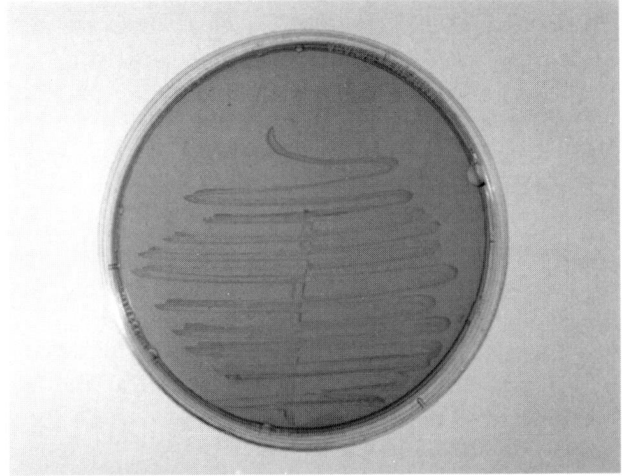

FIGURE 7-6
Mannitol salt agar showing negative fermentation of mannitol. Reaction is typical of *Staphylococcus epidermidis.*

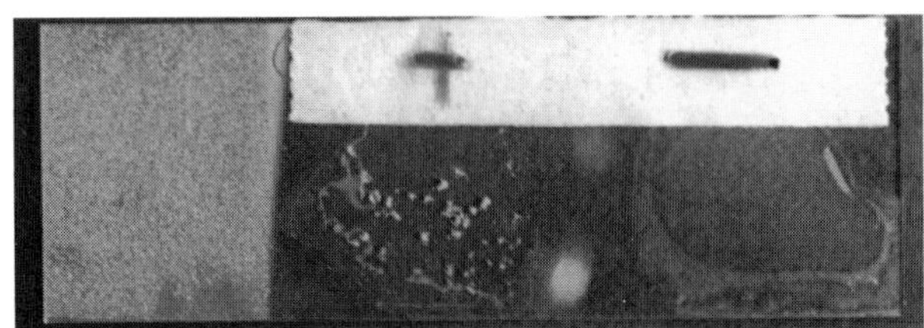

FIGURE 7-7
Coagulase slide test showing positive results with fibrin strands; the negative result shows a smooth suspension.

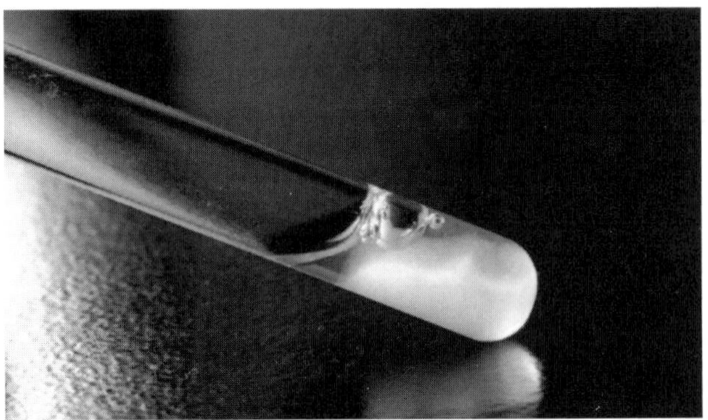

FIGURE 7-8
Tube coagulase test showing positive result with a solid fibrin gel.

hemolysis while some strains are nonhemolytic. Similar colonies are observed on CNA.

To differentiate *S. aureus* from other *Staphylococcus* species, the coagulase test is the most reliable procedure. *S. aureus* is the only staphylococcal species pathogenic to humans that produces coagulase. In the coagulase slide test, **bound coagulase** or clumping factor is measured. A small amount of bacterial growth is emulsified in sterile saline on a microscopic slide, and one drop of rabbit plasma is added. The suspension is mixed and observed for the appearance of white fibrin clots, indicating the conversion of **fibrinogen** to **fibrin,** which indicates a positive test (Figure 7-7).

If the slide test is negative, the tube coagulase test must be performed. The tube test detects **free coagulase,** an extracellular toxin that reacts in the presence of coagulase reacting factor (CRF), a compound normally found in plasma to form coagulase-CRF complex, which resembles thrombin and converts fibrinogen to fibrin. In the tube test, 0.5 ml of rabbit plasma is inoculated with the organism and incubated in a 35° to 37°C water bath and read for partial or complete clot lysis at 1 to 4 hours. The test should be checked at 30-minute intervals. Since some strains of *S. aureus* produce a **fibrinolysin** (staphylokinase), false-negative results can occur if the test is not periodically observed or if the test is only observed for clot formation at the end of 18 to 24 hours of incubation. Tests that are negative at 4 hours can be incubated at room temperature overnight for 16 to 18 hours for slower coagulase producers (Figure 7-8).

The traditional coagulase slide tests have been modified by many manufacturers to provide more accurate and rapid identification of *S. aureus.* In most of these tests, use of latex beads or red blood cells provides clear and rapid results. In latex agglutination techniques, such as the Staph Latex (Difco Laboratories) or Staphaurex (Wellcome Diagnostics), latex particles are coated with human plasma fibrinogen and immunoglobulin G (IgG), which will react with clumping factor and protein A of *S. aureus.* In the Staph Latex technique, the latex beads are colored yellow to facilitate the ease of reading the reaction (Figure 7-9 [Color Plate 18]). In the Staphyloslide (Becton Dickinson) and Hemastaph (Remel Laboratories) rapid hemagglutination techniques, sheep erythrocytes are coated with fibrinogen, which will likewise react with the clumping factor of *S. aureus.*

Other tests to identify *S. aureus* include growth and fermentation of MSA. The organism can grow in 6.5% to 10% NaCl and ferment the carbohydrate-alcohol mannitol. Fermentation is indicated by a yellow color in the medium as the phenol red indicator takes on its acidic color.

S. aureus also gives a positive DNase test reaction, as indicated by a clearing of the dye toluidine blue

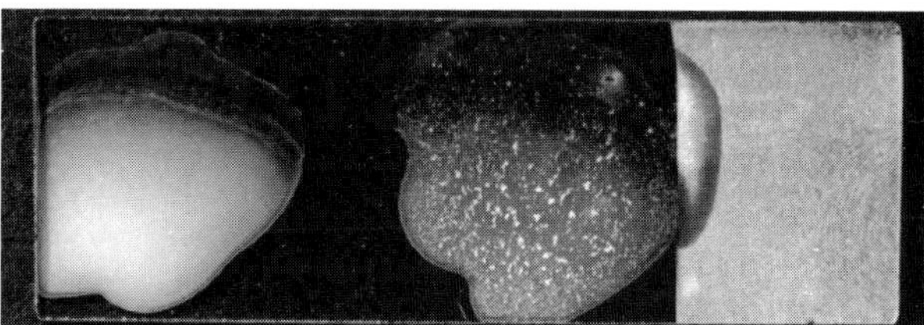

FIGURE 7-9

Bacto Staph Latex technique showing positive agglutination with yellow latex beads on the right with a negative smooth suspension on the left. A positive reaction indicates the presence of bound coagulase and/or protein A (Difco Laboratories, Detroit, Michigan.)

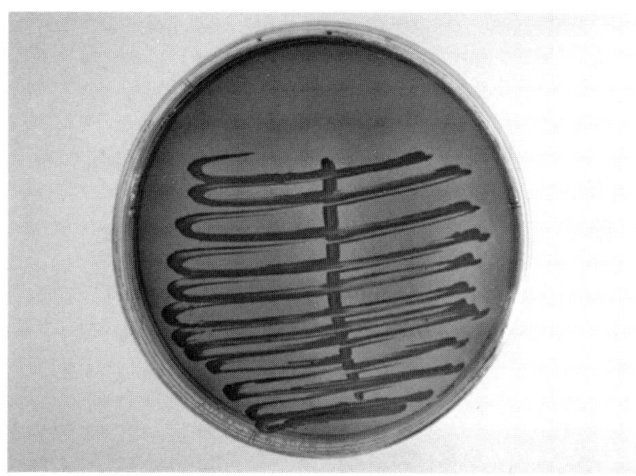

FIGURE 7-10

DNase test showing positive result, evidenced by clearing of medium.

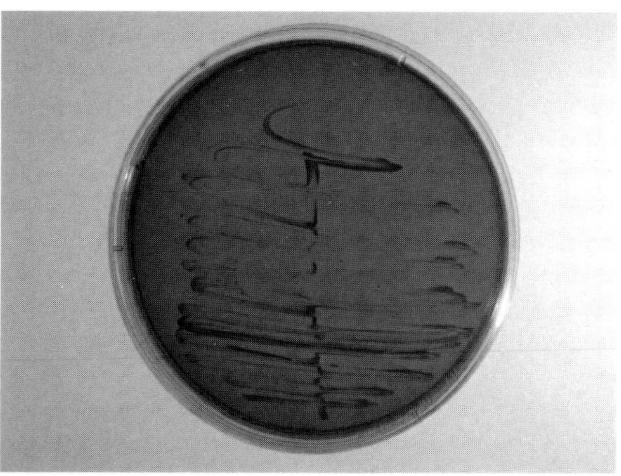

FIGURE 7-11

DNase test showing negative result, evidenced by lack of clearing of medium.

(Figures 7-10 and 7-11), which is incorporated into the nutrient agar-based medium. In a modification of the DNase test, the plate can be flooded with dilute hydrochloric acid after incubation. A change in color from blue-green to pink indicates a positive hydrolysis of deoxyribonucleic acid (DNA).

S. aureus is also thermostable nuclease positive. This enzyme is detected by boring small wells into DNase agar. The wells are then filled with a broth culture of the organism, which has been boiled in a water bath for 15 minutes. A positive reaction is indicated by the presence of pink halos surrounding the wells.

The important characteristics of *S. aureus* are as follows:

Medium to large, raised colonies on blood agar and CNA with cream to golden yellow pigmentation
Gram stain: gram-positive cocci arranged in clusters
Beta hemolytic or nonhemolytic on sheep blood agar
Bound coagulase (clumping factor): positive
Free coagulase: positive
MSA: growth and fermentation
DNase: positive
Thermostable nuclease: positive

S. aureus liberates a number of extracellular toxins and compounds, which lead to its significance as a serious pathogen. The organism is almost always infectious when isolated from patients. The exception is in the carrier state, when the organism can be carried asymptomatically in an individual without showing signs of being pathogenic. Approximately 10% to 15% of the general population may carry the organism asymptomatically in the anterior nares or on the skin. The carrier rate is even higher in the health care setting and serves as a source of nosocomial infection.

S. aureus forms many extracellular toxins and enzymes. These exotoxins are released from living cells into the extracellular environment. Some of the more significant examples of such toxins and enzymes are listed in the box below.

In addition, *S. aureus* possesses several surface characteristics that play a role in the establishment and course of infection, including:

Protein A: binds to the antibody molecule, which causes interference with phagocytosis and fixation of complement

Capsular polysaccharide: enables organism to resist phagocytosis

Peptidoglycan and teichoic acids: found in the cell wall; aid the organism's attachment to mucous membranes and enable organism to resist unfavorable environmental conditions

Staphylococcus aureus: Extracellular Enzymes and Toxins

Coagulases: conversion of fibrinogen to fibrin; may coat neutrophils with fibrin formed to protect organism from phagocytosis

Staphylokinase (fibrinolysin): dissolves fibrin clots and may enable infection to spread once clot is dissolved

Lipase: hydrolyzes lipids in plasma and skin; enables staphylococci to colonize certain body areas; is associated with initiation of skin infections, such as boils, carbuncles, and furuncles

Hyaluronidases: hydrolysis of hyaluronic acid present in connective tissue, which can result in the spread of infection

Deoxyribonuclease (DNase): degradation of DNA

Exfoliatins: hydrolyze tissue through cleavage of stratum granulosum; associated with **staphylococcal scalded skin syndrome**

Leukocidins: lysis of neutrophils and macrophages; inhibit phagocytosis

Hemolysins: group of alpha, beta, gamma, and delta hemolysins that lyse erythrocytes; in addition, alpha, gamma, and delta hemolysins may lyse leukocytes

Enterotoxins: group of seven heat-stable proteins: **A, B, C, C2, D, E,** and **F.** Most staphylococcal-related food poisonings are associated with enterotoxins A and B. Enterotoxin F is also known as **toxic shock syndrome toxin (TSST-1)**

Beta lactamase (penicillinase): hydrolysis and inactivation of penicillin antibiotics through breakdown of beta-lactam ring in penicillin molecule

Infections caused by *S. aureus* are characteristically pyogenic in nature. These infections are accompanied by swelling, redness, increase in temperature to the affected area, and accumulation of leukocytes. The most common staphylococcal infections include those of the skin, such as folliculitis (infection of the hair follicle), boils, furuncles, and carbuncles. Impetigo is found in newborns, infants, and young children. Scalded skin syndrome is produced through the effects of exfoliation; the epidermis peels away, leaving a red, moist area. Acne and postoperative wound infections are often attributed to *S. aureus* as well.

Staphylococcal food poisoning, the most common type of food poisoning in the United States, results from ingestion of preformed enterotoxin. Improper refrigeration of foods such as custards, cream puffs, potatoes, eggs, chicken salad, and processed meats is frequently the cause. The toxin is produced at room temperature but is inactive at refrigerated temperatures. Therefore the organism can multiply and produce additional toxin when the food product is handled improperly. Symptoms include the rapid onset of nausea, vomiting, and diarrhea approximately 2 to 6 hours after ingestion of the enterotoxin. There may also be abdominal pain and cramping. Recovery occurs within 6 to 8 hours in most affected individuals.

S. aureus is also an important cause of pneumonia in infants, debilitated individuals, and those in immunosuppressive states. Bacteremia is common and is often found in patients with cardiovascular disease, diabetes mellitus, and immunosuppressive conditions. Many cases of bacteremia are nosocomial. Bacteremia is also seen in patients who have prosthetic devices, such as plastic catheters. *S. aureus* bacteremia has recently been increasingly associated with intravenous drug use. A frequent complication of staphylococcal bacteremia is endocarditis.

Osteomyelitis is seen in children, as a complication in patients with diabetes mellitus or atherosclerosis, and as a result of trauma or surgery.

Toxic shock syndrome (TSS), a clinical syndrome characterized by hypotension, fever, desquamation of the palms and soles, fever, chills, headache, and vomiting was first characterized by Todd in 1978. Although primarily affecting young menstruating females, this multisystemic disease, attributed to the effects of TSS toxin 1, may also affect males and children, often in complications from staphylococcal infections such as abscesses and pneumonias. An apparent link between superabsorbent tampon use and the disease has been established.

Because many *S. aureus* isolates produce **beta lactamase** and are resistant to penicillin, penicillinase-resistant drugs are the drugs of choice in the treatment of most staphylococcal infections. Examples of penicillinase-resistant penicillins include oxacillin, cloxacillin, and methicillin. Patients hypersensitive to penicillin may be treated with the cephalosporins or vancomycin. There has been a growing resistance of staphylococci to methicillin, particularly in nosocomial outbreaks in debilitated patients. **Methicillin-resistant *Staphylococcus aureus* (MRSA)** may also be resistant to other semisynthetic penicillins and to the cephalosporins. In such cases, vancomycin alone or in combination with rifampin may be used.

A high carrier rate exists for *S. aureus*. As mentioned earlier, an estimated 10% to 15% of adults carry the organism asymptomatically on the skin, on mucosal surfaces, or in the anterior nares. This rate is estimated to be more than 50% in the hospital environment. The organism can survive in the air and on inanimate objects. For these reasons, *S. aureus* is a frequent isolate in the clinical laboratory. Proper personal hygiene and aseptic measures are essential to decrease the spread of staphylococcal infection in the health care environment.

COAGULASE-NEGATIVE STAPHYLOCOCCI

Frequently considered to be contaminants or normal flora, the **coagulase-negative staphylococci (CoNS)** are isolated with increasing frequency in patients. Today, at least 11 species of CoNS have been isolated from humans, of which *S. epidermidis* and *S. saprophyticus* are most significant.

Staphylococcus epidermidis

Staphylococcus epidermidis resembles *S. aureus* in morphology and in the Gram stain preparation. More than 50% of all clinical isolates containing CoNS contain *S. epidermidis.* Identifying characteristics of *S. epidermidis* include the following:

Gram-positive cocci in clusters
White, creamy, raised growth on blood agar
Nonhemolytic on blood agar
Positive growth on CNA
Growth, but lack of fermentation of MSA
Coagulase negative
DNase negative
Susceptible to novobiocin

To differentiate the organism from *S. aureus,* one relies on the coagulase test. *S. epidermidis* gives negative reactions for both the slide and tube coagulase tests. In addition, the organism cannot ferment mannitol, and the MSA plate remains pink in color. *S. epidermidis* is also DNase negative, failing to clear the dye from DNase agar.

S. epidermidis is normal flora of the skin and mucous membranes of humans and other animals. In the past the organism was considered to be nonpathogenic, but now it has been found with increasing frequency in immunosuppressed patients. The organism is associated with bacterial endocarditis, frequently

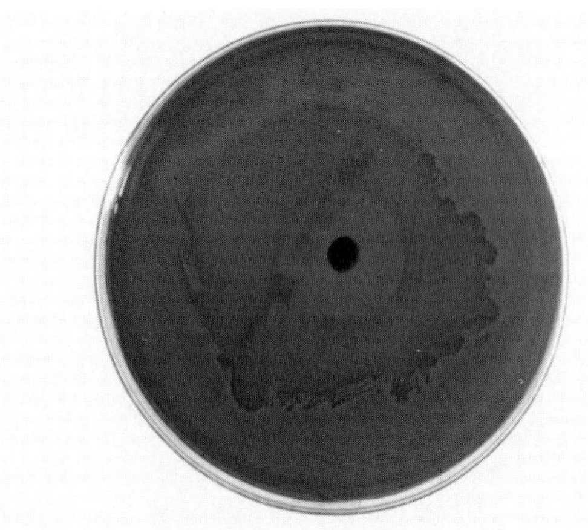

FIGURE 7-12
Novobiocin susceptibility evidenced by zone of inhibition greater than 16 mm surrounding novobiocin disk. Reaction is typical of *S. epidermidis* and other coagulase-negative staphylococci, other than *S. saprophyticus.*

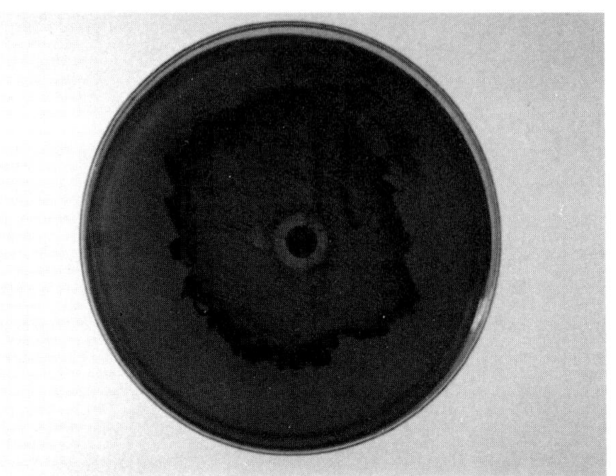

FIGURE 7-13
Novobiocin resistance evidenced by lack of zone of inhibition (or zone less than 16 mm) surrounding novobiocin disk. Reaction is typical of *S. saprophyticus.*

following the insertion of artificial heart valves. *S. epidermidis* can colonize prosthetic devices, including central nervous system shunts, intravascular catheters, and prosthetic orthopedic devices, resulting in infections such as bacteremia and septicemia. In addition, the organism has been found to cause urinary tract infections (UTIs) and wound infections. Frequently, these infections are found in immunosuppressed patients, such as those with malignancies, severe burns, or transplant patients. A great majority of *S. epidermidis* infections are nosocomial, and the route of infection may be from hospital personnel or contaminated surgical devices.

Staphylococcus saprophyticus

Staphylococcus saprophyticus, although considered a contaminant in the past, is an important cause of UTIs, associated with pyelonephritis and cystitis in young women and in older men who have indwelling catheters. The organism is coagulase negative, DNase negative, and nonhemolytic on blood agar. Fermentation of mannitol is variable, with some strains exhibiting positive fermentation. Initial colony counts to confirm the UTI usually run low, less than 1.0×10^5/ml. *S. saprophyticus* is resistant to novobiocin, and this principle is used to differentiate the organism from *S. epidermidis* and other clinically significant CoNS that are susceptible to novobiocin. A 0.5 McFarland standard of the suspect organism is prepared and streaked on a blood agar plate, and a 5μg novobiocin disk is applied. The plate is then incubated for 18 to 24 hours overnight at 35° to 37°C. *S. saprophyticus* will exhibit zone sizes of 6 to 12 mm, indicating resistance, while other CoNS will exhibit zone sizes of at least 16 mm. Figures 7-12 and 7-13 illustrate examples of novobiocin susceptibility and resistance. The box at right describes some rarely isolated CoNS.

Rarely Isolated Coagulase-Negative *Staphylococcus*

S. auricularis: normal flora of humans, rare pathogen

S. capitis: normal flora of human scalp; usually nonpathogenic

S. cohnii: normal flora of human skin; rare pathogen

S. haemolyticus: normal flora of human skin; etiologic agent in endocarditis, septicemia, and peritonitis; resistant to vancomycin

S. hominis: normal flora of human skin; rare pathogen

S. lugdunensis: opportunistic pathogen in septicemia, wound and skin infections, and endocarditis

S. saccharolyticus: normal flora of human mucous membranes; rare cause of endocarditis

S. schleiferi: rare human pathogen in wound infections and bacteremia

S. simulans: normal flora of human mucous membranes; rare pathogen

S. warneri: normal flora of humans; usually nonpathogenic

S. xylosus: normal flora of humans; rare cause of urinary tract infections

STOMATOCOCCUS

Stomatococcus mucilanginosus is an emerging pathogen in immunosuppressed patients. The organism has been isolated from blood cultures as the agent of endocarditis and bacteremia. *Stomatococcus* cannot grow in the presence of 5% NaCl as can *Staphylococcus* and *Micrococcus.* The organism also has a capsule, is weakly catalase positive, and coagulase negative.

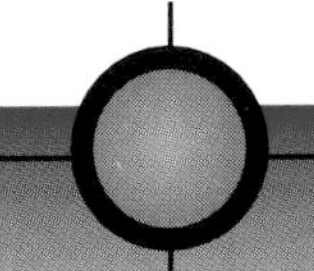

PROCEDURE
BLOOD AGAR

PURPOSE
Blood agar is an example of a nonselective enriched media.

PRINCIPLE
Blood agar is prepared through addition of 5% defibrinated sheep, horse, or rabbit blood to a base of either trypticase or tryptic soy agar. The soy provides peptones, which serve as a source of amino acids, carbon, nitrogen, and sulfur. Blood provides serum ingredients as well as erythrocytes, which enable detection of the hemolytic pattern. Because growth and hemolysis patterns may vary depending on the type of blood cells used, it is important to know the source of the cells.

The types of hemolysis are **alpha:** incomplete or partial lysis, with greening; **beta:** complete lysis, with a colorless, clear zone; **gamma:** nonhemolytic; and **alpha prime:** a wide zone of beta hemolysis surrounding a small zone of alpha hemolysis, which surrounds the colony. Blood agar plates should be observed for surface and subsurface hemolysis. The latter is detected by forcing a small amount of growth approximately one-half into the agar's depth by "stabbing" the medium. Subsurface hemolysis is caused by oxygen-labile **streptolysin O,** whereas surface hemolysis is caused by oxygen-stable **streptolysin S.** Both hemolysins are produced by various strains of *Streptococcus pyogenes.*

PROCEDURE
1. Streak the culture or specimen on blood agar to obtain isolated colonies.
2. Stab the media approximately one-half its depth in at least three different areas of the streak.
3. Incubate at 35°C for 18 to 24 hours.
4. Interpret growth and type of hemolysis according to above descriptions.

QUALITY CONTROL
Streptococcus pyogenes: growth, beta hemolysis
Streptococcus pneumoniae: growth, alpha hemolysis

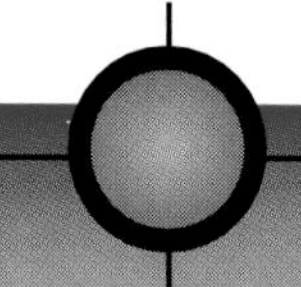

PROCEDURE
COLISTIN–NALIDIXIC ACID AGAR (CNA)

PURPOSE
CNA permits the selective recovery of gram-positive bacteria.

PRINCIPLE
CNA is a medium that selectively inhibits the growth of gram-negative bacteria. It is useful to isolate staphylococci and streptococci from clinical specimens containing mixed flora. Colistin (polymyxin E) disrupts the cell membrane of the gram-negative bacteria, while nalidixic acid blocks DNA replication and membrane integrity in many gram-negative bacteria. The medium is a blood agar base to which the antibiotics have been added.

PROCEDURE
1. Inoculate the CNA plate with the culture and streak for isolation.
2. Stab the media approximately one-half its depth in at least three different areas of the streak.
3. Incubate at 35°C for 18 to 24 hours. Interpret plate for growth and hemolysis.

QUALITY CONTROL
Escherichia coli: total inhibition
Proteus mirabilis: partial inhibition
Streptococcus pneumoniae: growth, alpha hemolysis
Streptococcus pyogenes: growth, beta hemolysis

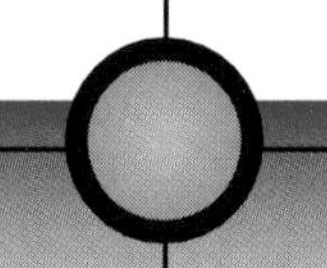

PROCEDURE
CATALASE

PURPOSE
Catalase enzymatically converts hydrogen peroxide into water and oxygen. Most aerobes and facultative anaerobes possess the enzyme. The test is useful in differentiation of members of the family Micrococcaceae (including *Staphylococcus*), which are catalase positive, from *Streptococcus* species, which are catalase negative.

PRINCIPLE
Catalase converts hydrogen peroxide (H_2O_2) into water and oxygen. A positive reaction is indicated by rapid and continuous bubble formation.

MATERIALS
3% Hydrogen peroxide (store in a dark bottle in refrigerator)
Microscope slides

PROCEDURE
1. Transfer a small portion of a well-isolated colony that is 18 to 24 hours old onto a clean microscope slide.
2. Add one to two drops of 3% hydrogen peroxide.
3. Observe for the formation of rapid and continuous bubbles.

INTERPRETATION
Positive: rapid and continuous bubbles
Negative: lack of bubble formation 30 seconds later

QUALITY CONTROL
Staphylococcus epidermidis: positive, bubbling
Streptococcus pyogenes: negative, no bubbling

NOTES
1. The order in the procedure should not be reversed. Do not add the organism to the reagent. This may lead to a false-positive reaction.
2. Since red blood cells also contain catalase, avoid inclusion of red cells from the medium into the test reaction. This may lead to false-positive reactions.

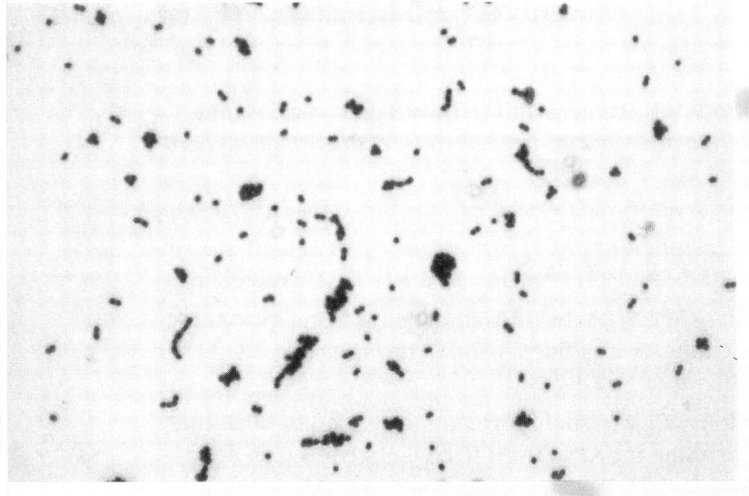

STREPTOCOCCUS PYOGENES

CHAPTER OUTLINE

- GROUP A *STREPTOCOCCUS*
- GROUP B *STREPTOCOCCUS*
- GROUP D *STREPTOCOCCUS* AND *ENTEROCOCCUS*
- MISCELLANEOUS LANCEFIELD GROUPS
- *VIRIDANS STREPTOCOCCI*
- *STREPTOCOCCUS PNEUMONIAE*
- NUTRITIONALLY VARIANT STREPTOCOCCI
- BACITRACIN AND SULFAMETHOXAZOLE-TRIMETHOPRIM SUSCEPTIBILITY TESTS
- CAMP REACTION
- BILE-ESCULIN AGAR
- 6.5% SALT BROTH
- PYRase
- OPTOCHIN

KEY TERMS

- BACITRACIN TEST
- BILE ESCULIN
- BROWN'S CLASSIFICATION
- CAMP REACTION
- LANCEFIELD GROUPING
- OPTOCHIN TEST
- PNEUMOLYSIN
- PYOGENIC EXOTOXIN A
- SALT TOLERANT
- STREPTOKINASE
- STREPTOLYSIN S AND O
- SXT
- VIRIDANS STREPTOCOCCI

Streptococci and Related Organisms

LEARNING OBJECTIVES

1. Describe characteristics of the genus *Streptococcus.*
2. List the media typically used to isolate streptococci.
3. List, recognize, and describe the four types of hemolysis.
4. Differentiate between streptolysin S and streptolysin O.
5. Give the Lancefield group and preliminary tests used to identify each of the following streptococcal species:
   a. *S. pyogenes*
   b. *S. agalactiae*
   c. *Enterococcus: E. faecalis, E. faecium, E. durans, E. avium*
   d. Non-*Enterococcus: S. bovis, S. equinus*
6. Differentiate between the *Enterococcus* and the non-*Enterococcus.*
7. State the principle and the purpose of the following tests. Perform and interpret each test without error.
   a. Bacitracin ("A" Disk)
   b. SXT
   c. CAMP reaction
   d. Bile-esculin
   e. 6.5% salt broth
   f. PYRase
8. Describe the principle of rapid tests for group A streptococci.
9. Discuss the clinical significance of infection caused by:
   a. Group A streptococci, including primary infection and sequelae
   b. Group B streptococci
   c. *Enterococcus*
   d. Non-*Enterococcus*
10. List antibiotics effective in the treatment of streptococcal infections.
11. List those species known as "viridans" streptococci, and discuss the clinical significance of their isolation.
12. Describe and recognize the appearance of *Streptococcus pneumoniae* on:
    a. Gram-stained smear
    b. Blood agar at 24-hour and 48-hour incubations
13. Differentiate between viridans *streptococcus* and *Streptococcus pneumoniae.*
14. State the principle of and perform and interpret the optochin test without error.

15. Describe the principle and use of the following in the identification of *Streptococcus pneumoniae*:
   a. Neufeld (quellung) reaction
   b. Latex agglutination

16. List infections associated with *Streptococcus pneumoniae.*

17. List antibiotics effective in treatment of pneumococcal infections.

18. Briefly discuss the significance of the following streptococci:
   a. Lancefield group C
   b. Lancefield group F
   c. Lancefield group G
   d. Nutritionally variant

This chapter discusses the following genera: *Aerococcus, Enterococcus, Gemella, Lactococcus, Leuconostoc, Pediococcus,* and *Streptococcus.*

Aerococcus viridans is rarely isolated as a cause of endocarditis and meningitis in immunosuppressed individuals. *Leuconostoc* species have been infrequently isolated from several clinical sites, including the blood, and from wounds and abscesses. *Pediococcus* is normal flora of the lower gastrointestinal (GI) tract and has been isolated occasionally from abscesses. *Leuconostoc* and *Pediococcus* are both resistant to vancomycin. *Lactococcus* is a rare human pathogen, and *Gemella* is a rare isolate of the upper respiratory tract.

The focus of this chapter is on *Streptococcus* and *Enterococcus,* which are frequently associated with a variety of human infections. The *Enterococcus* species were previously classified in the genus *Streptococcus* and have been elevated to the genus level of *Enterococcus.*

The genus *Streptococcus* contains a variety of species; some are nonpathogenic and normal flora for humans, whereas others are important human pathogens. Streptococci are widely distributed in the environment, in dairy products, and as normal flora of the human GI tract.

Streptococci are typically gram-positive cocci and are arranged in pairs or chains, since cell division occurs in one plane. The organisms are nonmotile and facultative anaerobes. An important biochemical distinction from *Staphylococcus* is the catalase reaction; *Streptococcus* species are catalase negative.

Some strains of *Streptococcus* are fastidious, and isolation is best achieved through enriched media, such as blood agar, Todd-Hewitt broth, or chocolate agar. Colonies are typically small, (0.5 to 2.0 μm in diameter), pinpoint, and translucent or clear. Frequently, large hemolytic zones are observed. Growth is enhanced when the blood agar plates are incubated under increased (5% to 10%) carbon dioxide. Since streptococci are facultative anaerobes, growth is observed both aerobically and anaerobically. Important characteristics of the genus *Streptococcus* are as follows:

- Gram-positive cocci occurring in pairs or chains
- Nonmotile
- Non-spore forming
- Facultative anaerobes
- Some species show enhanced growth under increased CO_2
- Require supportive or enriched media such as blood agar for growth
- Catalase negative
- Susceptible to vancomycin

Enhanced recovery of beta-hemolytic streptococci from clinical specimens may be accomplished through use of a selective blood agar medium that is inhibitory to other bacteria, including staphylococci and gram-negative bacilli. Blood agar containing the antibiotics trimethoprim and sulfamethoxazole is one example of such a medium available commercially for this purpose, which facilitates the isolation of beta-hemolytic streptococci.

Streptococci may be classified according to the type and pattern of hemolysis, by physiological divisions, and by antigenic character of a group-specific cell wall polysaccharide known as the **Lancefield grouping.** Physiological divisions are pyogenic, viridans, lactic, and enterococcal streptococci.

In 1933, Rebecca Lancefield identified several distinct antigenic streptococcal groups based on a specific cell wall polysaccharide. She named the first five groups A, B, C, D, and E. Today, there are almost 20 Lancefield groups, designated A through H and K through T. Serological methods are available whereby the cell wall antigen can be extracted and the organism serotyped to the specific Lancefield group. Clinically significant Lancefield groups include groups A, B, C, D, F, and G.

To initially identify an organism as a *Streptococcus*, one relies on the size and appearance of the colonies on primary plating media, as well as on the type and pattern of hemolysis on blood agar. It is important to remember that the type of hemolysis depends on the source of the blood agar. Traditional classifications of hemolytic patterns have been largely established on 5% sheep blood agar with a trypticase soy agar base. Other types of blood agar include horse, rabbit, and human blood agars. Hemolysis should always be determined by holding the plate directly in front of a light source. The box below presents the hemolytic patterns known as **Brown's classification.** Table 8-1 summarizes clinically important streptococci with Lancefield group and type of hemolysis.

Types of Hemolysis

Alpha (α): incomplete or partial hemolysis; green or brown color surrounding the colony. This pattern is seen with the viridans streptococci (the major normal flora of the oropharynx) and *Streptococcus pneumoniae* (an important cause of pneumonia).

Beta (β) complete hemolysis of red blood cells; clearing or colorless zone around colony. This pattern is best characterized by *Streptococcus pyogenes* (the agent of streptococcal pharyngitis).

Gamma (γ): lack of hemolysis; no apparent change in color of area surrounding colony. Most *Enterococcus* species of Lancefield group D are gamma hemolytic.

Alpha prime (α′): a small zone of alpha hemolysis surrounds the colony. A small zone of beta hemolysis surrounds the zone of alpha hemolysis.

Beta hemolysis results from the production of two hemolysins, streptolysin S and streptolysin O. **Streptolysin O** is antigenic, oxygen labile, and produced mainly by group A streptococci. Recent group A streptococcal infection can be diagnosed through the detection of **anti–streptolysin O,** an antibody, in the patient's serum. **Streptolysin S** is nonantigenic, oxygen stable, and thus noted as surface hemolysis. Because a small percentage of group A streptococci do not produce streptolysin S, blood agar should be "stabbed" several times to force some of the organism to grow in the reduced oxygen content. Stabs made approximately one-half the depth of the agar with the inoculating loop while streaking the culture will allow for the detection of streptolysin O.

GROUP A *STREPTOCOCCUS*

Group A *Streptococcus, Streptococcus pyogenes,* is best isolated on blood agar. Addition of trimethoprim and sulfamethoxazole **(SXT)** to the blood agar will enhance its recovery from highly contaminated or heavily grown specimens. After 18 to 24 hours of incubation at 35° to 37°C, growth is typically pinpoint (0.5 to 1.0 μm in diameter) and opalescent or gray in color. The colonies are usually surrounded by a large, wide zone of beta hemolysis. Figure 8-1 (Color Plate 19) illustrates group A *Streptococcus* on sheep blood agar. Group A streptococcal colonies may appear either smooth and glossy or round and mucoid, which indicates the presence of **M protein.** M protein or hyaluronic acid is found in encapsulated strains of *S. pyogenes,* and its presence is associated with virulence. M protein holds antiphagocytic properties, and therefore infection can be established in the absence of type-specific antibody.

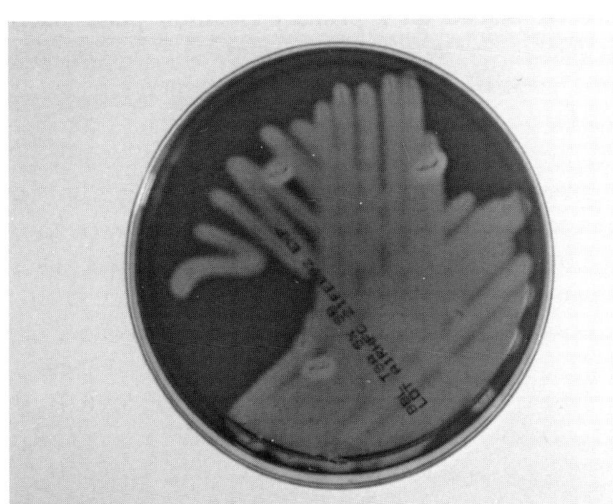

FIGURE 8–1
Group A beta-hemolytic *Streptococcus* on sheep blood agar showing small pinpoint colonies and wide zone of beta hemolysis.

infections, and erysipelas. Whereas impetigo is a superficial skin infection, cellulitis involves deeper tissue, and erysipelas is characterized by erythema and edema. Erysipelas may invade the skin and subcutaneous tissue and is most frequently seen on the face or legs. Puerpural sepsis, a once common infection, is infrequently attributed to group A *Streptococcus* today. Other infection associated with the organism include otitis media, pneumonia, and bacteremia.

All group A streptococcal infections require completion of the antibiotic course to eradicate the organism and prevent sequelae. Sequelae are believed to result from a cross-reacting antigen that attacks cardiac or renal tissue while attempting to destroy streptococci. Penicillin or erythromycin for penicillin-allergic patients is the drug of choice.

Untreated or partially treated streptococcal pharyngitis may be associated with acute rheumatic fever (ARF). ARF may occur 2 to 3 weeks after the onset of pharyngitis and is characterized by fever, arthralgia, and its most severe manifestation, cardiac valvular disease. This may lead to chronic rheumatic heart disease, which results in progressive degeneration of the heart. A resurgence of rheumatic fever in the United States was noted in 1985 in several areas, including Ohio, Pennsylvania, and Utah. Outbreaks were also noted in recruits in military camps in California and Missouri.

Acute glomerular nephritis (AGN) may be seen in patients following streptococcal pharyngitis or skin infections. Seen in children and teenagers, AGN is characterized by edema, hypertension, hematuria, proteinuria, and red blood cell casts in the urine. Group A *Streptococcus* is frequently isolated from the throat, and the ASO titer is elevated.

An increase in invasive group A beta-hemolytic streptococcal infections and bacteremia have been reported during recent years. These diseases were seen in several patient populations but more extensively in elderly nursing home patients and in children. In addition, these invasive infections were often associated with bacteremia and patients with underlying medical disorders, surgery, trauma, or disruptions to the skin barrier. The syndrome, now known as streptococcal toxic shock-like syndrome (TSLS), is a toxin-mediated disease that can affect several organs. Known to affect young to middle-aged adults with no medical predisposition, as well as elderly persons, the disease is characterized by severe pain and an abrupt onset. A prior history of the "flu" was noted in several patients. Other symptoms of TSLS include fever, hypotension, erythema, swelling, tachycardia, acute respiratory distress, renal impairment, shock, and mortality. Specific M protein types have been associated with these syndromes. Many of these effects can be attributed to **pyogenic exotoxin A,** the same toxin that has been associated with scarlet fever.

GROUP B *STREPTOCOCCUS*

Group B *Streptococcus, Streptococcus agalactiae,* is isolated on sheep blood agar. Colonies are pinpoint and clear and usually beta hemolytic while a few strains are nonhemolytic (Figure 8-6 [Color Plate 20]).

In the **CAMP reaction** (acronym for Christie, Atkins, Munch, Peterson—those individuals who first characterized the phenomena) an "arrowhead" zone of hemolysis forms when group B *Streptococcus* is streaked perpendicularly to a beta-hemolytic strain of *Staphylococcus aureus* (Figure 8-7). The CAMP factor is an extracellular, thermostable, antigenic protein produced by group B *Streptococcus.* A small percentage of group A *Streptococcus* give a positive reaction. Thus bacitracin

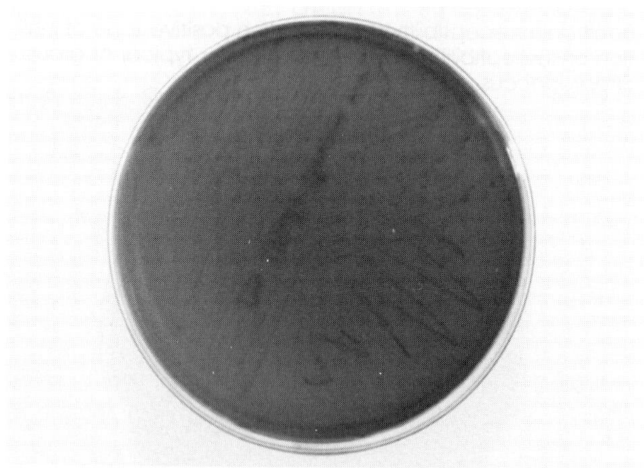

FIGURE 8–6

Group B *Streptococcus* on sheep blood agar. Colonies are pinpoint, clear, and either narrow-zone beta hemolytic or nonhemolytic.

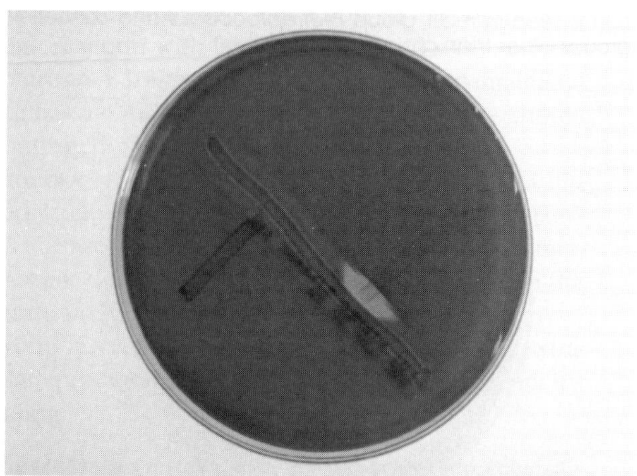

FIGURE 8–7

CAMP reaction. Streptococcal colonies are streaked at right angles to beta-hemolytic *Staphylococcus aureus.* Positive reaction is indicated by an arrowhead pattern, resulting from synergistic hemolysis between group B *Streptococcus* and *S. aureus.*

and SXT susceptibilities should be used in combination with the CAMP reaction in the identification of beta-hemolytic streptococci.

In the **hippurate reaction,** group B streptococci hydrolyze sodium hippurate to benzoic acid and glycine. Benzoic acid is detected with ferric chloride. Alternatively, glycine may be detected with Ninhydrin reagent.

Group B streptococci are resistant to bacitracin and are bile-esculin negative.

Group B *Streptococcus* is normal flora of the GI tract, pharynx, and vaginal tract. The organism is associated with neonatal infections, including pneumonia, meningitis, and bacteremia, and mortality. Approximately 15% to 25% of females carry the organism as normal vaginal flora, and transmission to the infant may occur during delivery. Group B *Streptococcus* typically causes early-onset infections in the newborn and is a leading cause of neonatal sepsis. The organism may also cause puerpural sepsis and maternal septicemia. Adult group B streptococcal infections include skin infections, bacteremia, urinary tract infections (UTIs), and endocarditis. These infections frequently involve an immunosuppressed host.

Infections are frequently treated with penicillin.

GROUP D *STREPTOCOCCUS* AND *ENTEROCOCCUS*

This Lancefield group possesses the group D antigen and is characterized by the ability to grow in 40% bile and hydrolyze esculin. Figures 8-8 and 8-9 illustrate positive and negative **bile esculin** reactions. Group D *Streptococcus* is divided into two subgroups: the *Enterococcus* and the non-*Enterococcus*. *Enterococcus* consists of several species, including the following, which may be associated with human infections:

***E. faecalis* (subsp. *faecalis, liquifaciens, zymogens*)**
E. faecium
E. durans
E. avium

E. faecalis is the most common *Enterococcus* isolated from human infection, accounting for approximately 80% to 85% of all isolates, while *E. faecium* is responsible for approximately 10%. *E. durans* and *E. avium,* as well as the numerous other species, are rarely associated with human infection.

The enterococci may be alpha hemolytic, beta hemolytic, or nonhemolytic on sheep blood agar (Figure 8-10 [Color Plate 21]); the most frequent type is nonhemolytic. These organisms are normal flora of the skin, upper respiratory tract, GI tract, and genitourinary tract.

The nonenterococci comprise only two species: *S. bovis* and *S. equinus*. *S. bovis* is the only species found in humans, whereas *S. equinus* is usually nonpathogenic for humans.

The enterococci are bile-esculin positive and can grow in 6.5% sodium chloride (NaCl) broth (are **salt tolerant**). The nonenterococci are bile-esculin positive but are unable to grow in 6.5% NaCl broth. Figure 8-11 illustrates positive and negative reactions for 6.5% NaCl broth. A rapid test for the enzyme pyrrolidonylarylamidase (PYRase) is positive for *Enterococcus* but negative for non-*Enterococcus* (Figure 8-12 [Color Plate 22]). These reactions are summarized in Table 8-2.

Enterococci are frequent causes of UTIs and wound infections, which may be polymicrobic in nature. Intraabdominal abscesses and septicemia are also

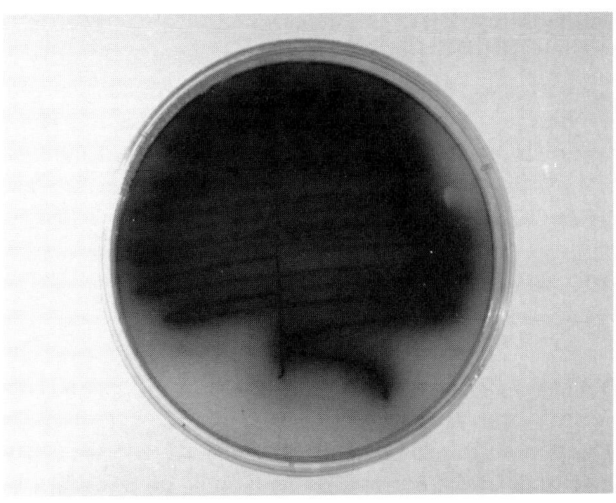

FIGURE 8–8
Bile-esculin agar indicating positive hydrolysis of bile esculin. Positive hydrolysis is characteristic of group D *Enterococcus* and group D *Streptococcus*.

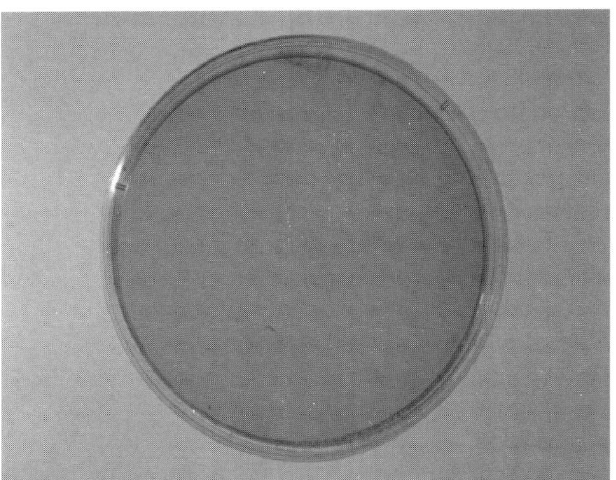

FIGURE 8–9
Bile-esculin agar indicating negative hydrolysis of bile esculin. Negative hydrolysis indicates a *Streptococcus* other than group D.

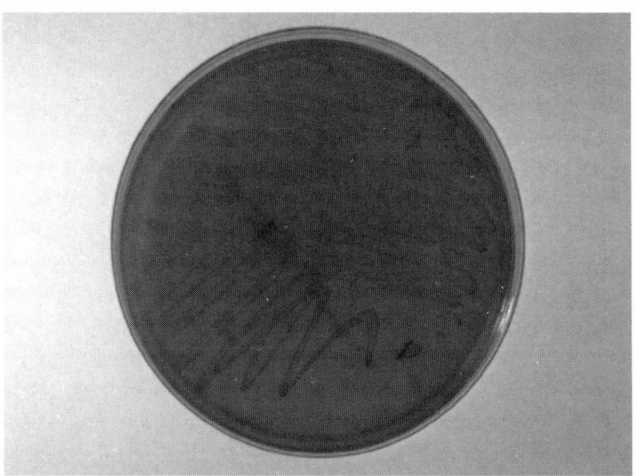

FIGURE 8-10

Enterococcus on sheep blood agar. Colonies are small, grayish, and may be alpha, beta, or nonhemolytic.

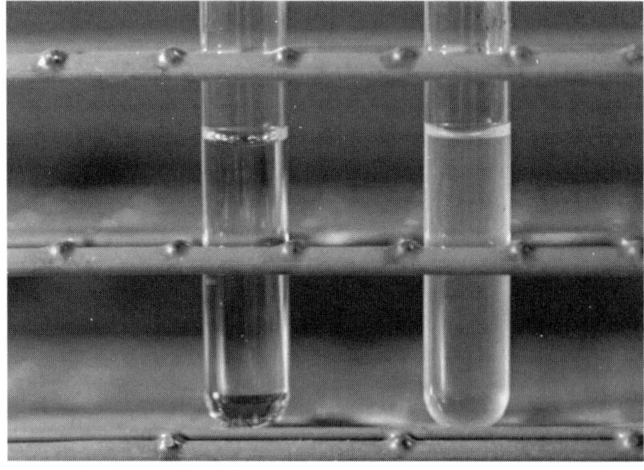

FIGURE 8-11

6.5% Salt broth test. Positive growth in 6.5% salt broth is characteristic of group D *Enterococcus,* whereas lack of growth is characteristic of group D non-*Enterococcus.* The reaction is used to differentiate these two groups.

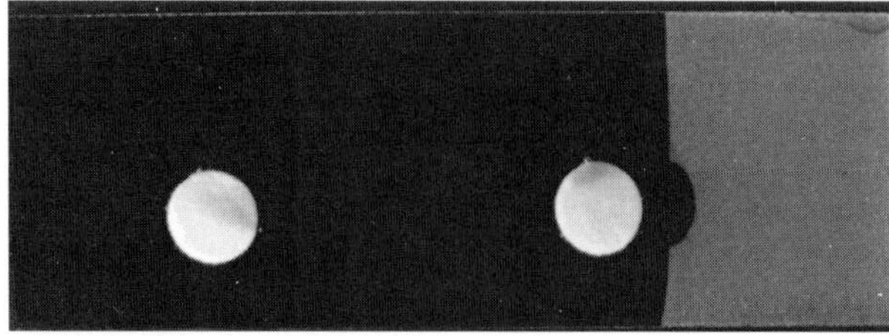

FIGURE 8-12

PYRase activity is positive for group D *Enterococcus* and group A *Streptococcus.* The reaction can be used to differentiate *Enterococcus* (+) from non-*Enterococcus* (−) and as an additional test to aid in the identification of group A *Streptococcus.*

associated with these bacteria. The enterococci may also cause endocarditis in elderly and debilitated persons. The nonenterococci are associated with UTIs, endocarditis, and septicemia. A possible association between *S. bovis* endocarditis and bacteremia and GI carcinoma has been identified. The organism has been found in the stool and blood of some patients with colon cancer.

Enterococcal strains are usually resistant to penicillin G and penicillinase-resistant penicillins. In fact, *Enterococcus* species are more resistant to penicillin, the cephalosporins, and aminoglycosides than are the non-*Enterococcus* species. Combining a penicillin product with an aminoglycoside, such as gentamycin, may be used for enterococcal infections. Vancomycin and erythromycin are also possible treatment choices. The nonenterococci can be treated with penicillin G.

MISCELLANEOUS LANCEFIELD GROUPS

Lancefield group C includes the following species of *Streptococcus: S. equisimilis, S. zooepidemicus, S. equi,* and *S. dysagalactiae. S. equisimilis* causes a severe pharyngitis that may be followed by bacteremia. It is an opportunistic pathogen that may also be associated with pneumonia, cellulitis, and abscesses. The organism is beta hemolytic and gives negative reactions for the CAMP factor, PYRase, and bile esculin and is susceptible to SXT.

S. anginosus is classified as Lancefield group F and is associated rarely with cellulitis, abscesses, and bacteremia. Particular strains of *S. anginosus* may also have A-, C-, or G-type Lancefield antigens.

Lancefield group G is found as normal flora of the human GI and vaginal tract and oropharynx. It has been implicated in otitis media, pharyngitis, and endocarditis.

Identification of Lancefield groups C, F, and G can be confirmed through reaction with type-specific antisera, as is the case for most Lancefield groups. After isolation of the bacteria, the cell wall antigen is extracted. This is then mixed with antisera specific for each Lancefield group. The antisera are usually tagged to latex beads to aid visualization. Agglutination should occur with only one antisera, thus identifying the Lancefield group.

VIRIDANS STREPTOCOCCI

The **viridans streptococci** are a group of streptococcal species characterized by alpha hemolysis on sheep blood agar. These organisms are not Lancefield grouped even though some strains possess specific Lancefield antigens. Some of the numerous species in this group include *S. mutans, S. uberis, S. mitis, S. sanguis I, S. sanguis II, S. salivarius, S. constellatus,* and *S. intermedius.* Most are normal flora of the human

TABLE 8–2

Differentiation of Group D Streptococci and Enterococci

	BILE-ESCULIN MEDIA	6.5% NaCl BROTH	PYRase
Group D *Enterococcus*	+	+	+
Group D non-*Enterococcus*	+	–	–
Not group D	–	–	–

oropharynx and are important agents of subacute bacterial endocarditis, frequently in patients with damaged valvular heart tissue, such as from rheumatic heart disease or a prolapsed mitral valve. The organism may enter the blood after dental procedures or genitourinary techniques and may cause bacteremia and septicemia. *S. mutans* is composed of a group of seven genospecies and is associated with dental caries. *S. constellatus* has been associated with abscesses and bacteremia.

Viridans streptococci are all resistant to surface active agents, such as bile, sodium desoxycholate, and optochin. In fact, viridans streptococci are often identified by "exclusion," which means that negative results are obtained for most presumptive tests used to identify streptococci. The organisms may be speciated based on specific biochemical reactions, such as carbohydrate fermentation. However, most clinical laboratories do not report to the species level.

STREPTOCOCCUS PNEUMONIAE

Streptococcus pneumoniae differs from other streptococci by its Gram-stained appearance, which is typically gram-positive diplococci, which tend to form chains. The organism is lancet or bullet shaped.

S. pneumoniae can be isolated on sheep blood agar and requires 5% to 10% CO_2. Thus primary isolation plates should be incubated in a candle jar or CO_2 chamber. At 24 hours' incubation at 35° to 37°C, encapsulated strains produce small, round, glistening, dome-shaped colonies that are transparent with an entire edge. Often the colonies will run together. Mucoid colonies indicate the presence of a capsule and contain M protein. A wide zone of alpha hemolysis surrounds the pneumococcal colony when incubated aerobically. The alpha hemolysis can be attributed to the production of **pneumolysin** by the organism. As the colonies age, **autolysis** occurs and the colonies "collapse," leaving an outer elevated margin and a centrally depressed region. Autolysis is usually seen after 48 hours of incubation.

The most common test used to identify *S. pneumoniae* is the **optochin test** ("P" disk). Optochin contains ethylhydrocupreine hydrochloride and selectively inhibits the growth of *S. pneumoniae* at low levels. A typical zone of inhibition around a 6 μm optochin disk for *S. pneumoniae* is a minimum of 14 mm. Other alpha-hemolytic streptococci, including viridans and enterococci, are resistant to optochin at this concentration. Figure 8-13 illustrates *S. pneumoniae's* susceptibility to optochin, and Figure 8-14 (Color Plate 23) illustrates the resistance of viridans streptococci to optochin.

In **bile solubility tests,** sodium desoxycholate and sodium taurocholate are able to lyse *S. pneumoniae* when grown in culture. On agar, colonies of the organism will characteristically lyse when exposed to either of these bile salts. Other alpha-hemolytic streptococci are resistant to the action of these bile salts.

More modern techniques include **antigen testing** for the **capsular polysaccharide.** In such techniques, antisera specific for *S. pneumoniae* are tagged with latex particles. Agglutination will occur in the presence of the corresponding capsular antigen. Such tests are rapid and can allow a decreased time for identification.

The **Neufeld reaction (Quellung, capsular swelling)** test can be used to identify the organism in direct body fluids, such as spinal fluid, synovial fluid, or sputum. When present in large numbers in a particular site, equal amounts of the body fluid can be mixed with *S. pneumoniae*-specific capsular antisera. If the reaction is positive, the antisera will bind to the capsular antigen, making the capsule "swell" or become more prominent.

Various extracellular products or antigenic compounds associated with *S. pneumoniae* contribute to its virulence, including:

Capsular antigens: antigenic polysaccharides that result in 84 different serogroups of the organism; resistant to phagocytosis and stimulate antibody production
M protein: type-specific protein antigens
Capsular polysaccharide: antiphagocytic
Pneumolysin: antiphagocytic, hemolytic

Because *S. pneumoniae* may be normal flora of the upper respiratory tract, it may be difficult to interpret its

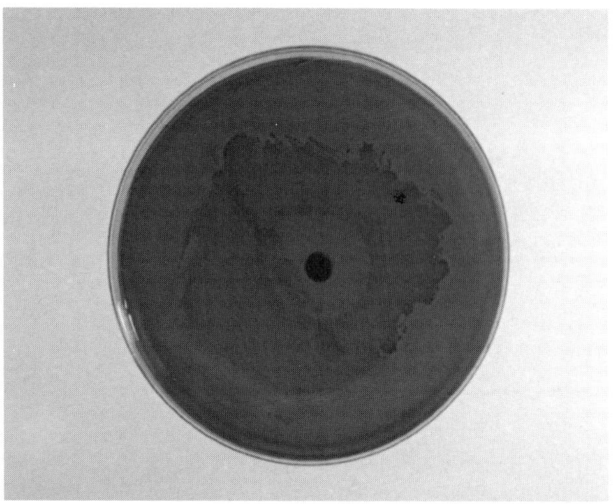

FIGURE 8–13

Optochin test for *S. pneumoniae.* Typical mucoid, alpha-hemolytic growth of the organism is seen with a zone of inhibition (exceeding 14 mm), indicating susceptibility of *S. pneumoniae* to 6 μg optochin.

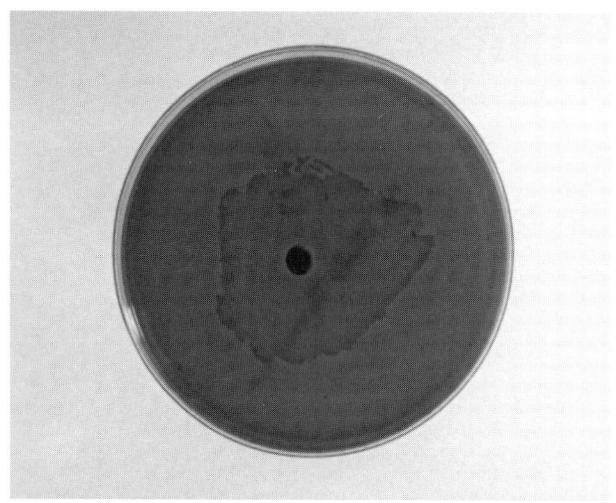

FIGURE 8–14

Optochin test for viridans streptococci indicating resistance of organism to 6 μg optochin. Reaction is characteristic of alpha-hemolytic streptococci other than *S. pneumoniae.*

recovery from sputum and lower respiratory tract cultures. Also, it is difficult to recover from clinical specimens, and many patients who are positive for infection may be culture negative. For that reason, the direct Gram stain is an important diagnostic tool. Bartlett's classification scheme discussed in Chapter 3 can be used to evaluate the suitability of the sputum sample.

Characteristically, patients with pneumococcal infections of the lower respiratory tract show a predominance of *S. pneumoniae* with a decrease or lack of normal oropharyngeal flora. A moderate to large amount of neutrophils also may be present, and the sputum may be rust tinged or bloody.

Infections attributed to *S. pneumoniae* include lobar pneumonia and community-acquired pneumonia. Acute pneumococcal pneumonia is especially prevalent in elderly, debilitated, and alcoholic patients. If the organism enters the blood, bacteremia and septicemia can result. Other complications include endocarditis, meningitis, and pericarditis.

S. pneumoniae is also a leading bacterial pathogen in infants and small children, accounting for numerous middle ear infections. It is also an important cause of meningitis in various age groups.

Penicillin has been the drug of choice for all pneumococcal infections. Since penicillin-resistant strains have been found and are increasing, isolates should be tested for penicillin susceptibility. Currently, a vaccination for immunity to *S. pneumoniae* is available and is recommended for those individuals at increased risk for infection.

NUTRITIONALLY VARIANT STREPTOCOCCI

Nutritionally variant streptococci are viridans streptococci that need cysteine or pyridoxal (Vitamin B_6) for growth. These organisms are also referred to as "satelliting" streptococci, thiol-requiring streptococci, or pyridoxal-requiring streptococci. When in a mixed culture with *Staphylococcus aureus,* the nutritionally variant streptococci "satellite" around the colonies of *S. aureus* because they provide the pyridoxal needed. *S. adjacens* and *S. defectivus* are classified as nutritionally variant streptococci. The organisms are normal flora of the upper respiratory tract and GI tract and have been implicated as agents in endocarditis.

The identification of clinically significant streptococci is shown in Figures 8-15 to 8-17.

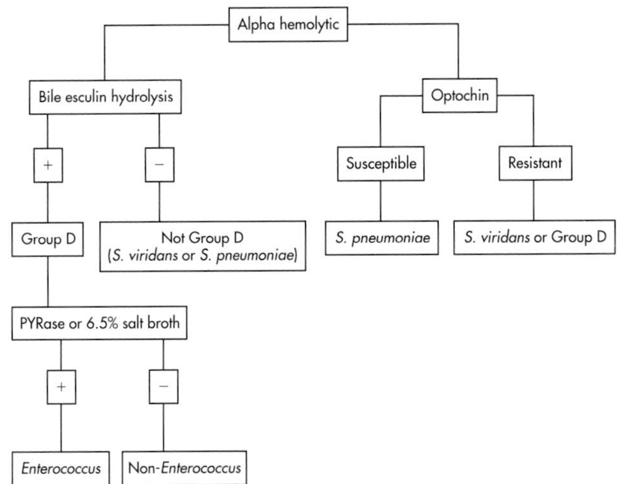

Group	Optochin	Bile esculin	6.5% salt broth	PYRase
D *Enterococcus*	R (−)	+	+	+
D non-*Enterococcus*	R (−)	+	−	−
S. pneumoniae	S (+)	−	−	−
S. viridans	R (−)	−	V	−

R, resistant; *S*, susceptible; *V*, variable.

FIGURE 8–15
Identification of alpha-hemolytic streptococci.

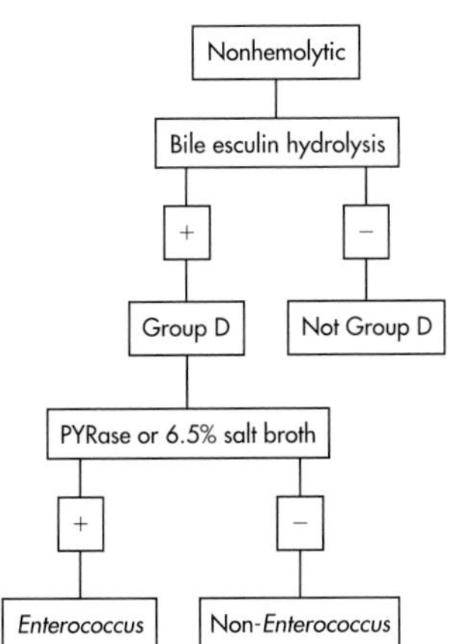

Group	Bile esculin	6.5% salt broth	PYRase
D *Enterococcus*	+	+	+
D non-*Enterococcus*	+	−	−

FIGURE 8–16
Identification of beta-hemolytic streptococci.

Group	Bacitracin	TS	CAMP	Bile esculin	6.5% salt broth	PYRase
A	S (+)	R (−)	−*	−	−	+
B	R (−)	R (−)	+	−	−	−
C, F, G	R (−)**	S (+)	−	−	−	−
D *Enterococcus*	R (−)	R (−)	−	+	+	+
D non-*Enterococcus*	R (−)	R (−)	−	+	−	−

TS, Trimethoprim sulfamethoxazole.
* A small percentage of Group A gives an intermediate positive CAMP reaction.
** A small percentage of Groups C, F, and G are susceptible to bacitracin.

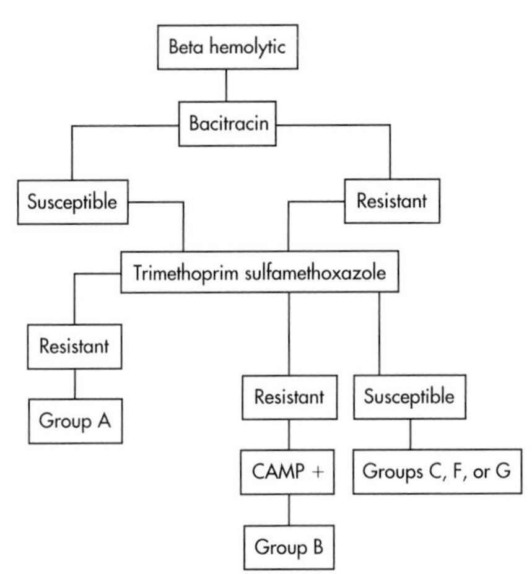

FIGURE 8–17
Identification of nonhemolytic streptococci.

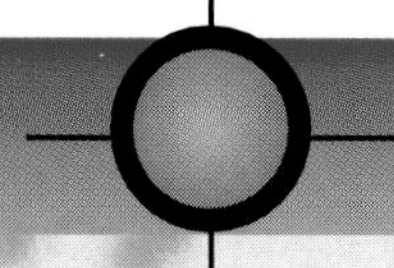

PROCEDURE

BACITRACIN AND SULFAMETHOXAZOLE-TRIMETHOPRIM SUSCEPTIBILITY TESTS

PURPOSE

Tests provide a mechanism to identify group A and group B beta-hemolytic streptococci.

PRINCIPLE

Group A beta-hemolytic streptococci *(S. pyogenes)* are susceptible to 0.04 U bacitracin but resistant to 1.25 μg sulfamethoxazole-trimethoprim (SXT). Group B beta-hemolytic streptococci are resistant to both bacitracin and SXT.

REAGENTS AND MATERIALS

Blood agar plates
0.04 U bacitracin disks
1.25 μg trimethoprim-sulfamethoxazide disks

PROCEDURE

1. Select a few of the beta-hemolytic streptococci to be tested and streak one-half the plate in three directions to obtain a lawn of growth.
2. Stab agar two or three times.
3. Using sterile forceps, place on bacitracin disk and SXT disk in the center of the streak. The disks should be spaced evenly so that zone diameters can be accurately interpreted. Tap gently with forceps.
4. Incubate 18 to 24 hours at 35° to 37°C.

INTERPRETATION

Any zone of inhibition around either disk indicates that the organism is susceptible.
Growth up to the disk (no zone of inhibition) indicates that the organism is resistant.

ORGANISM	BACITRACIN	SXT
Group A	*Susceptible*	*Resistant*
Group B	*Resistant*	*Resistant*
Not group A or B: possibly group C, F, or G	*Resistant*	*Susceptible*

QUALITY CONTROL

Group A *Streptococcus:* bacitracin susceptible and SXT resistant
Group B *Streptococcus:* bacitracin resistant and SXT resistant
Group C *Streptococcus:* bacitracin resistant and SXT susceptible

NOTE

A small percentage of Lancefield groups B, C, and F also give a positive bacitracin test; it is advisable also to perform a CAMP reaction.

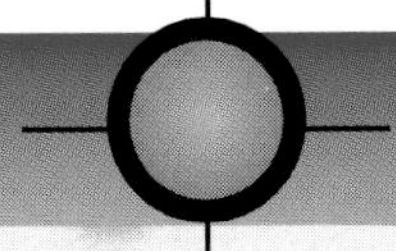

PROCEDURE
CAMP REACTION

PURPOSE
CAMP is an acronym for those individuals who first described the phenomena of synergistic hemolysis between group B *Streptococcus* and beta-hemolytic *Staphylococcus aureus.*

PRINCIPLE
The CAMP factor is a diffusible, proteinlike compound produced by *Streptococcus agalactiae.* A characteristic "arrowhead" hemolytic pattern results when the organism is streaked perpendicularly to beta-hemolytic *S. aureus.*

MATERIALS
5% sheep blood agar
Beta-hemolytic *S. aureus*

PROCEDURE
1. Streak *S. aureus* down the center of the blood agar plate.
2. At a right angle to the *S. aureus* streak, streak 18 to 24-hour culture to be tested. The two lines must not touch, even after incubation.
3. Incubate at 35° to 37°C for 24 hours. Do not incubate anaerobically or under increased CO_2 or false-positive results may occur.

INTERPRETATION
Positive: a zone of enhanced hemolysis given by an arrowhead appearance at the junction of the *Staphylococcus* and *Streptococcus* indicates the presence of group B *Streptococcus.* Report, "Group B *Streptococcus,* presumptive by CAMP reaction."
Negative: no zone of enhanced hemolysis; not group B *Streptococcus*

QUALITY CONTROL
Streptococcus agalactiae: positive; displays enhanced hemolysis in arrowhead pattern
Streptococcus bovis: negative; does not show an arrowhead

NOTE
Some strains of group A *Streptococcus* will show an intermediate positive reaction for the CAMP test. This is especially seen when incubation is at increased CO_2 or anaerobic. Incubation in ambient air is essential for accurate results.

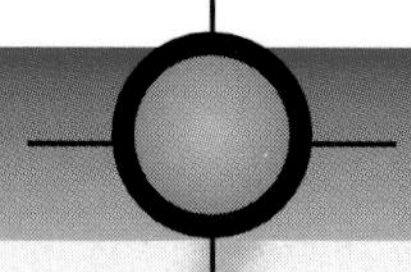

PROCEDURE
BILE-ESCULIN AGAR

PURPOSE
Bile-esculin agar (BEA) is used to distinguish group D *Streptococcus* and *Enterococcus* species. The group D *Streptococcus* can grow in 40% bile and hydrolyze esculin, while other Lancefield groups cannot.

PRINCIPLE
Esculin is a coumarin derivative of a glycoside that contains a glucose moiety and a glycone moiety. Differentiation is based on the organism's ability to grow in 40% bile and to hydrolyze esculin to produce esculetin. Esculetin reacts with ferric citrate to form a brown-black precipitate.

MATERIALS
Bile-esculin plates or agar slants

PROCEDURE
1. Touch the center of a well-isolated colony with a sterile loop and streak BEA plate or slant.
2. Incubate at 35° to 37°C for 24 to 48 hours.
3. Interpret plates for presence of growth and blackening.

INTERPRETATION
Positive: growth indicates tolerance to 40% bile (4% oxgall). Blackening indicates hydrolysis of esculin.
Negative: lack of growth indicates inability of organism to grow in 40% bile, and lack of color change indicates inability of organism to hydrolyze esculin.

QUALITY CONTROL
Enterococcus faecalis: growth with black color
Streptococcus viridans group: no growth

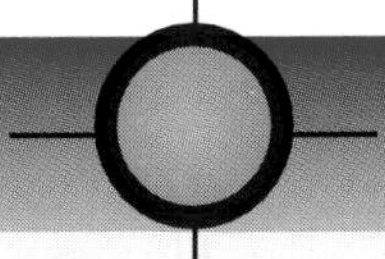

PROCEDURE
6.5% SALT BROTH

PURPOSE
Salt (NaCl) broth is useful for classifying bacteria based on their ability to grow in the presence of 6.5% NaCl. The ability to grow in 6.5% NaCl is characteristic of certain species of gram-positive cocci and gram-negative bacilli. The test is useful for differentiating the group D enterococci, which are salt tolerant, from the nonenterococci, which are intolerant.

PRINCIPLE
A medium without added salt is tested along with the 6.5% salt broth to serve as a growth control. If growth is equivalent in both media, the organism is tolerant of salt and a positive result is noted. However, if the growth on the salt-containing medium is very weak or absent but growth in the salt-free medium is good, a negative result is noted.

An indicator, such as bromcresol purple, can be incorporated into the medium to facilitate interpretation. A positive result is indicated by a change in the color of the indicator from purple to yellow or by the appearance of obvious growth.

MATERIALS
Trypticase soy broth or nutrient broth (control)
6.5% NaCl broth

PROCEDURE
1. Inoculate three to five colonies of the test organism to a tube of 6.5% NaCl and also to a tube of trypticase soy broth (or nutrient broth).
2. Incubate at 35° to 37°C for 24 to 72 hours.
3. Observe for growth, as evidenced by turbidity.

INTERPRETATION
Compare the degree of turbidity in the 6.5% NaCl tube to the control tube:
If growth is equivalent in both media, the organism is salt tolerant, indicating a positive result.
If growth is present in the control tube but scant or negative in the salt tube, the organism is salt intolerant, indicating a negative result.

QUALITY CONTROL
Enterococcus faecalis: positive; growth in both tubes
Streptococcus bovis: negative; no growth in NaCl tube, but growth in control tube

CASE STUDIES

1

An ambulatory patient with a temperature of 101°F and painful urination visits her physician, who orders a urine culture. A clean-catch midstream urine sample reveals numerous gram-positive cocci in chains in the Gram stain. The specimen is plated on blood agar and MacConkey. At 24 hours' incubation, flat, gray, nonhemolytic colonies are found on the blood agar. No growth is observed on MacConkey. Further testing revealed:

Bile-esculin agar: black precipitate
PYRase: pink color

Identify the organism: ____________________

2

Gram-positive diplococci are observed in the Gram stain of a sputum sample of a 72-year-old male patient. Numerous neutrophils are also observed. Sparse growth on blood agar at 24 hours reveals mucoid colonies with a wide zone of alpha hemolysis. An optochin test was performed using a 6 μg disk. A 20 mm zone of inhibition was noted.

This isolate is most likely: ____________________

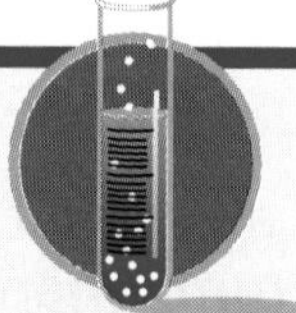

LABORATORY EXERCISES

1

Streak blood agar plates for each of the following species of *Streptococcus.* Remember to "stab" the media. Incubate at 35° to 37°C for 18 to 24 hours. Record your observations and interpret your results.

	Colonial Morphology	Hemolysis
Streptococcus pyogenes	____________	____________
Streptococcus agalactiae	____________	____________
Enterococcus faecalis	____________	____________
Streptococcus bovis	____________	____________
Streptococcus pneumoniae	____________	____________
Streptococcus mutans	____________	____________
Streptococcus equi	____________	____________

LABORATORY EXERCISES

(Continued)

2

Perform a Gram stain on the following streptococci. Record your observations.

S. pyogenes ____________________

E. faecalis ____________________

S. pneumoniae ____________________

3

Perform the bacitracin and sulfmethoxazole-trimethoprim (SXT) susceptibilit tests on the following streptococci. Measure each zone diameter, and interpret your results as susceptible or resistant.

	Bacitracin	**SXT**
S. pyogenes		
S. agalactiae		
S. equi		

4

Perform the bile-esculin, 6.5% salt broth, and PYRase procedures on the following streptococci. Record your observations.

	Bile-Esculin	**6.5% Salt Broth**	**PYRase**
E. faecalis			
S. bovis			
S. mutans			

5

Perform the optochin susceptibility test on the following *Streptococcus* species. Measure the zone diameters, and interpret and record your results.

S. pneumoniae ____________________

S. mutans ____________________

E. faecalis ____________________

LABORATORY EXERCISES

(Continued)

6

Draw a flow chart to indicate the proper identification scheme for:
a. Alpha-hemolytic streptococci b. Beta-hemolytic streptococci c. Nonhemolytic streptococci

7

Identify an unknown *Streptococcus.* Record all media used, procedures performed, observations, and results.

Unknown number: ______________________

Media ______________________

____

Morphology/Hemolysis ______________________

____

Procedure ______________________

____

Observations/Interpretation ______________________

____

Identification: ______________________

Explanation: ______________________

____

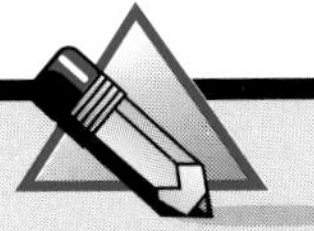

REVIEW QUESTIONS

MATCHING

Match the Lancefield group to the correct species:

_____ **1.** ***S. equisimilis***	a. A
_____ **2.** ***S. bovis***	b. B
_____ **3.** ***S. agalactiae***	c. C
_____ **4.** ***E. faecalis***	d. D, *Enterococcus*
_____ **5.** ***S. mutans***	e. D, Non-*Enterococcus*
_____ **6.** ***S. pyogenes***	f. F
_____ **7.** ***E. faecium***	g. G
_____ **8.** ***S. anginosus***	h. None of the above
_____ **9.** ***S. pneumoniae***	

MULTIPLE CHOICE

10. Lancefield's classification of *Streptococcus* is based on*:*
a. Type of hemolysis
b. Cell wall polysaccharide
c. Capsular antigens
d. M protein serotype

11. Streptolysin O is:
a. Oxygen stable
b. Antigenic
c. Observed as surface hemolysis
d. All the above

12. Which reaction is *incorrect* for *Entero-coccus?*
a. Positive growth in 6.5% salt broth
b. Positive hydrolysis of bile-esculin media
c. Negative catalase reaction
d. PYR negative

13. Sequelae of group ___ *Streptococcus* infection may lead to acute rheumatic fever of acute glomerular nephritis.
a. A
b. B
c. C
d. D, *Enterococcus*
e. D, Non-*Enterococcus*
d. *Plasmodium* and *Borrelia*

14. Colonies of *Streptococcus pneumoniae* at 24 hours are typically:
a. Mucoid and alpha hemolytic
b. Autolysed and alpha hemolytic
c. Mucoid and beta hemolytic
d. None of the above

15. Beta-hemolytic streptococci were isolated from the throat culture of a 15-year-old male. Select the *best* group of tests to identify this organism.
a. Bacitracin and SXT
b. Bacitracin and CAMP
c. Bile-esculin and PYRase
d. Optochin and CAMP

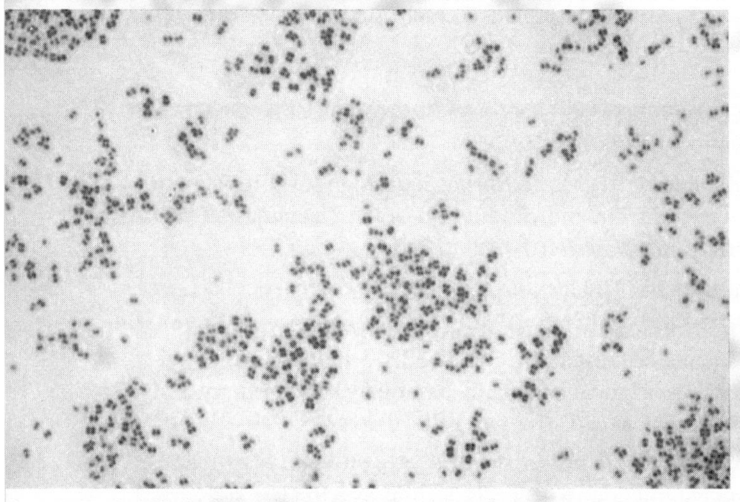

NEISSERIA SICCA

CHAPTER OUTLINE

NEISSERIA GONORRHOEAE
- Infectious Process
- Specimen Collection and Processing
- Identification
- Penicillin Resistance
- Auxotypes

NEISSERIA MENINGITIDIS
- Specimen Collection, Processing, and Identification
- Treatment and Prevention

MORAXELLA CATARRHALIS

MISCELLANEOUS *NEISSERIA*

CYTOCHROME OXIDASE

CYSTINE TRYPTICASE AGAR (CTA) SUGARS

QUADFERM+

KEY TERMS

AUXOTYPE

GONORRHEA

MENINGOCOCCEMIA

OPHTHALMIA NEONATORUM

PENICILLINASE-PRODUCING *N. GONORRHOEAE* (PPNG)

PILI

Neisseria

LEARNING OBJECTIVES

1. Describe the general morphological and biochemical characteristics of *Neisseria.* Explain the significance of pili.
2. List special growth requirements for the pathogenic *Neisseria.*
3. State the principle and purpose of the cytochrome oxidase reaction. Perform and interpret the reaction without error.
4. Describe the infections associated with *Neisseria gonorrhoeae.*
5. Explain the correct methods for specimen collection and processing for *N. gonorrhoeae.*
6. List and compare the media selective for isolation of *N. gonorrhoeae.*
7. Describe the use of the Gram stain in the workup of clinical specimens for *N. gonorrhoeae.*
8. Select, perform, and interpret the necessary media and procedures required to identify *N. gonorrhoeae.*
9. Describe how specimens for *Neisseria meningitidis* are cultured and processed.
10. Explain the infectious process of *N. meningitidis.*
11. Describe how *N. meningitidis* is isolated and identified.
12. Describe the isolation, identification, and clinical relevance of *Moraxella catarrhalis.*
13. Based on growth characteristics and biochemical reactions, differentiate among the following *Neisseria* and *Moraxella* species:
    a. *N. gonorrhoeae*
    b. *N. meningitidis*
    c. *M. catarrhalis*
    d. *N. lactamica*
    e. *N. cinerea*
    f. *N. sicca*
    g. *N. subflava*
    h. *N. flavescens*

The family Neisseriaceae consists of gram-negative aerobic cocci and rods. The family currently comprises the following genera: *Neisseria, Moraxella, Acinetobacter,* and *Kingella.*

The genus *Neisseria* is composed of 11 species, including the significant human pathogens, *Neisseria gonorrhoeae* and *Neisseria meningitidis.* Many of the other species are considered to be normal flora of the nasopharynx, pharynx, or other areas of the upper respiratory tract. These species are rarely associated with human infection. For example, *N. subflava* and *N. mucosa* may be occasionally associated with meningitis and endocarditis.

This chapter also discusses *Moraxella catarrhalis* (formerly *Branhamella catarrhalis*), which in the past had been considered nonpathogenic but has recently been implicated in an increasing number of upper and lower respiratory tract infections.

Organisms in the genus *Neisseria* are typically gram-negative diplococci with adjacent ends flattened, resembling tiny coffee beans or kidney beans on the Gram stain. Of special note is *N. elongata,* which is the only human pathogen that is rod shaped.

Neisseria species are obligate aerobes but prefer increased carbon dioxide (CO_2) and are thus termed **capnophilic.** A capnophilic environment of 3% to 10% CO_2 can be obtained through a candle jar, CO_2 Bio-Bag System (Becton Dickinson Microbiology Systems) or Pouch System (Difco Laboratories), or CO_2 incubator. A **candle jar** is an inexpensive and effective method to obtain an atmosphere with increased CO_2. Agar plates are placed in a large glass jar, and a small wax candle is lit. The lid is secured. When the oxygen in the jar has been used, the candle expires, providing an environment with 3% to 5% CO_2. In addition, the candle jar method also provides a humid environment that prevents the bacteria from drying.

The pathogenic *Neisseria* are very fastidious; *N. gonorrhoeae* requires chocolate agar and *N. meningitidis* and *M. catarrhalis* require blood agar as the minimal growth standard. Enriched media such as chocolate agar provide essential nutrients, including iron, hemin (X factor), and coenzyme I or nicotinamide adenine dinucleotide (NAD, V factor). In addition, *N. gonorrhoeae* requires the amino acid cysteine for growth. Furthermore, these organisms are very sensitive to temperature changes and should be protected from the cold. The pathogenic *Neisseria* grow optimally between 35° and 37°C. By contrast, most of the commensal *Neisseria* can grow on chocolate or blood agar at room temperature or on nutrient agar at 35° to 37°C.

All Neisseria are **cytochrome oxidase** positive. In this reaction a redox dye such as tetra-methyl-para-phenylenediamine dihydrochloride is reacted with the organism. The dye is colorless, and if the organism possesses the oxidase enzymes, the dye is oxidized and becomes blue to purple in color (Figure 9-1 [Color Plate 24]). In addition, all members of the *Neisseria* are catalase positive, except for *N. elongata.*

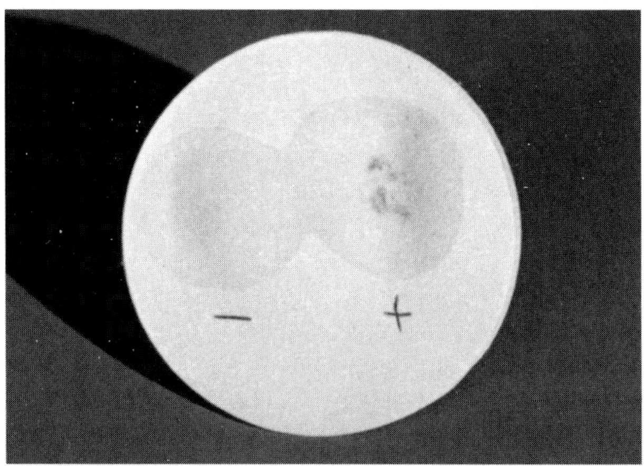

FIGURE 9–1
Cytochrome oxidase reaction illustrating positive violet color when a *Neisseria* organism is mixed with oxidase reagent (1% tetra-methyl-para-phenylenediamine dihydrochloride). Negative reaction is shown on the left.

The *Neisseria* organisms establish disease through attachment to the mucous membranes of the host through **pili,** hairlike structures on the bacterial cell that enable the bacteria to bind to human cells. Pili also participate in conjugation and the transfer of genetic material.

NEISSERIA GONORRHOEAE

Neisseria gonorrhoeae is the agent of **gonorrhea,** an acute pyogenic infection mainly of the mucous membranes of the endocervix in females and the urethra in males. In males the acute urethritis is associated with dysuria and a urethral discharge. Long-term effects of gonococcal infections in females may result in scarred fallopian tubes, ectopic pregnancy, and sterility. Oropharyngeal and rectal infections are seen in homosexual and bisexual males, as well as in females.

Because not all gonorrhea infections are symptomatic, it is necessary to culture both symptomatic and asymptomatic sexual contacts. Both males and females may be asymptomatic carriers. Today, it is recommended to screen those individuals who are at high risk. This includes individuals with multiple sex partners and those who are positive for other sexually transmittable diseases (STDs).

In the early 1980s an increased rate of gonorrhea was noted among the homosexual population. With the fear of acquired immunodeficiency syndrome (AIDS) and the practice of "safer sex" by the homosexual population, the rate has decreased. Today, the rate has increased in teenagers, young adults, urban drug abusers, prostitutes, and those who have a past history of gonorrhea or other STDs.

Extragenital infections include **ophthalmia neonatorum,** a conjunctivitis acquired by newborns from an infected mother during delivery. The condition may result in blindness if not treated. For this reason, all newborns are prophylactically treated with antibiotic drops or cream to prevent the infection from occurring. The use of antibiotics has virtually replaced the prior use of silver nitrate drops for this purpose.

N. gonorrhoeae infections can disseminate into the blood, causing **disseminated gonococcal infection (DGI),** a septicemia characterized by hemorrhagic skin eruptions; to the heart, causing **endocarditis;** and to the joints of the arms and legs, resulting in **gonococcal arthritis.**

Infectious Process

N. gonorrhoeae attaches by pili to susceptible cells of the mucous membranes, which initiates the infection. The pili also inhibit phagocytosis by interfering with the function of neutrophils. The gonococcus also has proteins associated with virulence, including **outer membrane proteins** that impart several biological activities, such as effects on antibody formation, leukocyte response, and cell-mediated immunity. **Lipopolysaccharide** produces endotoxic effects, whereas **protein I** allows for the organism to insert into host cells. **Protein II** is associated with virulence and allows the organism to attach to neutrophils and epithelial cells and to resist the effects of antibodies.

Specimen Collection and Processing

Proper specimen collection is paramount to obtain accurate results for the isolation of *N. gonorrhoeae.* Endocervical specimens are recommended for isolation in females, and urethral specimens are recommended for males. Anorectal, oropharyngeal, and conjunctival specimens may also be warranted based on the patient's age, symptoms, and medical history. In patients with suspected DGI, blood or synovial fluid may be cultured.

Since the organism is susceptible to drying, it is essential either to inoculate the appropriate agar immediately or to use a transport medium. In addition, the use of disinfectants on the patient before collection must be avoided because the organism is susceptible to these agents. Finally, the use of cotton swabs is discouraged because the fatty acids are toxic to the bacterium. Instead, Dacron, rayon, calcium alginate, or cotton swabs treated with charcoal to absorb the fatty acids should be used.

Ideally, specimens should be inoculated immediately onto an appropriate medium. The medium recommended is modified Thayer-Martin, Martin-Lewis, or New York City (NYC); all are selective for the isolation of *N. gonorrhoeae* (see descriptions of these media at the end of this chapter). In addition, some facilities prefer also to inoculate a chocolate agar plate for those rare strains of *N. gonorrhoeae* that are inhibited on the selective plates.

Since many specimens are collected in physicians' offices or clinics, a transport method is required. The **Transgrow** bottles, which consist of a flat bottle coated with modified Thayer-Martin and a bottle under increased CO_2, were once popular transport media for the gonococcus. However, their use is rare today due to a variable CO_2 content and the presence of contaminants. The **JEMBEC** plate (an acronym for John E. Martin Biological Environmental System) has virtually replaced the Transgrow system. The JEMBEC consists of a flat plastic dish containing a medium selective for gonococcus and a tablet that acts as a CO_2 generator. After inoculation of the agar, the tablet is placed in a well and the entire dish is placed into a plastic bag, incubated for 18 to 24 hours, and sent to the laboratory. The plate is observed for growth typical of *N. gonorrhoeae.* Negative plates are reincubated in a CO_2 incubator or candle jar and examined after an additional 24 hours' incubation.

Identification

The Gram stain is essential in the workup of *N. gonorrhoeae.* By "rolling the swab" over the slide, the morphology of the white blood cells and bacteria is better preserved. The Gram stain serves as a presumptive identification in smears prepared from the urethral exudate in male patients and is considered to be highly specific and sensitive in symptomatic males. The sensitivity and specificity are somewhat lower, and thus the Gram stain is somewhat less reliable, in the diagnosis of gonorrhea in female patients. This results from the presence of "look-alike" bacteria that are normally present in the female genital tract. These short gram-negative rods or coccobacilli, including *Moraxella* and *Acinetobacter,* may be mistaken for *N. gonorrhoeae* in a Gram-stained smear from a female patient.

On examination of the Gram stain for gonorrhea, one notes the approximate amount of polymorphonuclear neutrophils (PMNs) and the approximate amount of bacteria present. The report contains an estimate of each: "(Few, moderate, or many) gram-negative diplococci occurring (intracellularly or extracellularly) to (few, moderate, or many) PMNs." Figure 9-2 (Color Plate 25) illustrates gram-negative diplococci.

The specimen should be plated immediately both on a plate selective for *N. gonorrhoeae* and on chocolate agar, since the vancomycin present in the selective plates may also inhibit the gonococcus. Plates should be streaked in a "Z" motion by rolling the swab over the agar surface. Next, the plate is streaked with a loop for isolation. Plates are incubated at 35° to 37°C in the candle jar, CO_2 incubator, or plastic bag or pouch, providing an atmosphere of 3% to 5% CO_2.

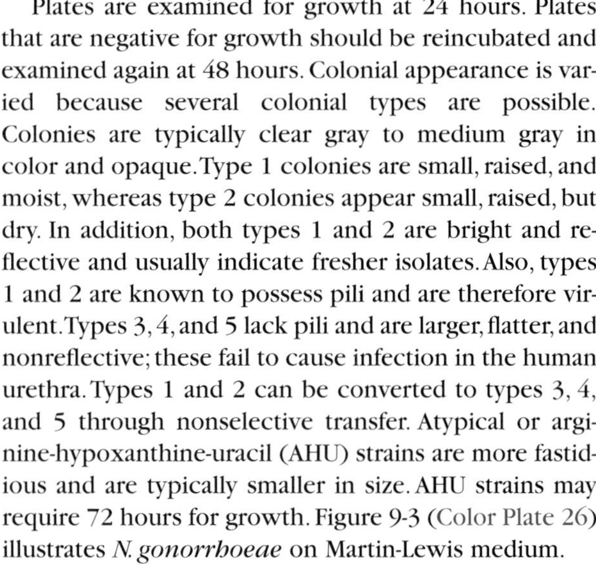

FIGURE 9–2

Gram stain illustrating gram-negative diplococci typical of *Neisseria* species.

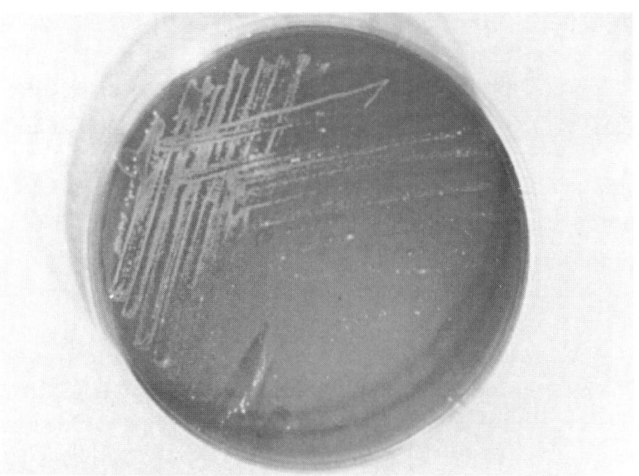

FIGURE 9–3

N. gonorrhoeae on Martin-Lewis medium showing typical gray, translucent, shiny colonies.

Plates are examined for growth at 24 hours. Plates that are negative for growth should be reincubated and examined again at 48 hours. Colonial appearance is varied because several colonial types are possible. Colonies are typically clear gray to medium gray in color and opaque. Type 1 colonies are small, raised, and moist, whereas type 2 colonies appear small, raised, but dry. In addition, both types 1 and 2 are bright and reflective and usually indicate fresher isolates. Also, types 1 and 2 are known to possess pili and are therefore virulent. Types 3, 4, and 5 lack pili and are larger, flatter, and nonreflective; these fail to cause infection in the human urethra. Types 1 and 2 can be converted to types 3, 4, and 5 through nonselective transfer. Atypical or arginine-hypoxanthine-uracil (AHU) strains are more fastidious and are typically smaller in size. AHU strains may require 72 hours for growth. Figure 9-3 (Color Plate 26) illustrates *N. gonorrhoeae* on Martin-Lewis medium.

The cytochrome oxidase test should be performed on any gram-negative diplococci found growing on media selective for *N. gonorrhoeae*. The previous criteria are useful for placing the organism in the genus *Neisseria* but should not be used for species identification.

Confirmatory tests rely on the ability of the organism to oxidize various carbohydrates with the production of acids. Traditionally, the cystine trypticase soy agar base (CTA) sugars have been used for this purpose. This medium supports the growth of the pathogenic *Neisseria*. The various carbohydrates are added to the agar in a 1% concentration. These carbohydrates include glucose, maltose, lactose, sucrose, and fructose. The tubes are inoculated with a heavy suspension of the organism and incubated in a non-CO_2 incubator for 24 hours. Tubes are examined for the production of acid, as indicated by a change to yellow in the pH indicator, phenol red. Negative tubes are reincubated and examined at 48 and 72 hours. All positive tubes should be Gram-stained or subcultured to check for purity of growth, since the CTA medium is very rich and supports the growth of many bacteria.

N. gonorrhoeae gives a positive reaction for glucose in the CTA sugar reactions.

Today, the CTA sugars have been virtually replaced by rapid methods of carbohydrate utilization due to the long incubation time necessary to identify certain strains of *N. gonorrhoeae*. In addition, the CTA system is prone to contamination, which may lead to false-positive reactions. Newer test systems rely on a heavy concentration of inoculum and a concentrated volume of carbohydrate. The rapid fermentation test (RFT) of Kellogg and Turner was one of the first systems designed for this purpose. Today, numerous test systems exist, including the Minitek (Becton-Dickinson Microbiological Systems), which uses carbohydrate-impregnated disks; the RapID NH, (Innovative Diagnostics Systems), which uses biochemical and substrate tests; the RIM-N Neisseria (Austin Biological Laboratories), which employs microtubes with carbohydrates; and the QuadFERM + (bioMerieux Vitek) (Figure 9-4 [Color Plate 27]), which determines carbohydrate utilization and production of beta-lactamase and deoxyribonuclease (DNase). Such systems can often be read in a shorter incubation time of 2 to 4 hours for results.

In addition, several methods for direct identification of *N. gonorrhoeae* from clinical specimens exist. Direct detection of the gonococcus can be accomplished through enzyme-linked immunosorbent assay (ELISA) performed on urethral swabs of male patients and endocervical swabs of female patients. The Gonozyme (Abbott Laboratories) allows for direct detection of the gonococcal antigen by absorbing the antigen from the swab onto a latex bead specific for *N. gonorrhoeae*.

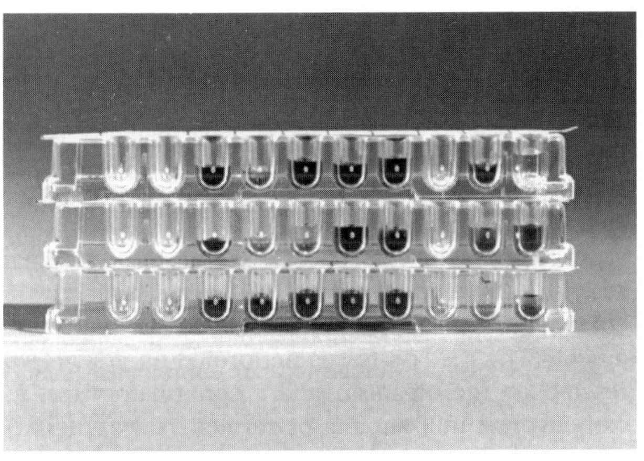

FIGURE 9–4

QuadFERM+ showing reactions typical of *N. gonorrhoeae* (note positive utilization of glucose only), *N. lactamica* (positive utilization of glucose, maltose, and lactose), and *Moraxella catarrhalis* (negative utilization of carbohydrates and positive DNase activity). (bioMérieux Vitek.)

After incubation and washing, antibodies to *N. gonorrhoeae* are added. After another incubation, immunoglobulin conjugated to horseradish peroxidase is added. Another incubation follows, and a chromogenic substrate is added. Positive specimens produce a color change that is proportional to the amount of gonococcus antigen present.

Other rapid methods available for direct detection include a nucleic acid probe. In this method the sample is collected and lysed, and a gene probe is added.

Serological methods used to detect *N. gonorrhoeae* from a primary culture plate include coagglutination methods. In the Phadebact Monoclonal GC OMNI (Karo-Bio Diagnostics AB) test, mouse monoclonal antibodies to the outer membrane proteins of the organism are used. In a positive test the antibodies bind to the gonococcal antigens. Fluorescent antibody techniques are also available, which use antisera specific for *N. gonorrhoeae* that will bind to the gonococcal antigens.

Penicillin Resistance

All *N. gonorrhoeae* isolates should be tested for production of beta-lactamase. Since penicillin has been used for almost 50 years in the treatment of gonorrhea, resistant strains have been found. Beta-lactamase hydrolyzes the beta-lactam ring of the penicillin molecule, enabling the organism to resist the effects of penicillin. In cases of penicillin resistance, alternative treatments include spectinomycin or ceftriaxone plus tetracycline, doxycycline, or erythromycin for **penicillinase-producing N. gonorrhoeae (PPNG).** Amoxicillin with probenecid, ampicillin with probenecid, or ceftriaxone can be used for uncomplicated cases.

Auxotypes

Nutritionally variant strains of *N. gonorrhoeae* exist. The **auxotype** refers to the strains that have different nutritional requirements to promote growth in artificial media. More than 30 auxotypes of the organism are currently known. The auxotype can also be used as a aid in determining the potential virulence, degree of invasiveness, and antibiotic resistance of the different strains of *N. gonorrhoeae.* For example, the auxotype AHU, which requires **a**rginine, **h**ypoxanthine, and **u**racil, is known to be sensitive to penicillin and is likely to cause urethritis in males, asymptomatic gonorrhea, and DGI in females. Auxotypes are of interest to those involved in research and are not routinely used in the identification of *N. gonorrhoeae* from clinical cultures.

NEISSERIA MENINGITIDIS

Neisseria meningitidis is a cause of bacterial meningitis and septicemia. The organism is carried by some individuals asymptomatically as normal flora in the nasopharynx. Most individuals form antibodies against the organism, and the infection remains limited as a minor respiratory tract infection. The inflammation may last for a few days to a few weeks.

The organism is encapsulated, and currently nine serogroups have been recognized and four have been proposed. The serogroup is based on the type of capsular polysaccharide. The recognized serogroups are groups A, B, C, D, X, Y, Z, 29E, and W135. The proposed serogroups are H, I, K, and L. The most serious types of infections in the United States are associated with serogroups A, B, C, and Y. The predominant serotypes in the United States are B, C, Y, and W135; group B is associated with approximately one half of all infections in the United States, and group Y has been found to cause approximately 20% of the cases reported. Group A has been associated with infections in underdeveloped countries and in areas of poverty, poor sanitation, and overcrowding. Group B has been found in endemic areas and as a cause of sporadic disease in developed countries. The presence of a capsule enables the organism to resist phagocytosis and is the principal virulence factor.

Asymptomatic carriers serve as the reservoir of infection, which is through aerosols that enter the nasopharynx of the new host. Individuals who cannot form antibodies are susceptible to serious infections, including infants less than 1 year old and those who cannot form antibodies. Others at increased risk include close contacts of carriers and individuals who live in overcrowded living conditions. Because of the close living quarters and fatigue associated with the military, new recruits have historically been susceptible to *N. meningitidis* infections.

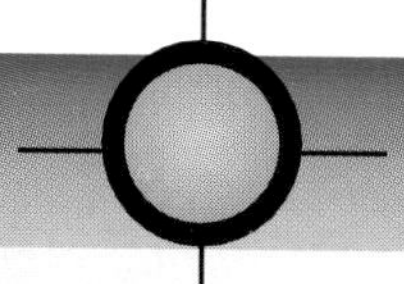

PROCEDURE
QuadFERM+

PURPOSE
The QuadFERM+ allows for the rapid detection of carbohydrate utilization and production of DNase and beta-lactamase by members of the genus *Neisseria.*

PRINCIPLE
The QuadFERM+ system consists of seven microcupules, carbohydrate control well, and glucose, maltose, lactose, sucrose, DNase, and penicillinase test wells. These microcupules are rehydrated with a bacterial suspension in 0.85% saline. The system uses an acidmetric method for detection of carbohydrate utilization and DNase and penicillinase activity. The carbohydrates and substrates are buffered systems containing the pH indicator, phenol red. Organisms that utilize carbohydrates will produce an acid environment that exceeds the buffering capacity of the substrates, resulting in a color change of the phenol red indicator. Organisms that produce DNase or penicillinase will likely cause a color change in the pH indicator.

REAGENTS AND MEDIA
Carbohydrate wells contain either 1% carbohydrates (glucose, lactose, sucrose) or 0.125% maltose and phenol red in a buffered solution.

Carbohydrate control well contains buffered phenol red.
DNase test well contains DNA and phenol red in a buffered solution.
Penicillinase well contains penicillin and phenol red in a phosphate-buffered solution.

NOTES
1. Store test system at 2° to 8°C on arrival.
2. For use, open pouches at one end and remove required number. Close, fold over twice, and secure opened end with tape.
3. Open pouches are stored at 2° to 8°C for up to 2 weeks or until expiration date, whichever comes first.

SPECIMEN COLLECTION AND PROCESSING
Regardless of source, specimens should be transported to the laboratory immediately after collection and processed as soon as possible following their receipt. Although methods for processing specimens may vary, proper selection of adequate plating media and conditions of incubation are very important.

MATERIALS
QuadFERM+ strips
Labeled tapes
Sterile Dacron swabs
Pasteur pipettes
Sterile saline

PROCEDURE
QuadFERM+
(Continued)

Test tubes
Test tube rack
Marking pen
Incubator (35° to 37°C, non-CO_2)

PROCEDURE

1. **Preparation of strips**
   a. Record patient's name or specimen number on sealing label.
   b. Open the pouch by carefully cutting on one end.
   c. Remove the QuadFERM+ strip from the sealed envelope.
   d. Return unused strips to pouch and seal.
   e. Allow strips to come to room temperature before use.
2. **Preparation of bacterial suspension**
   a. Add 2 ml sterile saline to a test tube.
   b. Use a sterile Dacron swab and inoculate saline with a pure bacterial culture. This inoculum should be taken from a fresh (18 to 24 hours) culture on recommended media for *Neisseria* (Modified Thayer-Martin, chocolate, Martin-Lewis). In cases of mixed bacterial flora, first isolate the suspected *Neisseria* colony and incubate for 18 to 24 hours.
   c. Transfer sufficient inoculum into the saline so that a heavy suspension (slurry of bacteria) is achieved. This turbidity should be equivalent to or greater than a no. 3 McFarland Turbidity Standard. Use bacterial suspension as quickly as possible after preparation (within 15 minutes)
3. **Inoculation of strips**
   a. Use a pipette to fill cupules 3, 4, 5, 6, 7, 9, and 10 with 200 μl of the suspension. Inoculated wells will be approximately two-thirds full. The other wells remain empty. The wells should be filled to the same height.
   b. Seal the strip by applying the label with patient's ID already recorded across the top of the wells. The sealing label should be placed over the strip so that the specimen number lines up with cupules 1 and 2.
   c. Gently shake the strip to resolubilize the contents by moving the strip from side to side.
4. **Incubation of strips.** After inoculation, incubate the strips for **2 hours** at 35°C to 37°C in a **non-CO_2** incubator.

INTERPRETATION

Contents of the wells are as follows:
#3—Carbohydrate control well
#4—Glucose (GLU)
#5—Maltose (MAL)
#6—Lactose (LAC)
#7—Sucrose (SUC)
#9—DNA (DNase)
#10—Penicillin (B-LAC)

Continued.

PROCEDURE
QuadFERM+
(Continued)

1. The strips should be read through the side, with the labels still attached across the top. Holding the strips against a white background may assist in reading the color reactions.
2. A positive reaction is indicated by a change in color from red to orange or yellow. A negative reaction remains red or is comparable to the carbohydrate control well.
3. DNase-positive organisms can be detected by a yellow or orange reaction in the DNase well (#9). A negative reaction remains red.
4. Penicillinase-producing organisms can be detected by a positive reaction in the penicillinase well (#10). A positive reaction ranges from yellow to orange. A negative reaction remains light-red to red.

Do not use the carbohydrate control well for comparison with the DNase and penicillinase reactions.

IDENTIFICATION
Identification of *Neisseria* and *Moraxella (Branhamella)* species may be accomplished through use of QuadFERM+ results as well as the Gram stain reaction, catalase, and oxidase tests.

Data from QuadFERM+ package insert, bioMérieux Vitek, Hazelwood, Mo.

Media Selective for *Neisseria gonorrhoeae*

All media are enriched agar bases with antibiotics added to suppress the normal flora or contaminating bacteria that may inhibit the isolation of *N. gonorrhoeae*. They selectively isolate *N. gonorrhoeae* from specimens that may contain contaminating bacteria or normal flora.

Modified Thayer-Martin

Media consists of a chocolate agar base (heated defibrinated sheep red blood cells) that contains hemin and nicotinamide adenine dinucleotide (NAD).

Vancomycin inhibits gram positive bacteria.

Colistin inhibits gram-negative bacteria other than *N. gonorrhoeae.*

Nystatin inhibits yeast and mold.

Trimethoprim lactate inhibits swarming of *Proteus.*

Martin-Lewis Media

Media consists of a chocolate agar base (heated defibrinated sheep red blood cells), containing hemin and NAD.

Vancomycin inhibits gram-positive bacteria.

Colistin inhibits gram-negative bacteria other than *N. gonorrhoeae.*

Anisomycin inhibits yeast and mold.

Trimethoprim lactate inhibits swarming of *Proteus.*

New York City

Clear peptone/cornstarch base with horse plasma, 3% hemoglobin, and yeast added

Vancomycin inhibits gram-positive bacteria.

Colistin inhibits gram-negative bacteria other than *N. gonorrhoeae.*

Amphotericin B inhibits yeast and mold.

Trimethoprim lactate inhibits swarming of *Proteus.*

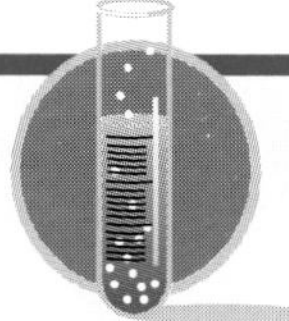

LABORATORY EXERCISES

1

Compare the growth of the following *Neisseria* species on the media (MTM, modified Thayer-Martin; ML, Martin-Lewis) and at the temperature listed.

Colonial Morphology	MTM (ML) 35°C	Chocolate 22°C	Nutrient 35°C
Neisseria gonorrhoeae			
Neisseria lactamica			
Neisseria sicca			
Moraxella catarrhalis			
Neisseria flavescens			

2

Perform the cytochrome oxidase test on the following bacteria and record your results. Explain why the oxidase test is useful in preliminary identification of bacteria. ______

N. gonorrhoeae ______

Proteus vulgaris ______

N. lactamica ______

M. catarrhalis ______

3

Perform the cystine trypticase agar (CTA) reactions on the bacteria listed and record your results. Why is it important to ensure a CO_2-free incubation environment? ______

	Glucose	Maltose	Lactose	Sucrose	Fructose
N. gonorrhoeae					
N. lactamica					
M. catarrhalis					
N. sicca					
N. flavescens					

4

Which species of *Neisseria* is typically DNase positive? ______

What specie(s) (one or more) should be tested for beta-lactamase activity? ______

REVIEW QUESTIONS

MULTIPLE CHOICE

1. **Pili antigens are associated with:**
   a. *Staphylococcus aureus*
   b. *Streptococcus pyogenes*
   c. *Streptococcus pneumoniae*
   d. *Neisseria gonorrhoeae*
2. **A gram-negative diplococcus isolated from a middle ear aspirate grew on chocolate agar but was inhibited on Martin-Lewis agar. The organism failed to produce acid from glucose, maltose, lactose, and sucrose. It was DNase positive and is most likely:**
   a. *Neisseria gonorrhoeae*
   b. *Neisseria meningitidis*
   c. *Neisseria lactamica*
   d. *Moraxella catarrhalis*
3. **All *Neisseria* species are positive for the enzyme:**
   a. Coagulase
   b. DNase
   c. Oxidase
   d. Penicillinase
4. **Cotton swabs are preferred for the culture and transport of specimens to be cultured for *Neisseria gonorrhoeae.***
   a. True
   b. False
5. **An isolate recovered from a blood culture specimen was subcultured onto chocolate agar and produced gram-negative diplococci that were oxidase positive and produced acid from glucose and maltose but not from lactose or sucrose. The isolate is most likely:**
   a. *Neisseria meningitidis*
   b. *Neisseria gonorrhoeae*
   c. *Moraxella catarrhalis*
   d. *Neisseria lactamica*
   e. *Neisseria sicca*
6. **An infant has been diagnosed with bacterial meningitis. Further testing of the spinal fluid would likely indicate:**
   a. Increased white blood cells with a predominance of lymphocytes, decreased glucose, and increased protein
   b. Increased white blood cells with a predominance of neutrophils, increased glucose, and decreased protein
   c. Decreased white blood cells, increased protein, and decreased glucose
   d. Increased white blood cells with a predominance of neutrophils, increased protein, and decreased glucose
7. **Gram-negative diplococci are isolated from a female genital tract specimen. Which of the following is the most appropriate action?**
   a. Report "*Neisseria gonorrhoeae* isolated" and perform susceptibility testing.
   b. Report amount of gram-negative diplococci (few, moderate, many) and estimate number of neutrophils present.
   c. Report "normal flora isolated" and discard specimen.
   d. Plate specimen on blood agar.
8. **Waterhouse-Friderichsen syndrome is associated with:**
   a. Autoimmune response to group A streptococcal infection
   b. Adrenal hemorrhage from *Neisseria meningitidis*
   c. Septicemia from *Neisseria gonorrhoeae*
   d. Hemolytic reaction from *Staphylococcus aureus*
9. **Which statement correctly describes the toxins associated with *Neisseria*?**
   a. The toxins are released by the living bacterial cell.
   b. The toxins are composed of lipopolysaccharide—components of the cell wall.
   c. The toxins are categorized as exotoxins.
   d. The toxins are similar to the enzymes of *Staphylococcus aureus.*

Use the following information for Questions 10 and 11.

A Gram stain from the purulent drainage of a synovial fluid reveals numerous gram-negative diplococci. The organism grew on chocolate agar and Martin-Lewis but failed to grow on blood agar or MacConkey. Further testing revealed the organism to be oxidase positive with positive carbohydrate utilization of glucose. All other carbohydrates were negative. The beta-lactamase result was positive.

REVIEW QUESTIONS

(Continued)

10. The organism is most likely:
a. *Streptococcus pneumoniae*
b. *Neisseria gonorrhoeae*
c. *Neisseria meningitidis*
d. *Staphylococcus aureus*
e. *Moraxella catarrhalis*

11. Based on the information provided, which antibiotic should definitely *not* be used to treat this infection?
a. Ceftriaxone
b. Spectinomycin
c. Penicillin
d. Tetracycline

12. *Neisseria meningitidis* can be carried _____, which serves as a reservoir for infection.
a. In the nasopharynx
b. In the blood
c. In the oral cavity
d. On the skin

13. There is only one type of capsular antigen for *Neisseria meningitidis*.
a. True
b. False

14. A gram-negative diplococcus isolated from a nasopharyngeal culture yielded the following results: blood agar—few, small, nonhemolytic colonies; chocolate agar—many small, grayish colonies; and oxidase—positive. The organism utilized glucose and maltose in the CTA reactions. Based on the information given, the organism is most likely:
a. *Streptococcus pneumoniae*
b. *Neisseria lactamica*
c. *Neisseria meningitidis*
d. *Moraxella catarrhalis*

15. Which statement correctly describes the mode of action of the antibiotic listed for modified Thayer-Martin medium?
a. Vancomycin inhibits gram-negative bacteria.
b. Colistin inhibits gram-positive bacteria.
c. Nystatin inhibits fungi and molds.
d. Trimethoprim lactate inhibits gram-positive bacteria.

16. *Neisseria meningitidis* cannot grow on blood agar.
a. True
b. False

17. Which of the following organisms is DNase positive?
a. *Neisseria gonorrhoeae*
b. *Neisseria meningitidis*
c. *Moraxella catarrhalis*
d. *Neisseria lactamica*
e. *Neisseria sicca*

18. Which of the following *Neisseria* fails to produce acid from glucose, maltose, lactose, and sucrose; produces yellow-pigmented colonies on blood and nutrient agar; and fails to produce DNase?
a. *Moraxella catarrhalis*
b. *Neisseria gonorrhoeae*
c. *Neisseria subflava*
d. *Neisseria flavescens*
e. *Neisseria sicca*

19. The Gram stain serves as the definite identification in cases of suspected gonorrhea in female patients.
a. True
b. False

BIBLIOGRAPHY

Baron EJ, Peterson LR, Finegold SM: Aerobic gram negative cocci (*Neisseria* and *Moraxella catarrhalis*). In *Bailey and Scott's diagnostic microbiology*, ed 9, St Louis, 1994, Mosby.

Bonin P, Tanino TT, Handsfield HH: Isolation of *Neisseria gonorrhoeae* on selective and nonselective media in a sexually transmitted disease clinic, *J Clin Microbiol* 19:218, 1984.

Boyce JM, Mitchell EB Jr: Difficulties in differentiating *Neisseria cinerea* from *Neisseria gonorrhoeae* in rapid systems used for identifying pathogenic *Neisseria* species, *J Clin Microbiol* 22:731, 1985.

Catlin BW: *Branhamella catarrhalis:* an organism gaining respect as a pathogen, *Clin Microbiol Rev* 3:293, 1990.

Evans KD, Peterson EM, Curry JI et al: Effect on holding temperature on isolation of *Neisseria gonorrhoeae*, *J Clin Microbiol* 24:1109, 1986.

Feldman HA: The meningococcus: a 20 year perspective, *Rev Infect Dis* 8:288, 1986.

Greenwood JR, Voss J, Smith RF: Comparative evaluation of New York City and modified Thayer Martin media for isolation of *Neisseria gonorrhoeae*, *J Clin Microbiol* 24:1111, 1986.

Hager H, Verghese A, Alverez S et al: *Branhamella catarrhalis* respiratory infections, *Rev Infec Dis* 9:1140, 1987.

Holt JG, King NR, Sneath PHA: *Bergey's manual of determinative bacteriology,* ed 9, Baltimore, 1992, Williams & Wilkins.

Hook EW III, Brady WE, Reichart CA et al: Determinations of emergence of antibiotic-resistant *Neisseria gonorrhoeae*, *J Infect Dis* 159:900, 1989.

Knapp JS: Historical perspectives and identification of *Neisseria* and related species, *Clin Microbiol Rev* 1:415, 1988.

Lossick JG, Smeltzer MP, Curan JW: The value of the cervical gram stain in the diagnosis of gonorrhea in women in a sexually transmitted diseases clinic, *Sex Transm Dis* 9:124, 1982.

Morello JA, Janda WM, Bohnhoff M: *Neisseria* and *Branhamella.* In Balows A et al, editors: *Manual of clinical microbiology,* ed 5, Washington, DC, 1991, American Society for Microbiology.

Schachter J, MacCormack WM, Smith RF et al: Enzyme immunoassay for diagnosis of gonorrhea, *J Clin Microbiol* 19:57, 1984.

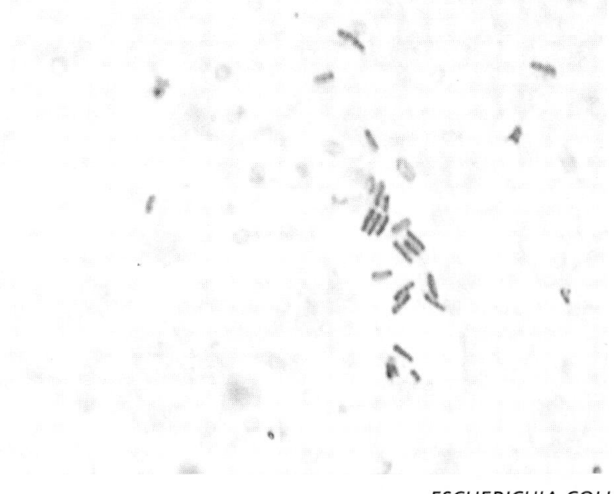

ESCHERICHIA COLI

CHAPTER OUTLINE

SEROLOGICAL CHARACTERISTICS
ISOLATION
IDENTIFICATION
IDENTIFICATION AND SIGNIFICANCE OF SELECTED ENTEROBACTERIACEAE
- *Escherichia coli*
- *Shigella*
- *Klebsiella-Enterobacter-Serratia-Hafnia* Group
- *Salmonella*
- Proteeae
- *Citrobacter*
- *Edwardsiella*
- *Yersinia*

MACCONKEY AGAR
EOSIN–METHYLENE BLUE (EMB) AGAR
HEKTOEN ENTERIC AGAR
XYLOSE-LYSINE-DESOXYCHOLATE (XLD) AGAR
SALMONELLA-SHIGELLA AGAR
TRIPLE SUGAR IRON (TSI) AGAR
INDOLE BROTH
METHYL RED–VOGES-PROSKAUER (MR-VP) TESTS
SIMMONS CITRATE REACTION
MOTILITY
DECARBOXYLASE REACTIONS
DEAMINASE REACTIONS
LYSINE-IRON AGAR (LIA)
ONPG REACTION
UREASE REACTION

KEY TERMS

ANAEROGENIC *E. COLI*
CARBOHYDRATE FERMENTATION
ENTEROHEMORRHAGIC *E. COLI*
ENTEROINVASIVE *E. COLI*
ENTEROPATHOGENIC *E. COLI*
ENTEROTOXIGENIC *E. COLI*
ENVELOPE ANTIGEN
FLAGELLAR ANTIGEN
KAUFFMAN WHITE CLASSIFICATION
LATE (SLOW) LACTOSE FERMENTERS
SHIGELLOSIS
SOMATIC ANTIGEN

Enterobacteriaceae

CHAPTER TEN

LEARNING OBJECTIVES

1. List and describe the serological characteristics of the members of Enterobacteriaceae.

2. Describe the biochemical reactions that are characteristic for the Enterobacteriaceae.

3. State the principle of each of the following biochemical techniques. Perform and interpret each test without error.

a. Carbohydrate fermentation
b. Triple sugar iron (TSI)
c. Indole
d. Methyl red
e. Voges-Proskauer
f. Citrate
g. Urease
h. Deaminase (phenylalanine)
i. Decarboxylase
j. ONPG
k. Hydrogen sulfide (H_2S)
l. Motility

4. Describe the isolation, identification, and infections of *Escherichia coli.*

5. Discuss the significance of ETEC, EIEC, EPEC, and VTEC.

6. Discuss the identification of the subgroups and species of *Shigella* and the infections associated with *Shigella.*

7. Describe the identification and infections of the *Klebsiella-Enterobacter-Serratia-Hafnia* group.

8. Describe the currently accepted method for classification of *Salmonella.*

a. Describe the types of *Salmonella* infections and indicate how each is acquired.
b. Identify *Salmonella* from a clinical specimen without error.

9. List the members of the tribe Proteeae (*Proteus* group).

a. State the important biochemical reactions of this group.
b. Identify clinically significant members of this tribe and state the clinical significance of each.

10. Explain how *Citrobacter* can be differentiated from *Salmonella.* Describe the identification and clinical significance of clinically important members of the genus *Citrobacter.*

11. Describe the identification and clinical significance of the isolation of *Edwardsiella tarda.*

Continued.

12. List the three species of *Yersinia* and discuss the identification and clinical significance of each.
13. Select and correctly streak the appropriate media for isolation for the following specimen sites when culturing for Enterobacteriaceae:
    a. Urine
    b. Blood
    c. Stool
    d. Wounds

The Enterobacteriaceae are a very large family of bacteria consisting of gram-negative bacilli and coccobacilli. The organisms are frequently encountered in the clinical laboratory and are associated with infections of almost every area of the human body. These bacteria are found in soil and water and on plants and are also considered to be normal flora of the gastrointestinal (GI) tract of many animals and humans. Infections are associated with lapses in personal hygiene via the fecal-oral route, poor sanitation in impoverished countries, and colonization of the skin and respiratory tract of hospitalized patients. These bacteria are known to cause disease in poultry, livestock, fish, and vegetable crops in addition to being significant human pathogens. Common types of infections attributed to the Enterobacteriaceae include urinary tract infections (UTIs), gastroenteritis, and septicemia.

More than 100 different species of Enterobacteriaceae exist in 27 different genera. Many different methods of classification exist, and changes in taxonomy occur frequently. In addition, the number of genera and species has increased in recent years. Early classification was based primarily on phenotypical characteristics, such as biochemical reactions. Later, deoxyribonucleic acid (DNA) relatedness or homology has also been used in the nomenclature scheme. In 1972 Edwards and Ewing described 11 genera and 26 species. In 1985 Farmer noted 22 genera with 69 species. Today, 27 genera are recognized, with more than 100 species and subspecies. This chapter focuses on those species that are most frequently found in human infections.

All Enterobacteriaceae are **glucose fermenters;** that is, glucose is utilized anaerobically, with an organic substrate serving as the final hydrogen ion acceptor. In addition, all members of the family are **cytochrome oxidase negative,** and most species, except for *Erwinia* and *Pantoea agglomerans,* (*Enterobacter agglomerans* group) reduce nitrates to nitrites. Most members of this family are motile with peritrichous flagella, and some species possess **pili** or **fimbrae,** which serve as structures for attachment.

The Enterobacteriaceae are facultative anaerobes and grow well in the presence or absence of air. These bacteria grow very well on blood agar, producing large, dull-gray colonies with variable hemolysis. Isolation is usually accomplished on a differential plate, such as MacConkey medium, with which determination of lactose fermentation can be made.

SEROLOGICAL CHARACTERISTICS

Members of the Enterobacteriaceae may possess three types of antigenic determinants, which can be used in the serological identification of a particular organism. These antigens are particularly useful in the characterization of *Escherichia coli, Klebsiella, Shigella,* and *Salmonella* and are useful for epidemiological purposes.

The **O** or **somatic antigen** is associated with the cell wall. It is heat stable and is the **lipopolysaccharide** of the cell wall, composing the **endotoxin** portion. There are 164 types of O antigen for *E. coli,* and specific types may be associated with particular diseases. For example, serotype O111 is associated with diarrhea in infants, while serotype O157 is associated with verocytotoxin production. Based on the nature of the O antigen, *Shigella* species have been grouped into four serotypes: A, B, C, and D. More than 60 different types of O antigen exist for *Salmonella.*

The **K** or **envelope antigen** consists of capsular polysaccharide that surrounds the cell wall. It is heat labile and covers the O antigen, thus inhibiting agglutination with type-specific O antisera. After determination of the K antigen, the organism must be boiled for 30 minutes and then retested to detect the O antigen.

Klebsiella, Salmonella, and *E. coli* are known to possess K antigens. The **Vi antigens** of *Salmonella typhi* are categorized as K antigens.

The **H** or **flagellar antigen** is only found in motile members of the Enterobacteriaceae. This antigen is found in the flagellum, is protein in nature, and is heat labile. The H antigen is used to serotype within species of *Salmonella* and other bacteria. *Salmonella* species are known to produce two different types of H antigens, called phase 1 and phase 2 antigens.

The **Kauffman-White classification** is used to classify **Salmonella** species based on their O and H antigens. Based on these reactions, more than 2000 different serovars (serotypes) of *Salmonella* exist. All *Salmonella* isolates should be tested with polyvalent O antisera. If the isolate is positive for the polyvalent antisera, specific monovalent tests should be done. Once the serogroup is determined, the particular serotype should be found, usually through testing at a reference laboratory. When agglutination does *not* occur with the polyvalent antisera, a suspension of the organism should be boiled for 15 minutes and retested. Heating destroys the capsular antigen, which may block the reactivity of the O antigen. Also, *S. typhi* will agglutinate with the Vi antisera before, but not after, boiling.

Four subgroups (A, B, C, D) of *Shigella* are possible, and specific serotypes are present in each subgroup. Specific serotypes of *E. coli* are associated with gastroenteritis. Isolates are usually serotyped in reference laboratories because of the procedure's complexity.

ISOLATION

The selection of media for isolation for Enterobacteriaceae depends on the clinical source of the specimen. A combination of MacConkey agar and blood agar is usually acceptable for specimens other than stool cultures. Alternatively, eosin-methylene blue (EMB) agar can be substituted for MacConkey agar.

Some initial observations on blood agar can be helpful in identification of the organism. For example, members of the genus *Proteus* produces characteristic "swarming motility" (Figure 10-1) and grow in thin waves over the surface of the agar. *Klebsiella pneumoniae,* which produces a capsule, appears as mucoid colonies (Figure 10-2). Organisms that are hydrogen sulfide (H_2S) positive often produce subsurface greening of the agar.

Stool specimens should be directly plated onto a differential plate (MacConkey or EMB) and onto a selective plate (Hektoen enteric or *Salmonella-Shigella*). In addition, an enrichment broth, such as gram-negative, selenite, or tetrathionate broth, should be inoculated. Such enrichment broths hold the normal flora coliforms such as *E. coli* in a lag period of growth while permitting the pathogenic *Salmonella* and *Shigella* to enter a logarithmic phase of growth. Each broth contains a high concentration of bile salts, which inhibit the multiplication of the normal flora coliforms. The selenite broth should be subcultured within 8 to 24 hours and gram-negative broth within 4 to 8 hours to a selective plate to ensure proper recovery of pathogens. These broths can be reincubated up to 24 hours if

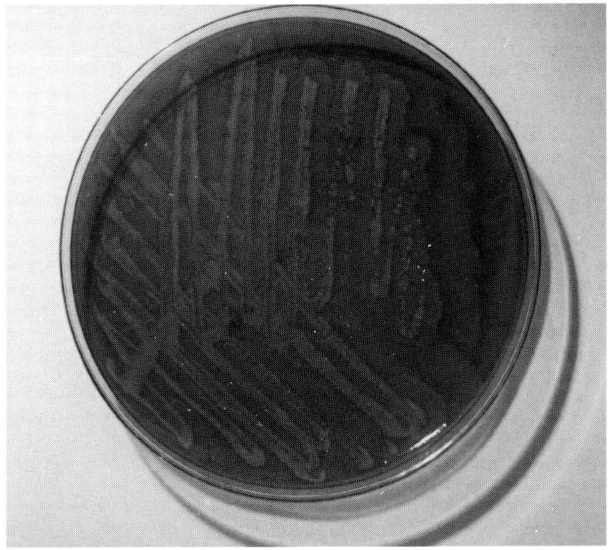

FIGURE 10–1
Swarming motility characteristic of *Proteus* on sheep blood agar; organism exhibits wavelike, concentric rings.

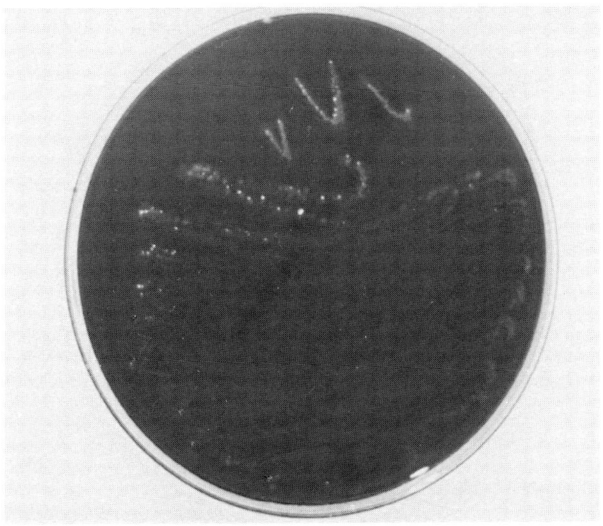

FIGURE 10–2
Mucoid morphology of *Klebsiella pneumoniae* on sheep blood agar; appearance is a result of the presence of a capsule.

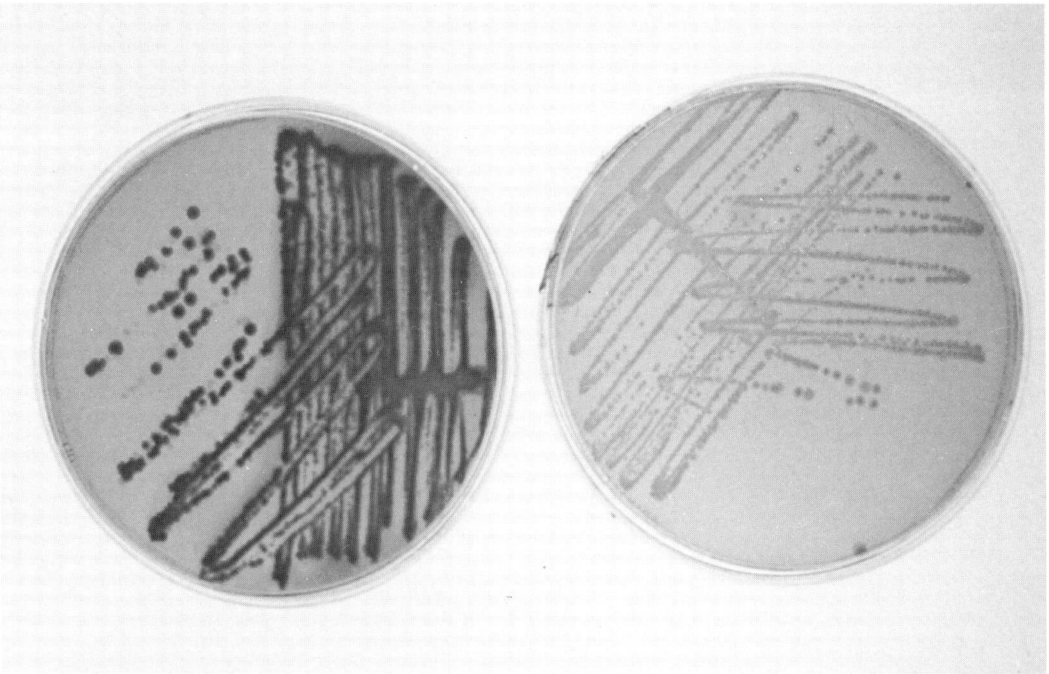

FIGURE 10-3

MacConkey agar showing pink colonies indicative of lactose fermentation and colorless colonies indicative of nonlactose fermenters. The plate isolates gram-negative bacteria and also differentiates lactose fermenters from those organisms that cannot ferment lactose.

desired. The normal flora coliforms appear as lactose-positive colonies on differential and selective plates, whereas the pathogenic Salmonella and Shigella appear as lactose-negative colonies. If enterotoxigenic E. coli is suspected, a blood agar plate should be inoculated as well. Also, if Yersinia enterocolitica is suspected, a cefsulodin-irgasan-novobiocin (CIN) medium should be inoculated and incubated at room temperature (22° to 26°C) for 24 hours to enhance its recovery.

For urine cultures, MacConkey and blood agars are a suitable combination. A colony count should be performed on all urine specimens. If a 1 μl (0.001 ml) calibrated loop is used to inoculate the plate, the number of colonies must be multiplied by 1000 to gain the colony count per milliliter of urine. For catheterized or suprapubic samples, a 10 μl loop may be used. In this case the number of colonies must be multiplied by 100 to determine the colony count per milliliter of urine. All counts for a single organism greater than 10^5/ml are considered to be positive for a UTI.

Figures 10-3 (Color Plate 28) and 10-4 (Color Plate 29) illustrate examples of characteristic reactions of the Enterobacteriaceae on MacConkey and Hektoen enteric agars. The box on p. 167 summarizes the media used to isolate Enterobacteriaceae.

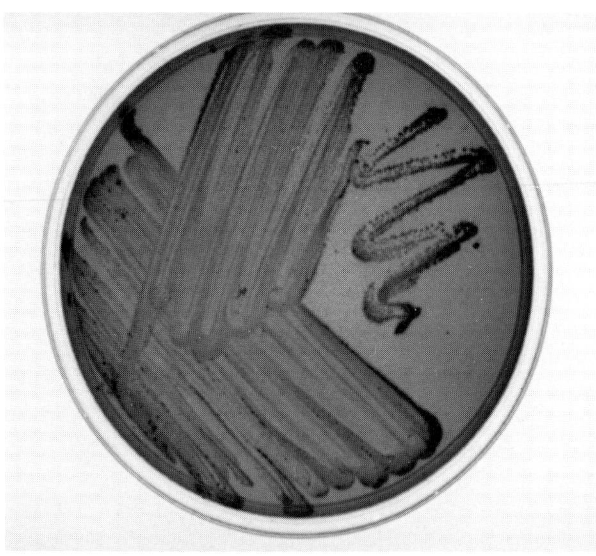

FIGURE 10-4

Hektoen-enteric agar is used to isolate and cultivate stool pathogens; the agar contains a high concentration of bile salts, which inhibits the growth of normal flora coliforms, such as *E. coli*, allowing for the isolation of pathogens such as *Salmonella* and *Shigella*. This illustration shows *Salmonella* species, which grows as an H_2S positive nonfermenter.

IDENTIFICATION

All Enterobacteriaceae grow well on MacConkey medium. After observation of growth on MacConkey,

Media Used for Isolation of Enterobacteriaceae

Cefsulodin-irgasan-novobiocin (CIN): agar selective for *Yersinia* species

Eosin–methylene blue (EMB): agar used for the isolation and differentiation of lactose fermenters from non–lactose fermenters

Gram-negative (GN) broth: enrichment broth used to enhance isolation of enteric pathogens

Hektoen enteric (HE): isolation and differentiation of *Salmonella* and *Shigella;* inhibition of normal flora coliforms

MacConkey: agar used for the isolation and differentiation of lactose fermenters from non–lactose fermenters

Salmonella-Shigella (SS): isolation and differentiation of *Salmonella* and *Shigella;* inhibition of normal flora coliforms

Selenite broth: enrichment broth used to enhance recovery of *Salmonella* and *Shigella*

Tetrathionate broth: enrichment broth used to enhance recovery of *Salmonella* and *Shigella*

Xylose-lysine-desoxycholate (XLD): agar used to isolate and differentiate *Salmonella* and *Shigella* from other Enterobacteriaceae

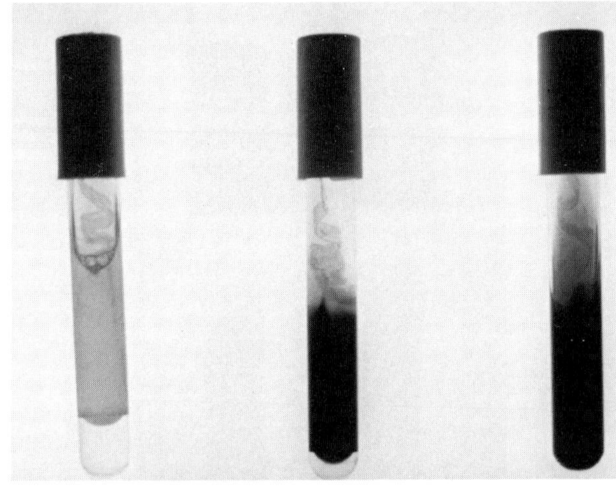

FIGURE 10–5

Triple sugar iron agar showing some characteristic reactions of the Enterobacteriaceae. A yellow deep indicates fermentation of glucose, wheras a yellow slant indicates fermentation of lactose and/or sucrose. Blackening in the deep indicates production of H_2S gas; cracks in the medium indicate production of gas during the fermentation process.

the oxidase test should be performed. Any oxidase-negative organism can be suspected of being a member of the Enterobacteriaceae. Identification now is based on a series of biochemical reactions. These reactions have historically been performed in various biochemical media prepared in test tubes. Today, most of the reactions are available as packaged test systems using small, concentrated reagent wells and coding indices to facilitate identification. The principles of both the tubed media and the packaged systems are generally the same. A brief summary of the significant biochemical reactions follows, with detailed experimental methods described at the end of this chapter.

The organism's pattern of **carbohydrate fermentation** is an important identifying characteristic for the Enterobacteriaceae. It has already been noted that all members of the Enterobacteriaceae ferment glucose. Through a series of steps, glucose is converted to pyruvic acid and then to lactic acid. The organism's ability to ferment lactose can be made through observation on MacConkey agar.

A variety of carbohydrates can be tested for fermentation and the results used in the identification of the organism. Frequently tested carbohydrates, in addition to lactose, include sucrose, mannose, sorbitol, mannitol, xylose, adonitol, cellobiose, dulcitol, and trehalose. In all tests to determine carbohydrate fermentation, the system must include a carbohydrate or sugar. Frequently, carbohydrate-like compounds or polyhedral alcohols are used to substitute for the carbohydrate. Such is the case with mannitol, which is actually a "sugar alcohol." The system must also contain a pH indicator that changes color as the pH changes from neutral or alkaline to acidic. A frequently used indicator is **phenol red,** which is orange-red in its original state and becomes yellow in an acidic environment of pH 6.8 or less. The change in indicator color shows that the carbohydrate has been fermented, resulting in the production of acidic end products. A particular pattern of fermentation of the carbohydrates tested assists in the identification of the organism.

Most members of the Enterobacteriaceae produce hydrogen and carbon dioxide (CO_2) gas during fermentation, which can be observed as cracks in the tubed media. Especially large amounts of gas are produced by members of *Klebsiella, Enterobacter, Hafnia,* and *Serratia.* Of special note is the genus *Shigella,* which cannot produce gas during fermentation of carbohydrates.

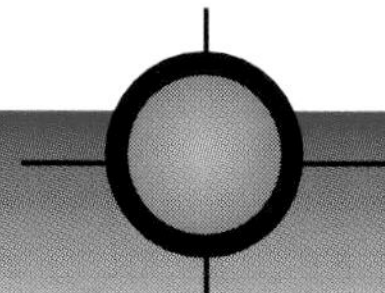

PROCEDURE
MACCONKEY AGAR

PURPOSE

MacConkey agar selects for gram-negative bacteria and also differentiates lactose fermenters (pink-red) from non–lactose fermenters (colorless).

PRINCIPLE

Bile salts inhibit gram-positive bacteria, which allows for the isolation of gram-negative bacteria. Neutral red and crystal violet further inhibit the gram-positive bacteria. Lactose is the only carbohydrate source. Neutral red indicator is brown in pH 6.8 to 8.0 and pink-red at pH less than 6.8.

PROCEDURE

1. Streak agar for isolation.
2. Incubate at 35°-37°C for 18 to 24 hours and observe for growth and color.

INTERPRETATION

If lactose is fermented, the medium is acidified, and bile salts are precipitated. The precipitated dye is absorbed, resulting in a pink-to-red complex.

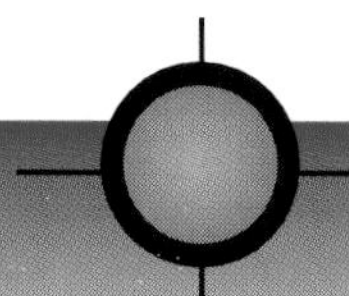

PROCEDURE
EOSIN–METHYLENE BLUE (EMB) AGAR

PURPOSE

The EMB medium selects for gram-negative bacteria and also differentiates lactose fermenters (purple color to "green metallic sheen") from non–lactose fermenters (colorless).

PRINCIPLE

Eosin and methylene blue are dyes that inhibit the gram-positive bacteria. Lactose is the only carbohydrate source in most formulations.

PROCEDURE

1. Streak agar for isolation.
2. Incubate at 35°-37°C for 18 to 24 hours and observe for growth and color.

INTERPRETATION

If lactose is fermented, precipitated eosin and methylene blue are absorbed, resulting in a purple color in the medium. A classical "green metallic sheen" is produced by *Escherichia coli,* which is a rapid lactose fermenter. Non–lactose fermenters produce colorless colonies on EMB.

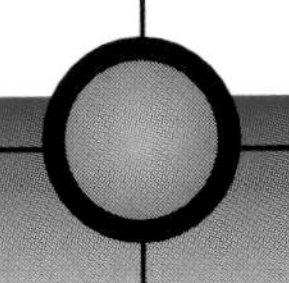

PROCEDURE
HEKTOEN ENTERIC AGAR

PURPOSE

Hektoen enteric medium selects for stool pathogens by inhibiting the normal flora coliforms of the lower GI tract.

PRINCIPLE

A high concentration of bile salts inhibits gram-positive bacteria and gram-negative coliforms. Lactose, sucrose, and salicin are carbohydrate sources. Bromthymol blue indicator has the following pH ranges:

Greater than 7.6—blue
6.0 to 7.6—green
Less than 6.0—yellow

Sodium thiosulfate is the sulfur source for H_2S detection. H_2S combines with ferric ammonium citrate to form ferric sulfide (FeS), which is represented by black-centered colonies. If one, two, or three of the carbohydrates are fermented, the colonies are orange in color. Nonfermenters produce green colonies.

PROCEDURE

1. Streak agar for isolation.
2. Incubate at 35°-37°C for 18 to 24 hours and observe for growth and color.

INTERPRETATION

Pathogens appear as green colonies or green colonies with black centers. Yellow colonies are considered normal flora except for *Yersinia enterocolitica,* which produces yellow colonies due to its fermentation of sucrose.

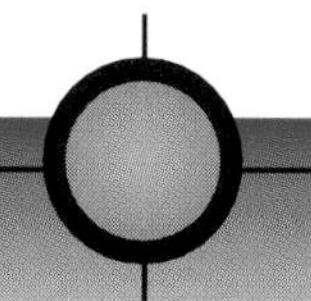

PROCEDURE
XYLOSE-LYSINE-DEOXYCHOLATE (XLD) AGAR

PURPOSE
The XLD medium is used for the isolation and differentiation of stool pathogens and inhibition of normal flora coliforms.

PRINCIPLE
Sodium deoxycholate inhibits gram-positive bacteria, partially inhibits the growth of *Escherichia coli,* and inhibits the swarming of *Proteus.*

Phenol red indicator becomes yellow in acidic environments. Fermentation of xylose results in yellow colonies. Most members of Enterobacteriaceae are xylose positive, except for *Shigella.* Most strains of *Shigella* cannot ferment lactose and thus produce red colonies. Lysine-positive bacteria first produce yellow colonies as xylose is fermented, followed by red colonies, indicating lysine decarboxylation. H_2S-positive colonies have black centers due to the reaction of H_2S with ferric ammonium citrate.

PROCEDURE
1. Streak agar for isolation.
2. Incubate at 35°-37°C for 18 to 24 hours and observe for growth and color.

INTERPRETATION
Salmonella typically produce red colonies with black centers, whereas *Citrobacter* and *Proteus* produce yellow colonies with black centers.

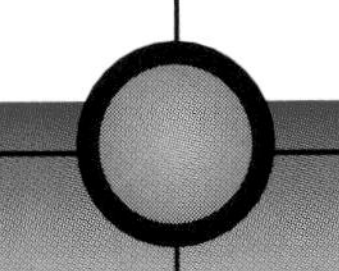

PROCEDURE

SALMONELLA-SHIGELLA AGAR

PURPOSE

Salmonella-Shigella medium provides for inhibition of normal flora coliforms and differentiation of stool pathogens.

PRINCIPLE

Bile salts inhibit gram-positive bacteria, and brilliant green agar and bile salts inhibit the gram-negative coliforms. Lactose is the sole carbohydrate source. Neutral red indicator is red in acidic conditions. Lactose fermenters appear pink-red, whereas non–lactose fermenters appear clear. To detect H_2S production, sodium thiosulfate serves as a sulfur source. When H_2S is formed, it combines with ferric ammonium citrate to form ferric sulfide (FeS), which is represented by black-centered colonies.

PROCEDURE

1. Streak agar for isolation.
2. Incubate at 35°-37°C for 18 to 24 hours and observe for growth and color.

INTERPRETATION

Normal flora coliforms appear as pink-to-red colonies.
Shigella appears as colorless colonies without black centers.
Salmonella appears as colorless colonies with black centers.

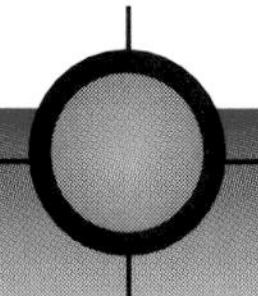

PROCEDURE
TRIPLE SUGAR IRON (TSI) AGAR

PURPOSE

TSI agar can be considered an initial step in the identification of the Enterobacteriaceae.

PRINCIPLE

The medium contains protein sources (beef extract, peptone, yeast extract, proteose peptone) that permit the growth of most bacterial strains. Lactose, sucrose, and glucose are present as well as phenol red indicator. Glucose is in a concentration one-tenth that of the other carbohydrates. Ferrous sulfate is present as an indicator of hydrogen sulfide (H_2S) production.

The TSI is a two-reaction chamber with an aerobic slant portion and an anaerobic deep portion. The slant portion of the tube is exposed to atmospheric oxygen and will become alkaline due to oxidative decarboxylation of peptides and amino acids. The slant tends to become and remain alkaline (red). Amino acid degradation is minimal in the deep (anaerobic) portion, and thus a small quantity of acid produced can be detected because few amines are being formed from amino acids.

Bacteria that ferment glucose, but not lactose or sucrose, only produce small quantities of acid and cannot counteract the degradation of amino acids at the slant, which results in an alkaline pH due to oxidative decarboxylation. Such organisms characteristically produce an alkaline slant over an acid deep (K/A).

Organisms that ferment both glucose and lactose and/or sucrose produce large quantities of acid, which overcome the alkaline reaction of the slant, yielding an acid slant over an acid deep (A/A).

An organism incapable of fermenting glucose produces no change in the indicator and is characterized by an alkaline slant over an alkaline deep (K/K).

A sulfur source, sodium thiosulfate, provides sulfur atoms to detect the production of H_2S gas. H_2S reacts with iron salts (ferrous sulfate or ferric ammonium citrate) to produce the black precipitate of ferrous sulfide.

The production of gas during fermentation is indicated by the presence of cracks in the medium or the "pulling away" of the medium from the walls of the test tube.

See Figure 10-5 for typical TSI reactions.

MATERIALS

Selected members of Enterobacteriaceae
Nonfermentative gram-negative bacilli
TSI slants

PROCEDURE
TRIPLE SUGAR IRON (TSI) AGAR
(Continued)

PROCEDURE

1. Use single, isolated 18- to 24-hour colony.
2. Select colony with sterile needle and stab within ½ inch of the bottom of the agar.
3. Streak colony up slant.
4. Leave cap on loosely and incubate at 35° to 37°C for 18 to 24 hours.
5. Read and interpret results.

A summary of TSI reactions follows:

REACTION*	CARBOHYDRATE FERMENTED	TYPICAL ORGANISMS
A/Ⓐ H_2S –	*Glucose with acid and gas* *Lactose and/or sucrose with acid and gas*	*Escherichia* *Klebsiella* *Enterobacter*
K/Ⓐ H_2S +	*Glucose with acid and gas* *Lactose or sucrose not fermented*	*Salmonella* *Proteus, Citrobacter*
K/A H_2S –	*Glucose with acid; no gas* *Lactose or sucrose not fermented*	*Shigella* *Providencia, Serratia, anaerogenic Escherichia coli*
K/K H_2S –	*Glucose not fermented* *Lactose or sucrose not fermented*	*Pseudomonas* *Alcaligenes*
A/Ⓐ H_2S +	*Glucose fermented with gas; lactose or sucrose fermented*	*Citrobacter freundii*

NOTE: Those species of Proteus that ferment sucrose may produce an acidic slant.
*A, Acid; Ⓐ, acid and gas; K, alkaline (no change).

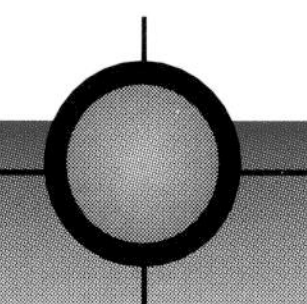

PROCEDURE
INDOLE BROTH

PURPOSE
Indole broth is used for distinguishing Enterobacteriaceae based on the ability to produce indole from tryptophan. The test is particularly useful for the identification of lactose-fermenting members of Enterobacteriaceae. *Escherichia coli* is indole positive, whereas *Enterobacter* and *Klebsiella* are indole negative. Indole is also useful in the speciation of *Proteus: P. mirabilis* is indole negative, whereas *P. vulgaris* is positive.

PRINCIPLE
Tryptophan present in peptone is oxidized by certain bacteria to indole, skatole, and indole–acetic acid. The intracellular enzymes that metabolize tryptophan are known as tryptophanase. Indole is detected in broth cultures of bacteria with an alcoholic p-dimethylaminobenzaldehyde reagent. Indole reacts with the aldehyde to form a red product. Two reagents may be used to detect indole, Kovac's and Ehrlich's. Ehrlich's reagent is believed to be more sensitive than Kovac's and is recommended for indole detection in anaerobes and nonfermentative bacteria. Kovac's reagent was initially used to classify members of the Enterobacteriaceae and should be used with these organisms.

$$\text{Tryptophan} \xrightarrow[\text{Tryptophanase}]{} \text{Indole} + \text{Pyruvic acid} + \text{Ammonia}$$

$$\text{Indole} + p\text{-Dimethylaminobenzaldehyde} \longrightarrow \text{Red}$$

REAGENTS AND MEDIA
Tryptophan (1%) broth
Kovac's reagent or Ehrlich's reagent
Xylene or chloroform for extraction if using Ehrlich's reagent

PROCEDURE
1. Inoculate indole broth.
2. Replace cap loosely and incubate at 35°C for 18 to 24 hours.
3. Add five drops of Kovac's reagent directly to the broth culture. Observe for a red color in the upper alcohol layer.
4. If using Ehrlich's reagent, first add 1 ml xylene or chloroform to the broth culture. Shake gently and then add five drops of reagent.

INTERPRETATION
Negative reaction: no color development
Positive reaction: red ring at the interface of reagent and broth (or reagent and xylene or chloroform)
Variable reaction: orange color, indicates production of skatole, a methylated intermediate that may be a precursor to indole production

QUALITY CONTROL
E. coli: positive control (red ring)
Enterobacter cloacae: negative control (no color development)

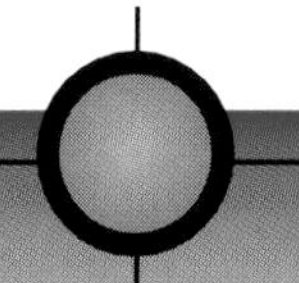

PROCEDURE

METHYL RED–VOGES-PROSKAUER (MR-VP) TESTS

PURPOSE

MR-VP broth is a dextrose broth medium buffered with peptone. Glucose is fermented to pyruvic acid by one of two pathways, which results in either a positive MR or a positive VP test. The tests are particularly useful for the lactose-fermenting Enterobacteriaceae. *Escherichia coli* is MR positive and VP negative, whereas most members of the *Klebsiella-Enterobacter-Serratia-Hafnia* group are VP positive.

PRINCIPLE

In the first pathway, mixed acid products (lactic, acetic, formic, and succinic) result, leading to a decrease in the pH of the medium and a positive MR test. The pH must drop to 4.4 or less for the MR indicator to take on its acidic red color.

In the second pathway, acetylmethyl carbinol (acetoin) is an intermediate product to butylene glycol. Acetoin is the neutral product detected in the VP reaction. The broth should be heavily inoculated, with a small volume of broth used for the VP test to obtain favorable results at 24 to 48 hours of incubation.

In the presence of oxygen and 40% potassium hydroxide (KOH), acetoin is converted to the diacetyl form, which results in a red color in the presence of alpha-naphthol.

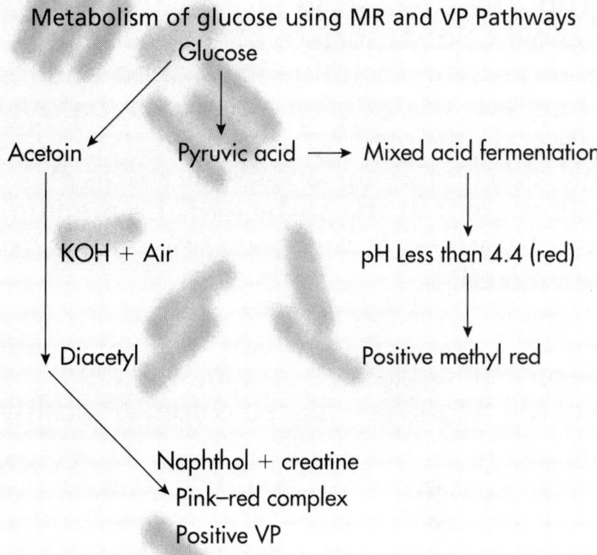

MEDIA AND REAGENTS

MR-VP broth: glucose base
MR pH indicator
5% alpha-naphthol in absolute methyl alcohol
40% KOH containing 0.3% creatine

Continued.

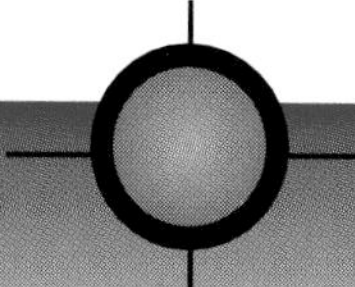

PROCEDURE
UREASE REACTION

PURPOSE

Urease is an enzyme that splits urea into alkaline end products. The reaction is useful in the identification of rapid urease producers, such as *Proteus* and *Morganella,* as well as weak urease producers, such as *Klebsiella pneumoniae* and some species of *Enterobacter.*

PRINCIPLE

Urease splits the urea molecule into ammonia (NH_3), carbon dioxide (CO_2), and water (H_2O). Ammonia reacts in solution to form an alkaline compound, ammonium carbonate, which results in an increased pH of the medium and a color change in the indicator to pink-red.

$$\text{Urea} + 2\,H_2O \xrightarrow[\text{Urease}]{} CO_2 + H_2O + 2\,NH_3 \rightleftarrows \underset{\text{ammonium carbonate}}{(NH_4)_2\,CO_3}$$

MEDIA AND REAGENTS

Christensen's (urea) agar tubes or Stuart urea broth

PROCEDURE

1. If using Stuart broth, dissolve one urea disk in 1 ml sterile distilled water.
2. Use single, isolated, 18- to 24-hour colony, and streak slant of agar tube or inoculate broth.
3. Replace cap loosely or parafilm broth.
4. Incubate at 35°C for 18 to 24 hours.

INTERPRETATION

Stuart broth

Positive: red color in medium
Negative: no color change (buff to pale yellow)
Strong positive reactions are seen only with *Proteus* species (*Proteus* and *Morganella*) and may be interpreted as early as after 4 hours of incubation.
Weakly positive reactions (pink to orange) may be seen with *K. pneumoniae* and other slow urease producers.

Christensen's agar

Positive (rapid urease activity): red throughout medium (seen only with *Proteus* and *Morganella*)
Positive (slow urease activity): red in slant *(K. pneumoniae)*
Negative (no urease activity): medium remains yellow

QUALITY CONTROL

Proteus vulgaris: positive—rapid urease producer
K. pneumoniae: positive—slow urease producer
Escherichia coli: negative—no urease production

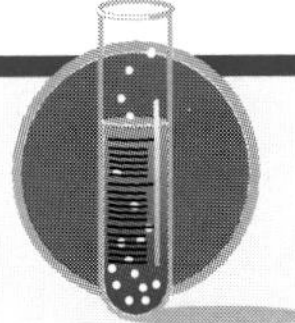

LABORATORY EXERCISES

1

1. Streak the organisms on the plates listed and incubate for 18 to 24 hours at 35° to 37° C. Describe the appearance of each of the following on the media listed. Interpret the reactions that have occurred.

	MacConkey	**Eosin-Methylene Blue**	**Hektoen Enteric**	**Sheep Blood Agar**
Escherichia coli				
Klebsiella pneumoniae				
Proteus mirabilis				
Salmonella enteritidis				

2. Perform a TSI on the following bacteria. Record your observations and interpret your results:
   Escherichia coli
   Observations: ______
   Interpretation: ______
   Klebsiella pneumoniae
   Observations: ______
   Interpretation: ______
   Salmonella enteritidis
   Observations: ______
   Interpretation: ______
   Proteus mirabilis
   Observations: ______
   Interpretation: ______
   Citrobacter freundii
   Observations: ______
   Interpretation: ______
   Shigella sonnei
   Observations: ______
   Interpretation: ______
3. Describe the appearance of a positive MR. ______
   Describe the appearance of a positive VP. ______
   Perform the MR-VP on the following bacteria. Record your observations and interpret your results.
   Escherichia coli
   MR: Observations: ______
   Interpretation: ______
   VP: Observations: ______
   Interpretation: ______

LABORATORY EXERCISES
(Continued)

Klebsiella pneumoniae
MR: Observations: ______
Interpretation: ______
VP: Observations: ______
Interpretation: ______
Proteus mirabilis
MR: Observations: ______
Interpretation: ______
VP: Observations: ______
Interpretation: ______
Enterobacter cloacae
MR: Observations: ______
Interpretation: ______
VP: Observations: ______
Interpretation: ______

4. Perform the indole reaction on the following bacteria. Record your observations and interpret your results.
Escherichia coli
Observations: ______
Interpretation: ______
Klebsiella pneumoniae
Observations: ______
Interpretation: ______
Proteus mirabilis
Observations: ______
Interpretation: ______
Proteus vulgaris
Observations: ______
Interpretation: ______
Enterobacter cloacae
Observations: ______
Interpretation: ______

5. Describe how a positive citrate reaction is indicated. ______
Perform the citrate test on the following bacteria; record your observations and interpret your results.
Escherichia coli
Observations: ______
Interpretation: ______
Klebsiella pneumoniae
Observations: ______
Interpretation: ______
Enterobacter cloacae
Observations: ______
Interpretation: ______

LABORATORY EXERCISES
(Continued)

Citrobacter freundii
Observations: ______
Interpretation: ______

6. What does a yellow color in a decarboxylase tube indicate? ______
Describe the appearance of a positive reaction. ______
Perform and interpret the following decarboxylase reactions. Record your observations and interpret your results. ______
Escherichia coli
ADH: Observations: ______
Interpretation: ______
ODC: Observations: ______
Interpretation: ______
LDC: Observations: ______
Interpretation: ______
Klebsiella pneumoniae
ADH: Observations: ______
Interpretation: ______
ODC: Observations: ______
Interpretation: ______
LDC: Observations: ______
Interpretation: ______
Enterobacter cloacae
ADH: Observations: ______
Interpretation: ______
ODC: Observations: ______
Interpretation: ______
LDC: Observations: ______
Interpretation: ______
Enterobacter aerogenes
ADH: Observations: ______
Interpretation: ______
ODC: Observations: ______
Interpretation: ______
LDC: Observations: ______
Interpretation: ______
Salmonella enteritidis
ADH: Observations: ______
Interpretation: ______
ODC: Observations: ______
Interpretation: ______
LDC: Observations: ______
Interpretation: ______

LABORATORY EXERCISES

(Continued)

7. What bacteria are strong urease producers?

   ____

   ____

   What bacteria are weak urease producers?

   ____

   ____

   Perform and interpret the urease reaction on the following bacteria.

   Escherichia coli
   Observations: ____________________
   Interpretation: ____________________

   Klebsiella pneumoniae
   Observations: ____________________
   Interpretation: ____________________

   Proteus vulgaris
   Observations: ____________________
   Interpretation: ____________________

   Proteus mirabilis
   Observations: ____________________
   Interpretation: ____________________

   Salmonella enteritidis
   Observations: ____________________
   Interpretation: ____________________

8. Explain how deaminase activity is determined and list those bacteria that are typically deaminase positive.

   ____

   ____

   Perform and interpret the deaminase reaction on the following bacteria.

   Escherichia coli
   Observations: ____________________
   Interpretation: ____________________

   Klebsiella pneumoniae
   Observations: ____________________
   Interpretation: ____________________

   Proteus mirabilis
   Observations: ____________________
   Interpretation: ____________________

   Providencia stuartii
   Observations: ____________________
   Interpretation: ____________________

LABORATORY EXERCISES
(Continued)

9. What is determined in the ONPG reaction?

   ____

   ____

   Perform and interpret the ONPG reaction on the following bacteria.

   Echerichia coli
   Observations: ____________________
   Interpretation: ____________________

   Salmonella enteritidis
   Observations: ____________________
   Interpretation: ____________________

   Citrobacter freundii
   Observations: ____________________
   Interpretation: ____________________

   Shigella sonnei
   Observations: ____________________
   Interpretation: ____________________

10. Describe how you would differentiate the following paired bacteria.
    a. *Escherichia coli* from *Enterobacter cloacae:*

    ____

    ____

    b. *Proteus mirabilis* from *Proteus vulgaris:*

    ____

    ____

    c. *Klebsiella pneumoniae* from *Enterobacter aerogenes:*

    ____

    ____

    d. *Shigella sonnei* from *Salmonella enteritidis:*

    ____

    ____

    e. *Proteus mirabilis* from *Salmonella enteritidis:*

    ____

    ____

    f. *Citrobacter freundii* from *Salmonella enteritidis:*

    ____

    ____

    g. *Proteus mirabilis* from *Providencia stuartii:*

    ____

    ____

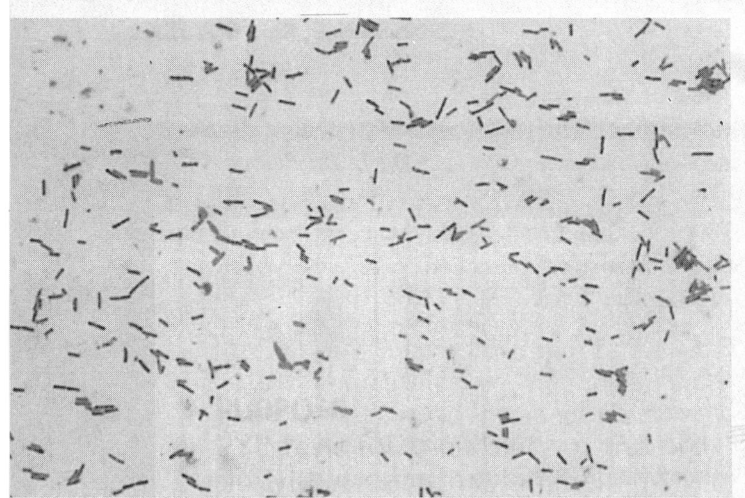

PSEUDOMONAS AERUGINOSA

CHAPTER OUTLINE

PSEUDOMONAS AERUGINOSA
OTHER *PSEUDOMONAS* SPECIES
ACINETOBACTER
ALCALIGENES
MORAXELLA
OLIGELLA
FLAVOBACTERIUM
EIKENELLA
KINGELLA
OXIDATIVE-FERMENTATIVE (OF) MEDIUM

KEY TERMS

ALGINATE
EXOTOXIN A
FERMENTATIVE
GLANDERS
MELIOIDOSIS
NONSACCHAROLYTIC
OXIDATIVE
PYOCYANIN
PYOVERDIN

Nonfermentative Gram-Negative Bacilli

CHAPTER ELEVEN

LEARNING OBJECTIVES

1. Describe the natural environment and types of infections attributed to the nonfermentative gram-negative bacilli.
2. Contrast the peptone-to-carbohydrate ratio in fermentative and oxidative-fermentative media and explain why this concentration is well suited for nonfermenters.
3. State the principle of, use, and interpret oxidative-fermentative medium. Differentiate nonfermenters, fermenters, and nonsaccharolytic organisms.
4. List those pseudomonads that are pyocyanin positive.
5. List two unique characteristics used in the identification of *Pseudomonas aeruginosa.*
   a. Explain how this organism is identified.
   b. Describe the types and sources of infections for this organism.
   c. List and describe at least three compounds produced by *P. aeruginosa* that are associated with its pathogenicity.
   d. Identify *P. aeruginosa* as an unknown without error.
6. Briefly discuss the identification and clinical significance of *Pseudomonas* species other than *P. aeruginosa,* including *P. cepacia.*
7. Describe the clinical significance of *Xanthomonas maltophilia,* and explain how it is identified.
8. State the characteristics of *Acinetobacter,* and differentiate *A. baumannii* from *A. calcoaceticus.*
   a. Differentiate *Acinetobacter* from *Neisseria.*
   b. Relate the clinical significance of *Acinetobacter.*
9. Describe the clinically significant *Alcaligenes,* and state the important morphological and biochemical characteristics.
10. Describe the clinically significant *Moraxella* and *Oligella,* and explain how each is identified in the laboratory.
11. State a unique trait of the genus *Flavobacterium*. Describe infections associated with *F. meningosepticum,* and explain how this organism is identified.
12. Identify an unknown gram-negative nonfermenter through biochemical reactions and morphological characteristics.

The nonfermentative (or **oxidative**) gram-negative bacilli oxidatively metabolize carbohydrates and require molecular oxygen as the final hydrogen ion acceptor. These organisms are unable to use glucose or other carbohydrates fermentatively in the absence of oxygen. This oxidative process results in the formation of very weak acids as end products of the reaction. Other gram-negative bacilli discussed in this chapter are termed **nonsaccharolytic** or **nonoxidizers.** These bacteria cannot utilize carbohydrates in the absence or presence of oxygen and must rely on compounds other than carbohydrates for sources of energy.

The nonfermentative gram-negative bacilli (Figure 11-1 [Color Plate 35]) are non-spore formers and obligate aerobes. Typically, the triple sugar iron (TSI) agar shows no reaction or K/K H_2S negative. Some of the bacteria can grow on the TSI slant where oxygen is present (Figure 11-2 [Color Plate 36]).

The bacteria are usually found in natural water sources as well as in contaminants in respiratory care equipment, water baths, and sinks. In addition, some nonfermenters can be found on the mucous membranes and skin of humans; others are known to contaminate intravenous solutions.

These organisms are opportunistic pathogens and can colonize and attach to the debilitated or immunosuppressed host. Those at particular risk include patients receiving prolonged antibiotic therapy or other powerful medications and those on prolonged or invasive instrumentation. The bacteria have an opportunity to gain access to normally sterile sites through trauma, burns, or wounds.

A nonfermenter should be suspected if an **oxidase-positive,** gram-negative bacillus is found growing better on blood than on MacConkey agar. A TSI showing K/K is a further clue toward the isolation of a nonfermenter. Differential reactions used to identify nonfermenters are as follows:

- Cellular morphology of the flagellum: type, number, and arrangement
- Modified indole test
- Growth on MacConkey agar (positive or negative)
- Motility
- Oxidative-fermentative carbohydrate utilization patterns
- Decarboxylation reactions
- Nitrate reduction
- Urease

In the modified indole test, small amounts of indole produced from the breakdown of tryptophan by tryptophanase in the nonfermenters must be extracted with xylene before detection. After inoculation of tryptone broth and incubation at 48 hours, 1.0 ml of xylene is added to the tube. The tube is shaken and left undisturbed until the solvent rises to the top. Next, 0.5 ml of Ehrlich's reagent is added gently down the sides of the tube, forming a ring between the test medium and solvent. In a positive reaction, a bright red ring forms just below the solvent layer after additions of Kovac's reagent. This is the recommended method to determine indole production by nonfermenters, since the amount of indole produced is very low.

TSI is not suitable to study carbohydrate use by the nonfermenters, since the bacteria are slow growing and only produce minimal amounts of acidic end

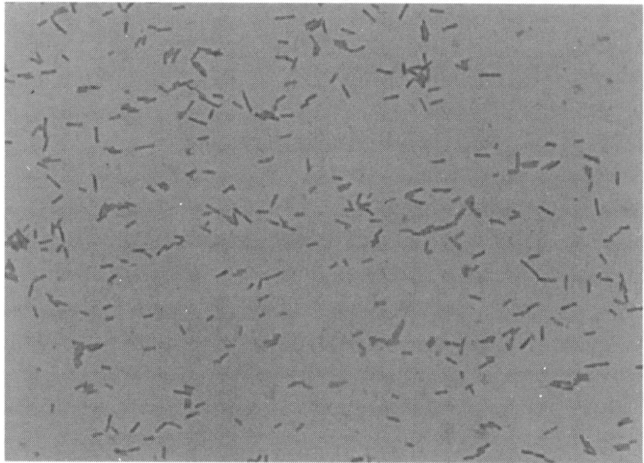

FIGURE 11-1

Photomicrograph of *Pseudomonas aeruginosa* illustrating long, narrow, non-spore-forming gram-negative bacillus.

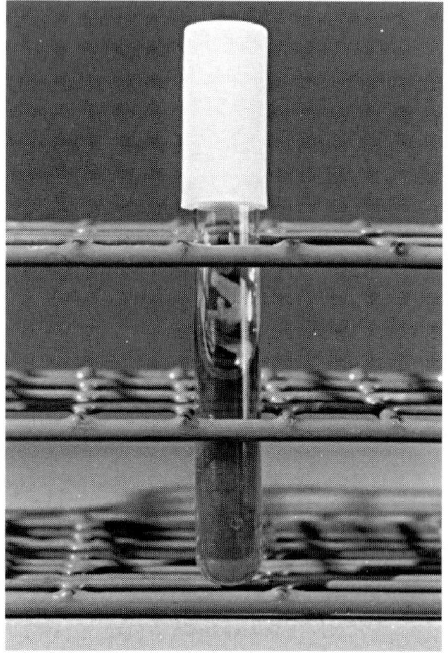

FIGURE 11-2

Triple sugar iron (TSI) agar. K/K indicates the organism's inability to ferment glucose or any carbohydrates in the TSI; this is the typical reaction of the nonfermenters. In addition, many nonfermenters are cytochrome oxidase positive.

products. A special medium for this purpose, the **oxidative-fermentative (OF) medium of Hugh and Leifson,** has been devised to study carbohydrate utilization by the nonfermenters. In OF medium, carbohydrate concentration is high at 1.0%, which enhances the production of acidic end products. The amount of peptone is low (0.2%), which decreases the formation of oxidative products and amino acids, tending to neutralize the pH and obscure a positive reaction. The concentration of peptone to carbohydrate is 1:5 in OF medium, whereas a concentration of 2:1 is used in other **fermentative** media.

In the OF determination, almost any carbohydrate can be tested, with glucose, maltose, and xylose traditionally used. The medium also contains bromthymol blue indicator, which is yellow in an acidic pH, indicating a positive reaction, and green to blue in an alkaline pH, indicating a negative reaction.

For each organism and carbohydrate to be tested, two tubes of that particular media are needed. One tube is exposed to the air (open tube), and the second tube is overlaid with mineral oil (closed tube), providing a fermentative environment. After inoculation and incubation, an organism can be classified into one of three categories:

Oxidative: positive (yellow) in the open tube and negative (green or blue-green) in the closed tube. The organism can only use the carbohydrate when oxygen is present (Figure 11-3 [Color Plate 37]).

Fermentative: positive (yellow) in both the open tube and the closed tube. Acid is produced in both tubes; this is typical of the Enterobacteriaceae, which indicates the activity of facultative anaerobes (Figure 11-4 [Color Plate 38]).

Nonsaccharolytic (nonoxidizer): no change or an alkaline (blue-green) reaction in both tubes. The organism cannot use the carbohydrate and must seek other sources of energy (Figure 11-5 [Color Plate 39]).

The reduction of nitrates (NO_3) to nitrites (NO_2) is another useful reaction for the identification of nonfermenters. Although some bacteria convert NO_3 to NO_2, others convert nitrates completely to nitrogen gas (N_2). N_2 can be detected by adding zinc to the final reaction. A red color with zinc indicates the presence of NO_3, and therefore a negative reaction for nitrogen reduction. No change with the addition of zinc indicates that nitrates have been completely reduced to N_2, which indicates a positive reaction.

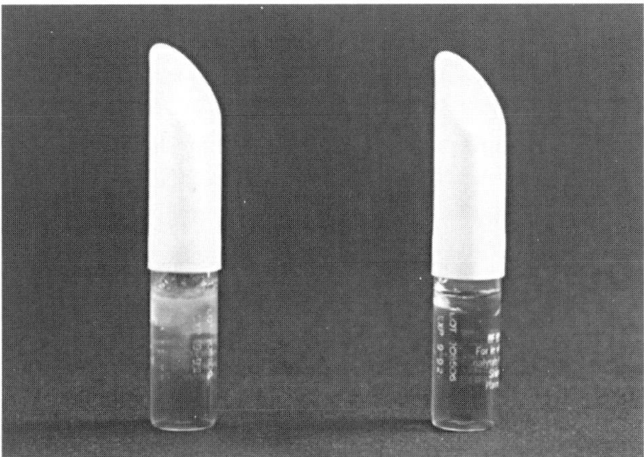

FIGURE 11–3

Oxidative-fermentative (OF) medium of Hugh and Leifson. Two tubes are inoculated, and one is overlaid with sterile mineral oil. The tube without mineral oil is known as the "open tube," and that with mineral oil is known as the "closed tube." Shown here is oxidation of glucose (yellow color), since the carbohydrate is utilized only in the open tube where oxygen is present.

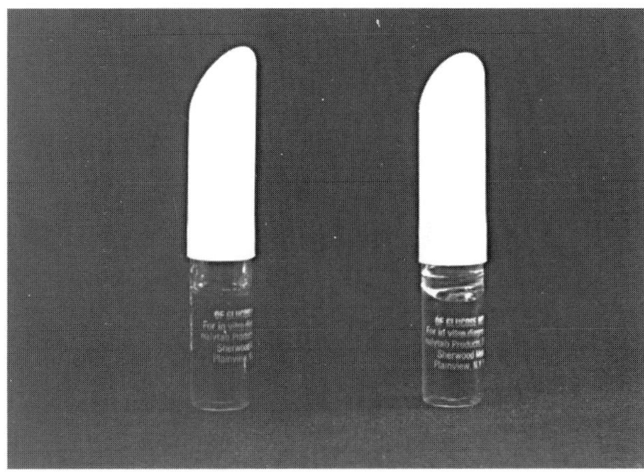

FIGURE 11–4

OF medium: fermentative. Fermentation of glucose is illustrated by utilization of the carbohydrate glucose (yellow color) in both the open and the closed tubes. Reaction is typical of members of the Enterobacteriaceae.

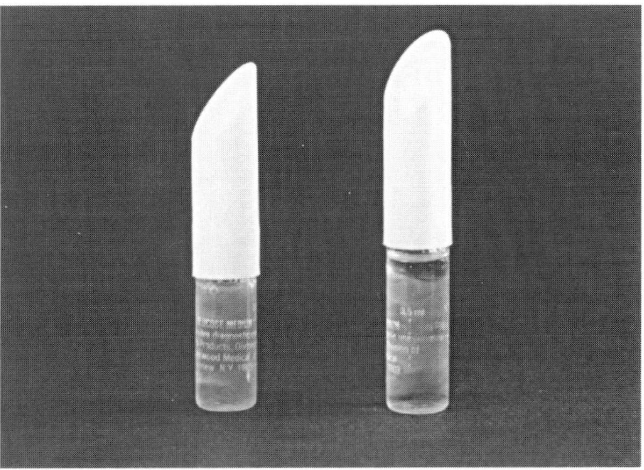

FIGURE 11–5

OF medium: nonsaccharolytic. Inability of organism to use carbohydrate either oxidatively or fermentatively is illustrated by negative (green to blue-green) reactions in both the open and the closed tubes.

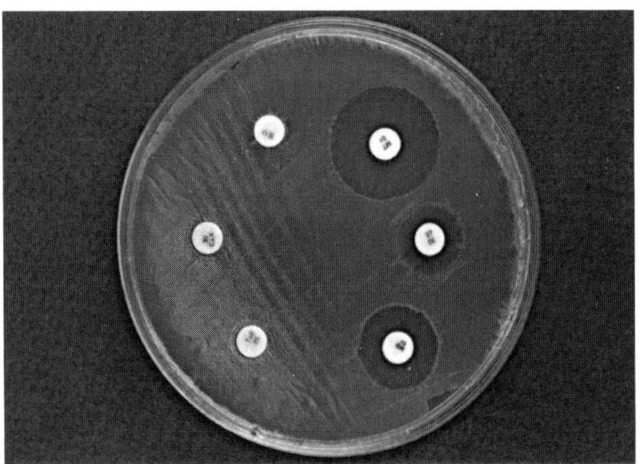

FIGURE 11-6
Pseudomonas aeruginosa on Mueller-Hinton medium illustrating its characteristic green to blue-green pigment.

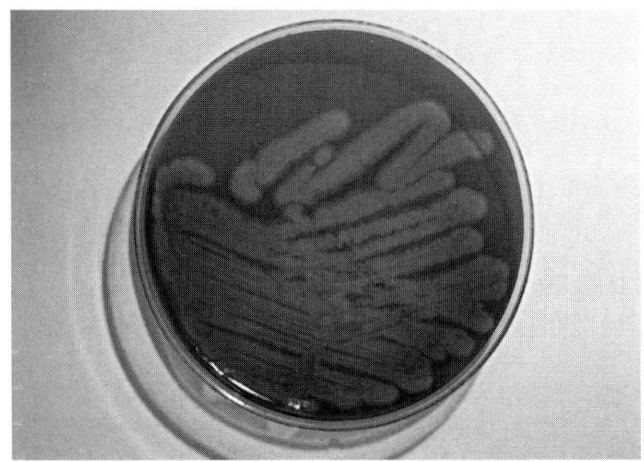

FIGURE 11-7
Pseudomonas aeruginosa on sheep blood agar with its typical large, dull, gray colonies that are beta hemolytic. Colonies typically have a "feathery edge" and may resemble ground glass.

PSEUDOMONAS AERUGINOSA

The most frequently isolated nonfermenter is *Pseudomonas aeruginosa,* an important opportunistic pathogen. In fact, this organism accounts for approximately 75% to 80% of all nonfermenters isolated from clinical specimens. *P. aeruginosa* is a strict aerobe. Identification of the organism is usually aided by its characteristic pigments of **pyocyanin,** a water-soluble blue pigment, and **fluorescein** or **pyoverdin,** a yellow fluorescing pigment that results in the typical blue-green color of *P. aeruginosa* (Figure 11-6 [Color Plate 40]). The pyocyanin can be extracted with chloroform; it is responsible for the blue exudate often seen with *P. aeruginosa* wound infections. Fluorescein must be visualized using an ultraviolet light. These pigments are visible on most clear agars, and their colors can be enhanced through use of *Flo (Pseudomonas F)* and *Tech (Pseudomonas P)* Agars (Becton Dickinson Microbiology Systems) or *Pseudomonas Agar F* (fluorescein) and *Pseudomonas Agar P* (pyocyanin) (Difco Laboratories).

Another significant characteristic of *P. aeruginosa* is its grapelike or "corn tortilla-like" odor resulting from the production of 2-aminoacetophenone. Other important factors include the organism's ability to grow at 42°C, as well as at room temperature and at 35°C. The organism is motile with a single, polar flagellum.

P. aeruginosa grows very well on MacConkey agar and eosin-methylene blue (EMB) as a lactose-negative organism. On blood agar the bacterium typically produces large, rough, dull grayish, spreading colonies with a feathery edge that may be beta hemolytic (Figure 11-7 [Color Plate 41]).

Although it will grow on the TSI slant, no reactions are observed in the TSI. *P. aeruginosa* is oxidase positive and oxidizes glucose but not maltose in the OF medium. The box on p. 211 lists important reactions to identify *P. aeruginosa.*

P. aeruginosa is an important pathogen, especially in the compromised host. Infections typically occur at sites where water or moisture accumulate, such as in the ears, eyes, indwelling catheters, and most often at sites of burns and wounds. The organism is found throughout the environment and nature and is known to cause infections in mammals, insects, birds, fish, and plants. It is able to survive the harsh environment of soap solutions, water faucets, disinfectants, and whirlpools and has even been isolated on flowers and plants in patients' rooms! Thus the organism is often associated with nosocomial infections, such as whirlpool-associated dermatitis, wound infections, and lower respiratory tract infections following respiratory ventilation in patients with preexisting lung disorders. The incidence of nosocomial infections caused by *P. aeruginosa* has been increasing in recent years.

Common infections attributed to *P. aeruginosa* are as follows:

Severe wound infections in burn patients
Urinary tract infections
Nosocomial pneumonia
Septicemia in immunosuppressed patients and infants
Chronic lung infections in patients with cystic fibrosis
Septic arthritis in intravenous drug abusers
Septicemia
Destructive eye infections (keratitis, corneal ulcers) in contact lens wearers
Swimmer's ear

A mucoid strain of *P. aeruginosa* has been found to cause a severe pneumonia in patients with cystic fibro-

Identification of *Pseudomonas aeruginosa*

Oxidase: positive

Pyocyanin: positive

Fluorescein (pyoverdin): positive

Oxidizes glucose, fructose, and xylose in oxidative-fermentative (OF) medium

Cannot utilize maltose, sucrose, or lactose in OF medium

Grows well on MacConkey agar

Ornithine decarboxylase: negative

Lysine decarboxylase: negative

Arginine dehydrolase: positive

Acidamide: positive

Nitrates are denitrified to nitrites

Citrate: positive

Urease: variable

Indole: negative

Growth at 42°C: positive

Motile by one or two polar flagella

Resistant to kanamycin

Susceptible to carbenicillin

sis. Patients with cystic fibrosis activate the alginate gene, resulting in the production of alginate, which surrounds the bacterial cell wall and protects it from phagocytosis.

P. aeruginosa has several characteristics and also produces a number of compounds that lead to these devastating infections. A very significant characteristic is the organism's resistance to most antibiotics used to treat gram-negative infections. For this reason, treatment has been largely limited to aminoglycosides: tobramycin and gentamycin, as well as carbenicillin and ticarcillin.

P. aeruginosa possesses fimbriae that enable it to attach to respiratory epithelial cells. **Pili** enable the organism to adhere to host cells, and **alginate** is associated with inhibition of **chemotaxis** and **phagocytosis. Elastase,** which digests elastin of the arterial walls; **collagenase,** which breaks down collagen; and **protease,** which degrades protein, are all important enzymes produced by the organism that facilitate the spread of disease to other sites of the body. The pigment pyocyanin is known to inhibit other bacteria, and **exotoxin A** inhibits protein synthesis, which leads to tissue destruction and an aggravated host immune response. Finally, hemolysins and endotoxin are also associated with *P. aeruginosa* infections.

Summary of Reactions for *Pseudomonas fluorescens* and *Pseudomonas putida*

Oxidase: positive

Motile by a polar tuft of flagella

Oxidize glucose in OF medium

Pyocyanin: negative

Pyoverdin: positive

Arginine dehydrolase: positive

Resistant to carbenicillin

Susceptible to kanamycin

Growth at 42°C: positive

Acetamide: negative

OTHER *PSEUDOMONAS* SPECIES

P. fluorescens and P. putida are mainly considered to be normal flora, cause few clinical diseases, and are associated with rare opportunistic infections. *P. fluorescens* is found in the soil and water as an environmental contaminant and is associated with food spoilage and plant infections. It is also a rare cause of urinary tract infections (UTIs) and wound infections, while *P. putida* has been associated with isolated cases of septicemia and infections of the arms and legs. The organisms have also been isolated from hospital environmental sources, such as in sinks. The box above lists important reactions of *P. fluorescens and P. putida.*

Important reactions to differentiate the pair include the fact that *P. fluorescens* is proteolytic and can hydrolyze gelatin, whereas *P. putida* is nonproteolytic and cannot hydrolyze gelatin.

P. stutzeri, P. mendocina, and CDC group Vb-3 are described as "soil denitrifiers" since these bacteria use ammonium (NH_4) as the sole nitrogen source and acetate as the sole carbon source and grow anaerobically and produce nitrogen gas. *P. stutzeri* is found in soil, marine water, sewage, and stagnant water, as well as in hospital instrumentation. It is a rare cause of otitis media, conjunctivitis, and septic arthritis. Colonies are dry and wrinkled with a buff or light-brown color. The colonies are often tough and adherent. The organism is arginine dehydrolase (ADH) negative and positive for starch hydrolysis.

P. mendocina, another rare clinical isolate, appears as smooth, buttery, flat, unwrinkled colonies on blood agar. It is motile by polar monotrichous flagella, grows at 42°C, is ADH positive, and is negative for starch hydrolysis.

P. mallei is the cause of **glanders,** an infectious disease of horses, goats, sheep, and donkeys. Although extremely rare, humans can acquire the infection by direct contact, trauma, or inhalation. The infection is found most frequently in Asia, Africa, and the Middle East. *P. mallei* is the only nonmotile pseudomonad and is resistant to polymyxin B. Colonies are smooth and cream to white on blood agar. The organism is weakly oxidase positive and fails to grow at 42°C.

P. pseudomallei is the agent of **melioidosis,** a glanderslike disease found in humans and animals in Southeast Asia and Australia. It is rarely found in the United States or other western parts of the world. The infection is characterized by an acute and severe pneumonia that can lead to septicemia. The organism is found in the natural environment, including water, soil, fruit, and vegetables of Southeast Asia and was associated with infections in American soldiers during the Vietnam conflict. This bacterium is easily aerosolized, and infections in the United States may be laboratory acquired. Colonies appear cream to tan and wrinkled. The organism is oxidase positive and motile via a polar tuft of multitrichous flagella and is ADH positive. It is highly oxidative and can oxidize glucose, maltose, lactose, mannitol, and cellobiose. The wrinkled colonies may be confused with *P. stutzeri,* which is ADH negative and susceptible to polymyxin.

P. cepacia, the cause of onion bulb rot in plants and foot rot in humans, is found near water sources, including environmental sources of water, and in intravenous fluids, detergents, and disinfectants, including chlorhexidine. It is being found with increasing frequency as an opportunistic and nosocomial pathogen, causing pneumonia, UTIs, septicemia, and endocarditis in patients with contaminated heart valves. Of particular significance is a severe pneumonia of *P. cepacia* seen with increasing frequency in patients with cystic fibrosis. The organism is resistant to the aminoglycosides and must be treated with sulfamethoxazole, chloramphenicol, or the third-generation cephalosporins. *P. cepacia* produces yellow, serrated colonies that are weakly oxidase positive. This bacterium acidifies the open glucose, maltose, lactose, and mannitol tubes and is ADH negative and lysine decarboxylase (LDC) positive.

Xanthomonas (formerly *Pseudomonas*) *maltophilia* is present in nature in food and water sources, soil, animals, and plants. It has also been isolated from a variety of clinical sites and is considered to be a contaminant or commensal on humans. It is a part of the transient flora that a patient acquires while in the hospital. Infections include pneumonia and a variety of nosocomial infections, such as septicemia, UTIs, wound infections, and meningitis. The organism is resistant to many antibiotics, including the aminoglycosides and betalactams, and is susceptible to trimethoprim-sulfamethoxazole. It is described as an emerging pathogen, found increasingly in immunosuppressed hosts, with infections being nosocomial in nature.

X. maltophilia produces large colonies with yellow-tan pigment on trypticase soy agar (TSA) and a lavender-green pigment on blood agar. It will grow at 42°C and is unique in being oxidase negative. The organism produces a weakly positive OF glucose in the open tube and a positive reaction in the open OF maltose tube. Pyoverdin is not produced, and an ammonia-like odor is sometimes produced by the bacterium. The box below lists important reactions of *X. maltophilia.*

Table 11-1 summarizes the biochemical reactions used to identify *Pseudomonas species.*

Important Reactions of *Xanthomonas maltophilia*

Yellow-tan pigment on trypticase soy agar

Lavender-green pigment on sheep blood agar

Growth at 42°C: positive

Oxidase: negative

Oxidizes glucose in OF medium: weakly positive

Oxidizes maltose in OF medium: strongly positive

Pyoverdin: negative

ONPG*: positive

Deoxyribonuclease: positive

Nitrates are not reduced to nitrogen gas

Lysine decarboxylase: slowly positive

Arginine dehydrolase: negative

Ornithine decarboxylase: negative

*o-Nitrophenyl-beta-d-galactopyranoside.

TABLE 11–1

Identification of Important *Pseudomonas* and Xanthomonas Species

	MENDOCINA	CEPACIA	PSEUDOMALLEI	XANTHOMONAS MALTOPHILIA	AERUGINOSA	FLUORESCENS	PUTIDA	STUTZERI
Oxidase	+	Weak +	+	−	+	+	+	+
Motility	+	+	+	+	+	+	+	+
Pyoverdin	−	−	−	−	+	+	+	−
Oxidation of:								
Glucose	+	+	+	Weak +	+	+	+	+
Maltose	−	+	+	Strong +	−	V	V	+
Lactose	−	+	+	+	−	−	−	−
Mannitol	−	+	+	−	+	+	−	V
Arginine hydrolase	+	−	+	−	+	+	+	−
Lysine decarboxylase	−	+	−	Slow +	−	−	−	−
Nitrate to nitrite	+	V	+	V	+	V	−	+
Nitrate to nitrogen gas	+	−	+	−	V	−	−	+
Deoxyribonuclease	−	−	−	+	−	−	−	−
Polymyxin susceptibility	S	R	R	S	S	S	S	S

+, most strains positive; −, most strains negative, V, variable reaction; S, susceptible; R, resistant.

REVIEW QUESTIONS

MULTIPLE CHOICE

1. **The nonfermentative gram-negative bacilli are generally opportunistic pathogens.**
   a. True
   b. False
2. **Oxidative-fermentative (OF) medium of Hugh and Leifson is well suited for nonferementers because of a:**
   a. High concentration of peptone and low concentration of carbohydrate
   b. High concentration of both peptone and carbohydrate
   c. High concentration of carbohydrate and low concentration of peptone
   d. Low concentration of both peptone and carbohydrate
3. **An organism producing a yellow color in the open tube and a blue-green color in the closed tube of an OF glucose determination is said to:**
   a. Ferment glucose
   b. Oxidize glucose
   c. Be unable to utilize carbohydrates
4. **Which reaction is incorrect for Pseudomonas aeruginosa?**
   a. Produces pyocyanin pigment
   b. Produces pyoverdin pigment
   c. Positive alkalinization of acidamide
   d. Fails to grow at 42°C
5. **Which statement most correctly describes infections attributed to Pseudomonas aeruginosa?**
   a. Common cause of wound infections in burn patients
   b. Resistant to many antibiotics typically used to treat gram-negative infections
   c. Cause of pneumonia in patients with cystic fibrosis
   d. Both a and b are correct
   e. All are correct
6. **Which of the following does not produce pyoverdin pigment?**
   a. *Pseudomonas aeruginosa*
   b. *Pseudomonas cepacia*
   c. *Pseudomonas fluorescens*
   d. *Pseudomonas putida*
7. **Pseudomonas mallei is the causative agent in:**
   a. Glanders
   b. Melloidosis
   c. Neonatal sepsis
   d. Onion bulb rot
8. **Which of the following correctly lists the characteristics of Xanthomonas maltophilia?**
   a. Blue-green pigment, oxidase positive, oxidizes glucose
   b. Yellow pigment, oxidase positive, oxidizes maltose
   c. Nonpigmented, oxidase negative, deoxyribonuclease positive
   d. Yellow pigment, oxidase negative, oxidizes maltose
9. **Acinetobacter baumannii is:**
   a. Oxidase positive
   b. Nonsaccharolytic
   c. Resistant to penicillin
   d. Motile
10. **Acinetobacter can be differentiated from Neisseria by:**
    a. A positive oxidase reaction for *Neisseria*
    b. Gram stain
    c. Carbohydrate utilization patterns
    d. Pigment production
11. **A yellow-pigmented gram-negative bacillus, isolated from a sink in a neonatal nursery where an outbreak of meningitis occurred, oxidized glucose but failed to oxidize mannitol in the OF reactions. It produced tiny pinpoint colonies on MacConkey agar. The organism is most likely:**
    a. *Xanthomonas maltophilia*
    b. *Pseudomonas aeruginosa*
    c. *Flavobacterium meningosepticum*
    d. *Alcaligenes faecalis*

BIBLIOGRAPHY

Applebaum PC, Leathers DH: Evaluation of the rapid NFT system for identification of gram-negative nonfermenting rods, *J Clin Microbiol* 20:730, 1984.

Applebaum PC, Stavitz J, Bentz MS et al: Four methods of identification of gram negative nonfermenting rods: organisms more commonly encountered in clinical specimens, *J Clin Microbiol* 12:271, 1980.

Bodey GP, Bolivar R, Fainstein V et al: Infections caused by *Pseudomonas aeruginosa, Rev Infect Dis* 5:279, 1983.

Burdash NM, Bannister ER, Manos JP et al: A comparison of four commercial systems for the identification of nonfermentative gram-negative bacilli, *Am J Clin Pathol* 73:564, 1980.

Clark WA, Hollis DG, Weaver RE et al: Identification of unusual pathogenic gram-negative aerobic and facultatively anaerobic bacteria, Atlanta, 1984, US Department of Health and Human Services, Centers for Disease Control.

Dance DAB: Melioidosis: the tip of the iceberg? *Clin Microbiol Rev* 4:52, 1991.

Gilardi GL: Pseudomonas and related genera. In Balows A, editor: *Manual of clinical microbiology,* ed 5, Washington, DC, 1991, The American Society of Microbiology.

Gilardi GL: Update on taxonomy of nonfastidious, glucose-nonfermenting gram-negative bacilli, *Clin Microbiol Newslett* 12:73, 1990.

Hofherr L, Votava H, Blazevic DJ: Comparison of three methods for identifying nonfermenting gram-negative rods, *Can J Microbiol* 24:1140, 1978.

Holmes B: The identification of *Pseudomonas cepacia* and its occurrence in clinical material, *J Appl Bacteriol* 61:299, 1986.

Holmes B: Identification and distribution of *Flavobacterium meningosepticum* in clinical material, *J Appl Bacteriol* 62:29, 1987.

Holmes B, Lapage SD, Easterling BG: Distribution in clinical material and identification of *Pseudomonas aeruginosa, J Clin Path* 32:66, 1979.

McKevitt AI, Woods DE: Characterization of *Pseudomonas cepacia* isolates from patients with cystic fibrosis, *J Clin Microbiol* 19:291, 1984.

Moss CW, Wallace PL, Hollis DG et al: Cultural and chemical characterization of CDC groups EO-2, M-5, and M-6, *Moraxella* species, *Acinetobacter* species, Oligella, and *Psychrocter immobilis, J Clin Microbiol* 26:484, 1988.

Oberhofer TR: Characteristics of human isolates of unidentified fluorescent pseudomonas capable of growth at 42° C, *J Clin Microbiol* 14:492, 1981.

Pickett MJ, Hollis DG, Bottone EJ: Miscellaneous gram negative bacteria. In Balows A, editor: *Manual of clinical microbiology,* ed 5, Washington, DC, 1991, American Society for Microbiology.

Schreckenberger PC: Classification of nonfermenting gram-negative bacilli, Clinical Microbiology Update, 1992, Western Pennsylvania Society for Clinical Microbiology.

Shewan JM, McMeekin TA: Taxonomy (and ecology) of *Flavobacterium* and related genera, *Ann Rev Microbiol* 37:233, 1983.

Suwanagool S, Rothkopf NM, Smith SM et al: Pathogenicity of *Eikenella corrodens* in humans, *Arch Intern Med* 143:2265, 1983.

Vasil ML: *Psuedomonas aeruginosa:* biology, mechanisms of virulence, epidemiology, *J Pediatr* 108:800, 1986.

Zuravleff JJ, Yu VL: Infections caused by *Pseudomonas maltophilia* with emphasis on bacteremia: case reports and a review of the literature, *Rev Infect Dis* 4:1236, 1982.

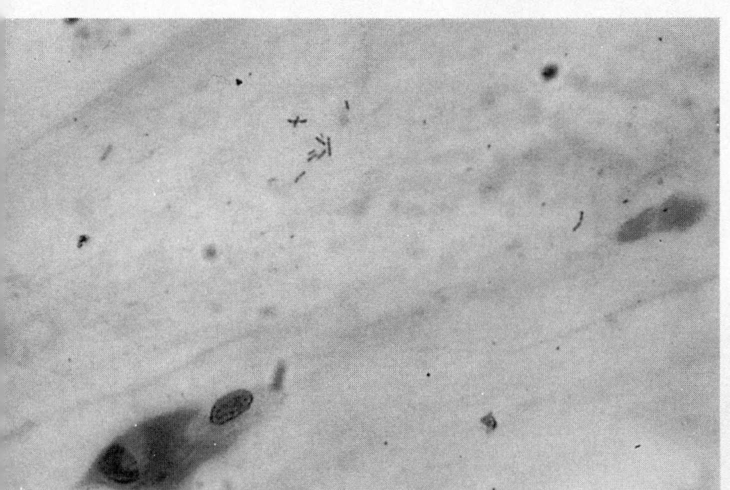

HAEMOPHILUS INFLUENZAE

CHAPTER OUTLINE

ISOLATION
IDENTIFICATION
HAEMOPHILUS INFLUENZAE
MISCELLANEOUS *HAEMOPHILUS* SPECIES
STAPHYLOCOCCUS STREAK
X AND V FACTORS
HAEMOPHILUS ID QUAD PLATES

KEY TERMS

CHANCROID
DELTA-AMINOLEVULINIC ACID
HAEMOPHILUS INFLUENZAE SEROTYPE B
HEMATIN
NICOTINAMIDE-ADENINE DINUCLEOTIDE (NAD)
SATELLITISM

Haemophilus

LEARNING OBJECTIVES

1. Describe the general morphological and biochemical characteristics of *Haemophilus.*
2. Describe X and V factors and indicate a source for each. Perform and interpret the test for X and V factors.
3. List the media used to isolate Haemophilus, and indicate why sheep blood agar is usually not acceptable.
4. Describe the principle of satellitism.
5. State the principle of the delta-aminolevulinic acid (ALA) test.
6. Explain how *H. influenzae* is identified from a clinical specimen.
   a. State the correct results for the following reactions: hemolysis, requirement for X and V factors, ALA, and fermentation of glucose, sucrose, lactose, and fructose.
   b. Identify *H. influenzae* in a clinical sample or stock culture.
7. List the serotypes of *H. influenzae,* and indicate which is found most frequently in human infection.
8. Describe how the capsular antigen is used to identify *H. influenzae.*
9. List the infections associated with *H. influenzae*, and indicate which population is most affected.
10. Briefly describe the identification and clinical relevance of:
    a. *H. ducreyi*
    b. *H. aegyptius*
    c. *H. parainfluenzae*
    d. *H. aphrophilus*
    e. *H. paraphrophilus*
    f. *H. haemolyticus*

TABLE 13–3

Differentiation of *Bordetella* Species

	UREASE	NITRATE	MOTILITY	OXIDASE
B. pertussis	−	−	−	+
B. parapertussis	+ (18 hours)	−	−	−
B. bronchiseptica	Strong + (4 hours)	+	+	+

The organism can be directly identified from nasopharyngeal specimens by using the DFA stain, which is the preferred method. In this technique, a smear is made from a nasopharyngeal specimen (swab or aspirate). Next, fluorescein-isothiocyanate-conjugated *B. pertussis* antibodies are added. After incubation, the slide is washed and examined under the fluorescent microscope. Some recommend that identification of *B. pertussis* include both culture and DFA.

B. parapertussis produces a brown pigment on B-G agar. It is nonmotile and has been associated with a pertussis-like syndrome that is a milder infection than seen with *B. pertussis.*

B. bronchiseptica is motile with peritrichous flagella and has been found to be a cause of a variety of infections, including septicemia and meningitis in immunosuppressed hosts. It is a rapid urease producer.

Some common biochemical reactions used to speciate *Bordetella* are found in Table 13-3.

BRUCELLA

Brucella organisms are catalase-positive, oxidase-positive, nonsaccharolytic, strictly aerobic gram-negative bacilli. The organisms are normal flora of the urinary and gastrointestinal tracts of goats, pigs, cows, and dogs. The organisms are agents of brucellosis in animals. Humans acquire *Brucella* infections through the ingestion of contaminated animal products, including meats and milk. Farmers can directly acquire *Brucella* infections through direct animal contact.

Brucella species are obligate parasites and can survive intracellularly in the reticuloendothelial system, bone, liver, and central nervous system of humans. The organism causes **undulant fever (brucellosis),** which is a chronic and recurring fever. The infection is characterized by weight loss and anorexia. Granulomatous infections occur in the reticuloendothelial system and in the bone. The infections become chronic because the organism resides intracellularly, protected from cell-mediated immunity.

Brucella can be isolated from blood cultures, which are positive the first 2 weeks of febrile illness. Blood cultures will become negative after the acute symptoms subside, since antibody production will begin. Although *Brucella* grows on blood and chocolate agar, *Brucella* agar plus 5% horse or rabbit serum is the recommended medium for isolation. *Brucella* agar contains a pancreatic digest of casein, a peptic digest of animal tissue, yeast, and sodium bisulfite. Plates are incubated in 5% to 10% CO_2 and are held for 3 weeks. Castañeda bottles are a biphasic system containing both agar and broth that can also be used to culture *Brucella.* In Gram-stained smears, *Brucella* organisms are tiny, gram-negative coccobacilli that may appear intracellular in tissue specimens. Carbolfuchsin should be substituted for safranin O to improve the quality of the Gram stain.

The "gold standard" for *Brucella* identification is **febrile agglutinins,** which is a serological test for antibodies in the patient's serum that react with antigen of killed *Brucella.* A fourfold increase between the acute and convalescent titer is considered significant.

Brucella is a type 3 biohazard that involves common and unusual pathogens. A biological safety cabinet must be used to prevent the generation of aerosols. All positive results should be sent to the state or another reference laboratory for confirmation. Most identifications are made in reference laboratories.

The species of *Brucella* can be identified using the biochemical reactions in Table 13-4.

PASTEURELLA

Pasteurella are nonmotile, oxidase-positive, fermentative, facultative, anaerobic gram-negative bacilli. The most important human species is *P. multocida,* which is the etiologic agent of pasteurellosis. *Pasteurella* is encapsulated, which enables it to resist phagocytosis. The organism is carried in the oral cavity and respiratory and gastrointestinal tracts of healthy domestic cats and dogs and also is normally found in many other animals, including rodents, rabbits, and birds. It is the agent of "shipping fever" in cattle, a hemorrhagic septicemia. Humans may acquire the infection following contact with domestic animals that harbor the bacterium. Most frequently the route of infection is from the bite or scratch of an infected animal, usually a cat. Local wound infections are the most common type of *Pasteurella* infection or **pasteurellosis,** which is characterized by pain, redness, swelling, cellulitis, and a purulent discharge. There is a rapid onset of inflammation, with a fever developing 3 to 5 days after the infection is acquired. Complications of pasteurellosis include osteomyelitis, meningitis, and joint infections. Bacteremia can result from the primary bite infection. A second route of infection is inhalation of the bacterium, which can lead to pneumonia, bronchitis, or sinusitis. Those at

Haemophilus

LEARNING OBJECTIVES

1. Describe the general morphological and biochemical characteristics of *Haemophilus.*
2. Describe X and V factors and indicate a source for each. Perform and interpret the test for X and V factors.
3. List the media used to isolate Haemophilus, and indicate why sheep blood agar is usually not acceptable.
4. Describe the principle of satellitism.
5. State the principle of the delta-aminolevulinic acid (ALA) test.
6. Explain how *H. influenzae* is identified from a clinical specimen.
   a. State the correct results for the following reactions: hemolysis, requirement for X and V factors, ALA, and fermentation of glucose, sucrose, lactose, and fructose.
   b. Identify *H. influenzae* in a clinical sample or stock culture.
7. List the serotypes of *H. influenzae,* and indicate which is found most frequently in human infection.
8. Describe how the capsular antigen is used to identify *H. influenzae.*
9. List the infections associated with *H. influenzae*, and indicate which population is most affected.
10. Briefly describe the identification and clinical relevance of:
    a. *H. ducreyi*
    b. *H. aegyptius*
    c. *H. parainfluenzae*
    d. *H. aphrophilus*
    e. *H. paraphrophilus*
    f. *H. haemolyticus*

The genus *Haemophilus* consists of tiny gram-negative coccobacilli that are nonmotile and non-spore forming. In clinical cultures the organisms may form long threadlike or filamentous strands. The organisms are facultative anaerobes, reduce nitrates, and utilize carbohydrates either fermentatively or with oxygen as the final hydrogen ion acceptor. Most species are oxidase and catalase positive and prefer incubation temperatures of 35° to 37°C with 5% to 10% carbon dioxide (CO_2). *Haemophilus* species are very prone to drying and chilling; thus abrupt fluctuations in temperature must be avoided.

Most species of *Haemophilus* are nonpathogenic or opportunistic pathogens, except for *H. influenzae* and *H. ducreyi.* Many species are considered to be indigenous flora of the mucous membranes of the upper respiratory tract and oral cavity.

Haemophilus, which means "blood loving," has particular growth requirements, which include a group of iron-containing compounds known as hemin or hematin. **Hemin** and **hematin,** also known as **X factor,** are heat-stable products that are released with the degradation of hemoglobin. Another requirement of some species is **nicotinamide-adenine dinucleotide (NAD)** or **coenzyme I,** also known as **V factor.** NAD is a heat-labile compound produced by certain bacteria and yeast. It also can be obtained through exogenous sources, such as potato or yeast extracts.

ISOLATION

Because of the requirement of NAD, sheep blood agar is usually not adequate to isolate *Haemophilus* species. Sheep red blood cells release NADase, which inactivates NAD present in the medium. Horse or rabbit blood agar can be used to isolate *Haemophilus* since neither contains NADase. However, these media are not usually maintained in the laboratory. For these reasons, chocolate agar is the preferred isolation medium. Chocolate agar is prepared by either heating sheep red blood cells to at least 80°C or using enzyme treatment. Either method will release hematin (X factor) and inactivate NADase. Additional cofactors and supplements can then be added to the medium. Synthetic chocolate agar is also available and contains NAD, iron, vitamin B_{12}, thiamin, iron, magnesium, glucose, cysteine, and glutamine.

The **"staph streak"** can also be used for primary isolation. In this technique the culture is heavily streaked onto a sheep blood agar plate. Next, a single streak of beta-hemolytic *Staphylococcus aureus* is streaked through the inoculum. Because many bacteria, including *S. aureus,* synthesize NAD (V factor), and because of the beta hemolysis that results from the release of hemin, both growth requirements are met for *Haemophilus* species. *Haemophilus* species that require both X and V factors appear as tiny **satellite** colonies around the *S. aureus* after incubation. Other organisms also produce NAD and allow satelliting. **Satellitism** is illustrated in Figure 12-1 (Color Plate 45).

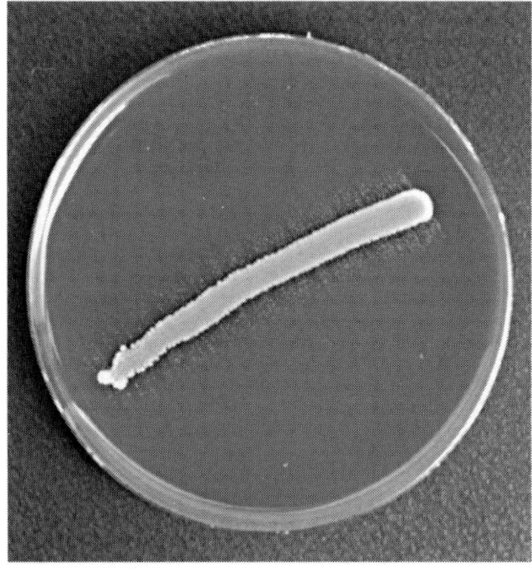

FIGURE 12-1
Satellitism on *Haemophilus influenzae* around beta-hemolytic *Staphylococcus aureus.*

Haemophilus isolation media such as horse blood-bacitracin agar can also be used. This medium contains beef heart infusion, peptone, yeast, 5% defibrinated horse blood (which provides X and V factors), and 300 mg/L of bacitracin. The bacitracin inhibits the normal flora, which enhances the recovery of *Haemophilus* species. In addition, hemolytic reactions can be observed on such media.

Levinthal agar is a clear medium containing X and V factors and other growth factors. Encapsulated colonies of *H. influenzae* appear iridescent when viewed with an oblique light, whereas nonencapsulated strains appear transparent, bluish, and noniridescent.

IDENTIFICATION

Haemophilus species are identified through hemolytic reactions on horse blood agar and through growth requirements for X and V factors. X and V factors are impregnated onto filter paper strips. The suspected organism is inoculated onto a medium deficient in these factors. Media such as Mueller-Hinton and trypticase soy agar are acceptable. The strips are then applied, and the plate is incubated under increased CO_2 at 35°C for 24 hours, at which time the plate is examined for growth. If growth occurs only around the X strip, the organism requires only X factor for growth. If growth occurs only around the V strip, the organism requires only V factor for growth. If growth occurs between the X and V strips, the organism requires both X and V factors.

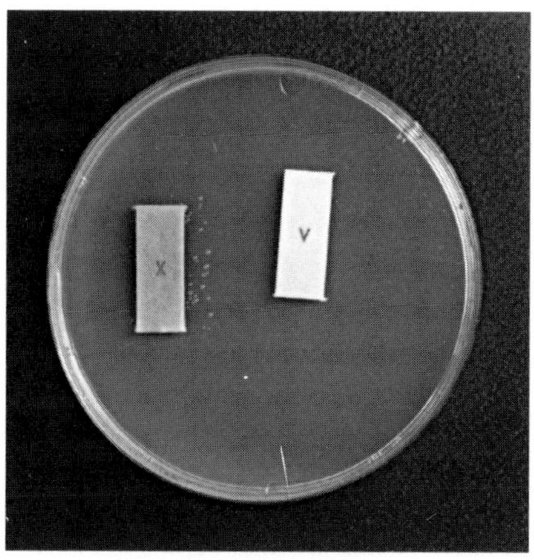

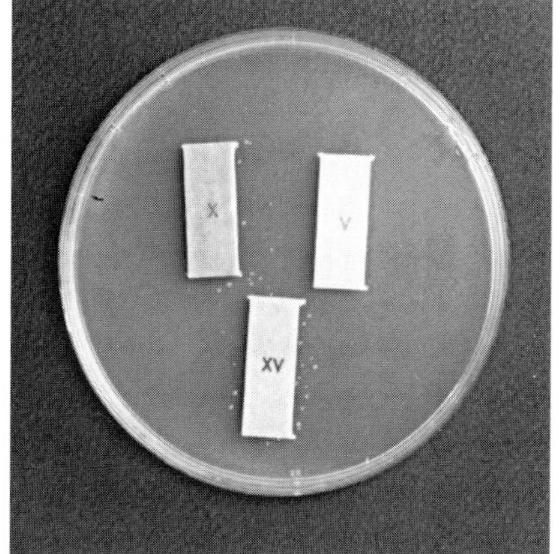

FIGURE 12-2

X and V factor strips for *Haemophilus influenzae* illustrating organism's requirement for both X and V factors.

In performing the test for X and V factors, it is essential not to transfer any chocolate-containing or blood-containing medium to prevent carry-over of the factors, which could lead to false results. X and V factor strips for *H. influenzae* are illustrated in Figure 12-2.

The **delta-aminolevulinic acid test (ALA porphyrin test)** can also be used to determine the requirement for X factor. The ALA porphyrin test is not affected by carry-over as is X factor testing. In this procedure the synthesis of protoporphyrin from the substrate ALA is determined. Species such as *H. parainfluenzae,* which do not require exogenous X factor, are ALA positive because they possess the necessary enzymes to convert ALA to porphobilinogen and porphyrin to hemin. Species that require exogenous X factor for growth, such as *H. influenzae,* are ALA negative.

Haemophilus identification plates are available commercially from several manufacturers. These *Haemophilus* identification plates contain one quadrant each for horse blood to determine growth and hemolysis, X factor–enriched medium, V factor–enriched medium, and both X and V factors–enriched medium. The plate can be used instead of the technique for X and V factors. Reactions for *H. influenzae* and *H. parainfluenzae* on *Haemophilus* identification plates are illustrated in Figures 12-3 (Color Plate 46) and 12-4.

Haemophilus speciation is also based on carbohydrate fermentation reactions. Table 12-1 summarizes the biochemical reactions of the clinically important *Haemophilus.*

Rapid identification kits are available commercially. These kits allow for determination of ALA and carbohydrate fermentation and include the RIM-H (Austin Biological Laboratories) and RapIDNH (Innovative Diagnostics).

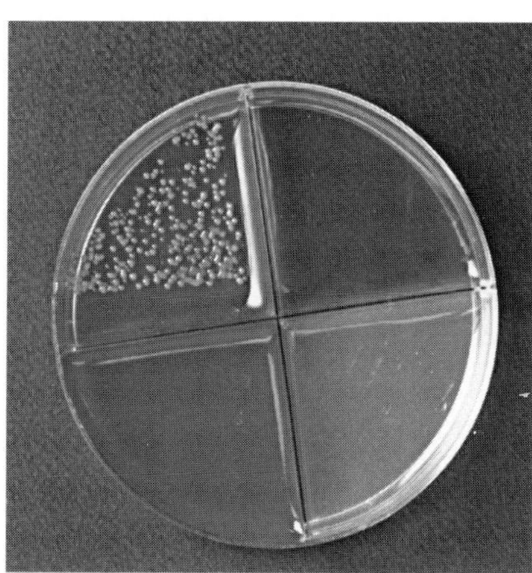

FIGURE 12-3

Haemophilus influenzae on *Haemophilus* ID plate. Plate contains four sections for X factor (quadrant I), V factor (quadrant II), both X and V factors (quadrant III), and horse blood with V factor (quadrant IV). *H. influenzae* will grow in quadrant III with both X and V factors and is nonhemolytic on horse blood.

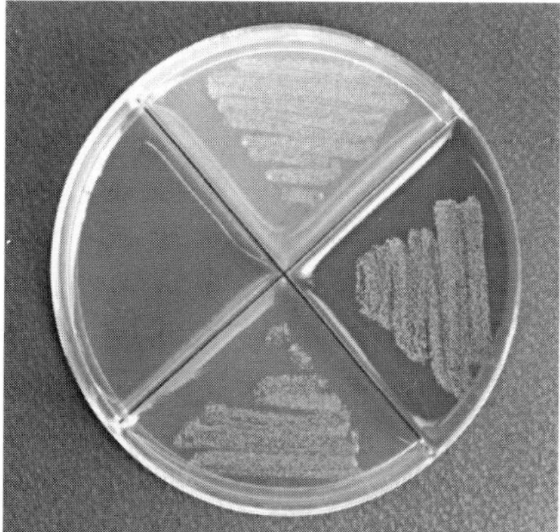

FIGURE 12-4

Haemophilus parainfluenzae on *Haemophilus* ID plate. *H. parainfluenzae* grows in quadrants II (V factor present) and III (X and V factors present) and is nonhemolytic on horse blood agar.

HAEMOPHILUS INFLUENZAE

The most frequent clinically isolated *Haemophilus* is *H. influenzae,* formerly known as "Pfeiffer's bacillus." There are six serotypes of *H. influenzae:* a, b, c, d, e, and f. **Serotype b** is encountered most frequently in infections. Serotyping is based on the characteristics of the capsule. The serotype can be determined through identification of the distinct capsular antigen through latex agglutination, capsular swelling, or immunofluorescence.

There are also currently eight biotypes of *H. influenzae:* I, II, III, IV, V, VI, VII, and VIII. Biotypes are based on biochemical reactions, including carbohydrate fermentation, indole, urease, and ornithine decarboxylase (ODC). The box below lists biochemical reactions used to identify the biotypes of *H. influenzae.*

H. influenzae is carried as normal flora of the upper respiratory tract. The nonencapsulated strain may be carried asymptomatically by more than 50% of the general population. The nonencapsulated strain is generally not virulent. The carrier rate is estimated to be 30% to 50% in children. Encapsulated strains are pathogenic and produce rapid, devastating disease in children less than 3 years of age. The capsule holds antiphagocytic properties, and children do not develop antibodies until age 2 to 3 years.

Before the mid-1980s, when the first vaccine was available, *H. influenzae* was the main cause of meningitis in children less than 5 years of age. Between ages 2 and 6 years, *H. influenzae* and *Neisseria meningitidis* occur with the same frequency. The infection is very contagious among siblings, since infection is spread by person-to-person contact through respiratory droplets. The organism spreads from the nasopharynx to the regional lymph nodes to the blood and finally to the meninges. Although some children may become asymptomatic carriers, others develop severe infections. Adults who develop *H. influenzae* meningitis may have a predisposing condition, such as chronic sinus infection, alcoholism, head trauma, diabetes, ear infections, or heart valve disease. More than 90% of the cases of meningitis are caused by serotype b.

H. influenzae is also associated with respiratory conditions, including epiglottitis, which is seen in children ages 2 to 4 years. This acute respiratory disease is characterized by a swollen, red, edematous epiglottis, and death may occur from suffocation. Other respiratory infections include acute sinusitis, chronic bronchitis, and pneumonia.

Systemic infections include bacteremia, septicemia, and endocarditis. The most common serological type in all cases is b. These infections are seen in children and immunosuppressed adults. Several cases have been reported in patients over age 60. Nonencapsulated strains of *H. influenzae* are associated with upper respiratory tract infections and bronchitis in immunosuppressed adults.

Because *H. influenzae* is very fastidious and adversely affected by changes in temperature and drying, specimens suspected of harboring the organism should be held at room temperature and inoculated onto enriched media as soon as possible. Swabs should be premoistened, or a transport medium such as modified Stuart's or Amie's charcoal should be used when it is not possible to inoculate the agar in a reasonable time.

Identification of *Haemophilus Influenzae* Biotypes

Biotypes are based on the biochemical reactions with indole, urease, and ornithine decarboxylase (ODC).

Certain biotypes more frequently cause certain diseases. For example, biotype I is found most often in human infections and is associated with meningitis and septicemia. Biotypes II and III have been found in the eye and respiratory tract, and biotypes IV and V have been found in the ear and respiratory tract.

BIOTYPE	INDOLE	UREASE	ODC
I	+	+	+
II	+	+	−
III	−	+	−
IV	−	+	+
V	+	−	+
VI	−	−	+
VII	+	−	−
VIII	−	−	−

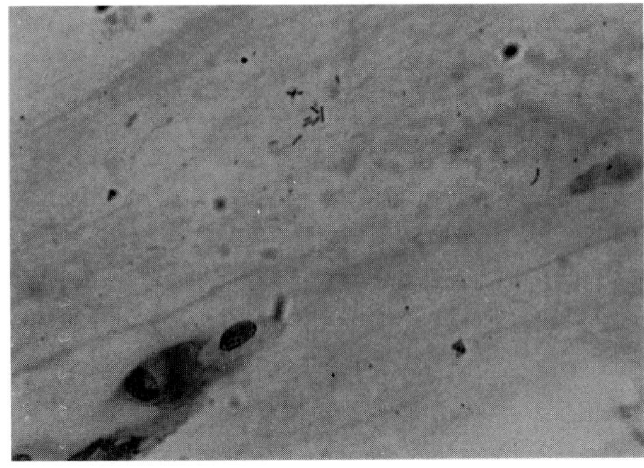

FIGURE 12–5

Gram stain of *Haemophilus influenzae* in a sputum specimen showing small, gram-negative coccobacilli.

Specimen type is dictated by the type of infection. Possible sites include the following: blood, cerebrospinal fluid (CSF), middle ear aspirate, infected joint fluid, nasopharyngeal swabs, and eye swabs.

H. influenzae identification begins with a Gram stain of the infected area. CSF smears are centrifuged, concentrated, and Gram-stained. The organism appears in CSF and blood smears as small, gram-negative coccobacilli; it may also appear pleomorphic or tangled. A Gram-stained smear of *H. influenzae* is shown in Figure 12-5 (Color Plate 47).

Rapid direct identification of the capsular antigen can be accomplished through the Neufeld reaction (Quellung, capsular swelling), in which antisera react with the antigens in the capsule of the organism, making the capsule more prominent. Other methods for direct antigen detection include staphylococcal coagglutination, latex agglutination, and enzyme-linked immunosorbent assay (ELISA). The capsular antigen can be detected in CSF, serum, or urine. In each method the capsular antigen reacts with antisera specific to serotype b. Antibodies against *H. influenzae* type b capsular material are fixed to latex beads or staphylococcal bacteria. The specimen is mixed with the sensitized reagent, with agglutination indicative of a positive result. Current tests available include Bactigen *H. influenzae* type b (Wampole Laboratories) and the Directigen Meningitis (Becton-Dickinson Microbiology Systems).

Specimens should be plated on chocolate agar, and a "staph streak" may also be performed on blood agar. Plates should be incubated at 35°C to 37°C under 5% to 10% CO_2 with increased humidity. The extremely fastidious *H. ducreyi* and *H. aegyptius* require Mueller-Hinton–based chocolate medium plus 10% IsoVitaleX for enhanced and more rapid growth. This medium also serves to enhance the growth of *H. influenzae.*

Reactions to identify *H. influenzae* can be found in Table 12-1 and the box on p. 228. A summary of important reactions is as follows:

Fails to grow on sheep blood agar
Nonhemolytic on rabbit or horse blood agar
ALA (porphyrin) negative
Carbohydrate fermentation
  Positive: glucose, ribose, xylose
  Negative: sucrose, lactose, fructose, mannose
Indole, urease, ODC: variable based on biotype

All *H. influenzae* isolates should be tested for beta lactamase, an extracellular enzyme produced by certain *H. influenzae* that hydrolyzes the amide bond in penicillin to penicillic acid. Ampicillin was the drug of choice for *H. influenzae* infections until 1974, when resistance was first observed. Ampicillin remains the drug of choice for ampicillin-susceptible *H. influenzae* meningitis. In resistant cases, chloramphenicol may be used, as well as cefotaxime or ceftriaxone, although chloramphenicol resistance is also possible.

Vaccines are available for *H. influenzae.* In 1985 the first vaccine for *H. influenzae,* the PRP (purified polyribosyl ribitol phosphate), was available. The vaccine was prepared from capsular material from *H. influenzae* type b strains. This vaccine was recommended for children over 18 months of age. In 1989, conjugated PRP vaccines were available that stimulated an enhanced immunological response. Earlier versions of *Haemophilus* vaccines were administered as early as age 15 months. Since 1990, upgraded versions of the vaccines have been licensed for use in infants at 2, 4, and 6 months, with a booster given at 15 months or older.

The administration of *Haemophilus* vaccines to infants and children has greatly reduced primary infections, such as meningitis and epiglottitis, thus reducing long-term neurological effects and the mortality rate.

TABLE 12–1

Identification of *Haemophilus* Species

	REQUIREMENT FOR				FERMENTATION OF:			
SPECIES	**X FACTOR**	**V FACTOR**	**BETA HEMOLYSIS**	**ALA**	**GLUCOSE**	**SUCROSE**	**LACTOSE**	**FRUCTOSE**
H. influenzae	+	+	−	−	+	−	−	−
H. parainfluenzae	−	+	−	+	+	+	−	+
H. haemolyticus	+	+	+	−	+	−	−	wk+
H. parahaemolyticus	−	+	+	+	+	+	−	+
H. aegyptius	+	+	−	−	+	−	−	−
H. aphrophilus	−	−	−	+	+	+	+	+
H. paraphrophilus	−	+	−	+	+	+	+	+
H. ducreyi	+	−	−	−	−	−	−	−

ALA, Delta-aminolevulinic acid; +, positive reaction; −, negative reaction; wk+, weakly positive.

MISCELLANEOUS *HAEMOPHILUS* SPECIES

Haemophilus aegyptius, formerly known as Koch-Weeks bacillus, closely resembles *H. influenzae* biotype III (*H. influenzae* subspecies *aegyptius*). The organism causes "pink eye," a very contagious conjunctivitis spread through the sharing of handkerchiefs and towels. The infection occurs in seasonal epidemics, especially in the warmer climates.

Haemophilus ducreyi is the infective agent of **chancroid**, a soft chancre venereal disease characterized by the appearance of a ragged, painful ulcer on the genitalia. Chancroid is found more frequently in Africa, Asia, and the tropics and less frequently in Europe and North America. The organism appears as tiny gram-negative bacilli (intracellular to polymorphonuclear neutrophils) on direct examination of the genital ulcer, and is said to resemble "schools of fish." The organism is very fastidious, requiring freshly clotted rabbit, sheep, or human blood to grow. Alternatively, it can be cultured on chocolate agar supplemented with 1% IsoVitaleX or *Gonococcus* agar with 1% to 2% hemoglobin, 5% bovine fetal serum, and 3 μg/ml vancomycin. *H. ducreyi* requires X but not V factor.

Haemophilus haemolyticus is occasional normal flora of the upper respiratory cavity. It requires both X and V factors and shows a wide zone of beta hemolysis on horse blood agar. It may be mistaken for group A *Streptococcus* on the blood agar plate; the differentiation can be made through the Gram stain.

Haemophilus parainfluenzae is normal flora of the upper respiratory tract. It is rarely infectious and requires only the V factor. Other *Haemophilus* species that are normal flora of the oral cavity include *H. aphrophilus* and *H. paraphrophilus*. The organisms are found in dental plaque and are very rarely associated with endocarditis.

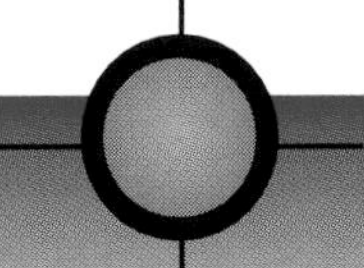

PROCEDURE
STAPHYLOCOCCUS STREAK

PURPOSE

Haemophilus can be isolated on blood agar by streaking the culture with beta-hemolytic *Staphylococcus aureus* and observing for satellitism.

PRINCIPLE

Many microorganisms, including *S. aureus, Neisseria,* and certain yeasts, are capable of synthesizing NAD (V factor). When these organisms appear in mixed culture, those species of *Haemophilus* that require V factor appear as small, "dewdrop" colonies around those bacterial colonies producing NAD. This phenomena is known as satellitism. When grown on sheep blood agar, beta-hemolytic strains of *S. aureus* release X factor (hemin) as the red cells are hemolyzed.

MATERIALS AND MEDIA

Sheep blood agar plate
S. aureus (beta-hemolytic strain)
Species of culture suspected of containing *Haemophilus*

PROCEDURE

1. Streak the *"Haemophilus"* culture heavily on the sheep blood agar plate. Use a swab if necessary.
2. Make a single, narrow streak of *S. aureus* through the area where the *Haemophilus* was streaked.
3. Incubate at 35° to 37°C under 3% to 10% CO_2 for 18 to 24 hours.

INTERPRETATION

Observe the plate for satellitism. *Haemophilus* colonies appear as moist, small, dewdrop colonies adjacent to the *S. aureus* colonies. The plate can also be observed for hemolysis and growth in the hemolyzed areas, indicating that the species requires factor X.

QUALITY CONTROL

Haemophilus influenzae: growth in beta-hemolytic zone surrounding *S. aureus*

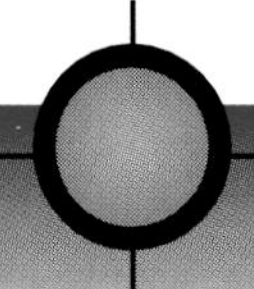

PROCEDURE
X AND V FACTORS

PURPOSE

Haemophilus organisms can be speciated based on their specific growth requirements for X and V factors.

PRINCIPLE

X factor (hemin or hematin) is derived from the digestion or degradation of blood. V factor (coenzyme I or NAD) is obtained from yeast or potato extract and is also produced by some bacteria, such as *Staphylococcus aureus.* These factors are required either singly or in combination by various *Haemophilus* species and are thus used as a method of species differentiation. The growth requirements are tested through use of filter paper strips impregnated with X factor and V factor and both X and V factors. A nutrient-poor medium such as Mueller-Hinton agar is used.

MATERIALS AND MEDIA

Mueller-Hinton agar
Brain-heart infusion broth or trypticase soy broth
X factor and V factor filter paper disks.

PROCEDURE

1. From a pure *Haemophilus* isolate, prepare a light suspension in brain-heart infusion broth or trypticase soy broth. It is important not to carry any chocolate agar over into the broth, since this may lead to inaccurate results.
2. Inoculate the Mueller-Hinton plate with a sterile swab. Streak the plate for maximum growth in three directions to obtain a lawn of growth.
3. Using sterile forceps, place the filter paper disks on the agar surface approximately 20 mm apart. Gently tap into place.
4. Incubate 18 to 24 hours under 3% to 10% CO_2 at 35° to 37°C.
5. Observe the plates for visible growth about each filter paper disk.

INTERPRETATION

Growth about X factor and XV: X factor is required
Growth about V factor and XV: V factor is required
Growth about XV: both X and V factors are required

EXPECTED RESULTS

	GROWTH ALONG STRIP		
HAEMOPHILUS SPECIES	XV	X	V
H. influenzae	+	−	−
H. parainfluenzae	+	−	+
H. haemolyticus	+	−	−
H. parahaemolyticus	+	−	+

QUALITY CONTROL

H. influenzae: growth about XV strip
H. parainfluenzae: growth around V and XV strips

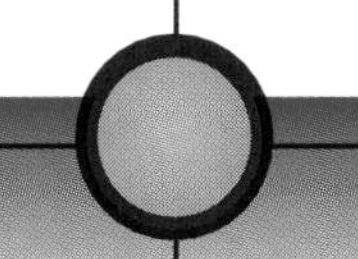

PROCEDURE
HAEMOPHILUS ID QUAD PLATES

PURPOSE

The *Haemophilus* identification plate is used to determine the hemolytic properties and requirements for X and V factors for particular *Haemophilus* species.

PRINCIPLE

The plate consists of four quadrants:

Quadrant I: brain-heart infusion agar (BHIA) and hemin (X)
Quadrant II: BHIA and Isovitale (V)
Quadrant III: BHIA with hemin (X) and Isovitale (V)
Quadrant IV: Horse blood agar (X) with NAD (V)

Presence or absence of growth in each quadrant and hemolytic properties are used to speciate *Haemophilus.* Hemolysis is observed in quadrant IV.

REAGENTS AND MEDIA

Haemophilus ID plate (Hemo ID QUAD available through Becton-Dickinson Microbiology Systems).
Trypticase soy broth

PROCEDURE

1. Pick several colonies of suspected organisms with a sterile inoculating needle or sterile cotton swab.
2. Suspend organism in trypticase soy broth until a turbidity of 0.5 McFarland is obtained.
3. Streak one loopful of this suspension on each quadrant of the plate. Streak the entire quadrant. Stab blood agar quadrant. Sterilize loop between quadrants, or use a new disposable loop for each quadrant.
4. Incubate plate in 3% to 10% CO_2 at 35°C for 24 to 48 hours.

INTERPRETATION

1. Interpret plate for visible growth and hemolysis. The organism should grow in quadrants III and IV. Read quadrant IV for hemolysis. Growth in quadrants II, III, and IV indicates requirement for X factor. Growth in quadrants I, III, and IV indicates requirement for X factor. Growth only in quadrants III and IV indicates requirement for both X and V factors.
2. Perform a Gram stain to obtain expected results to ensure purity and to obtain morphological characteristics of *Haemophilus.*

Continued.

PROCEDURE
HAEMOPHILUS ID QUAD PLATES
(Continued)

EXPECTED RESULTS

HAEMOPHILUS SPECIES	GROWTH ON QUADRANTS I (X)	II (V)	III (XV)	IV (HEMOLYSIS)
H. influenzae	−	−	+	−
H. parainfluenzae	−	+	+	−
H. haemolyticus	−	−	+	+
H. parahaemolyticus	−	+	+	+

QUALITY CONTROL

H. influenzae: nonhemolytic; growth in quadrants III and IV
H. parainfluenzae: nonhemolytic: growth in quadrants II, III, and IV

(Package insert, Hemo ID QUAD, Becton Dickinson Microbiology Systems.)

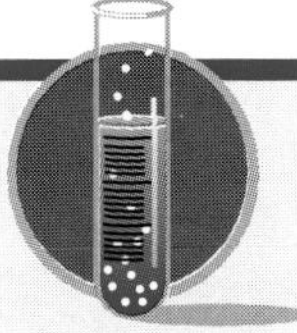

LABORATORY EXERCISES

1

Perform the tests for X and V factors for *Haemophilus influenzae* and *Haemophilus parainfluenzae*. Record your results.

		Observation	***Interpretation***
H. influenzae	X:		
	V:		
H. parainfluenzae	X:		
	V:		

2

Perform the "staph streak" on *H. influenzae* and *H. parainfluenzae*. Describe your results.

H. influenzae ______________________________

____

H. parainfluenzae ______________________________

____

3

Using a *Haemophilus* ID plate, identify an unknown *Haemophilus* provided by the instructor.
Unknown number: ______________

Observations

Quadrant I ______________________________

Quadrant II ______________________________

Quadrant III ______________________________

Quadrant IV ______________________________

Interpretation: ______________________________

____

Identification: ______________________________

REVIEW QUESTIONS

MATCHING

Identify the *Haemophilus* species by matching each with its correct biochemical reactions.

	Requirement for:				Fermentation of:			
	X factor	V factor	Hemolysis	ALA	Glucose	Sucrose	Lactose	Fructose
1.	−	+	−	+	+	+	−	+
2.	+	+	−	−	+	−	−	−
3.	+	−	−	−	−	−	−	−

a. *H. influenzae*
b. *H. parainfluenzae*
c. *H. haemolyticus*
d. *H. parahaemolyticus*
e. *H. ducreyi*

MULTIPLE CHOICE

4. Which statement correctly describes X factor?
a. Heat labile
b. Known as hemin or hematin
c. Derived from yeast and potato extract
d. Produced by *Staphylococcus aureus*

5. The medium most frequently used to isolate *Haemophilus* is:
a. Sheep blood agar
b. Rabbit blood agar
c. Chocolate agar
d. CNA

6. In the "staph streak," colonies of *S. aureus* satellite around a streak of *Haemophilus influenzae.*
a. True
b. False

Use the following information for questions 7 and 8.

In a determination of requirements for X and V factors, a suspected *Haemophilus* species grew only between the X and V strips.

7. This *Haemophilus* species requires:
a. Only V factor
b. Only X factor
c. Both X and V factors
d. Neither X nor V factor

8. Which of the following is *not* a possible species for these results?
a. *H. influenzae*
b. *H. aegyptius*
c. *H. parainfluenzae*
d. *H. hemolyticus*

9. Those *Haemophilus* species that are porphyrin positive:
a. Require exogenous NAD
b. Do not require exogenous NAD
c. Require exogenous hemin
d. Do not require exogenous hemin

10. The serotype of *H. influenzae* found most frequently in infections is:
a. a
b. b
c. c
d. d
e. e

11. The population most frequently infected by *H. influenzae* is:
a. Newborns
b. Nonimmunized infants and children less than 3 years of age
c. Nonimmunized preschool-age children, ages 3 to 5 years
d. School-age children, ages 6 to 10 years
e. Immunosuppressed adults

12. The infectious agent of chancroid is:
a. *H. aegyptius*
b. *H. haemolyticus*
c. *H. ducreyi*
d. *H. influenzae* biotype V

BIBLIOGRAPHY

Albritton WL, Penner S, Slaney L et al: Biochemical characteristics of *Haemophilus influenzae* in relationship to source of isolation and antibiotic resistance, *J Clin Microbiol* 7:519, 1978.

Doern GV, Chapin KC: Laboratory identification of Haemophilus influenzae: effects of basal media on the results of the satellitism test and evaluation of the rapid NH system, *J Clin Microbiol* 20:599, 1984.

Edberg SC, Melton E, Singer JM: Rapid biochemical characterization of Haemophilus species by using the Micro-ID, *J Clin Microbiol* 11:22, 1980.

Hilian M: *Haemophilus*. In Lennette EH, editor: Manual of clinical microbiology, ed 4, Washington, DC, 1985, American Society for Microbiology.

Mangum ME: *Haemophilus*. In Howard BJ, editor: *Clinical and pathogenic microbiology,* ed 2, St Louis, 1994, Mosby.

Marcon MJ, Hamoudi AC, Cannon HJ: Comparative laboratory evaluation of three antigen detection methods for diagnosis of *Haemophilus influenzae* type b disease, *J Clin Microbiol* 19:333, 1984.

Oberhofer TR, Back AE: Biotypes of Haemophilus encountered in clinical laboratories, *J Clin Microbiol* 10:168, 1979.

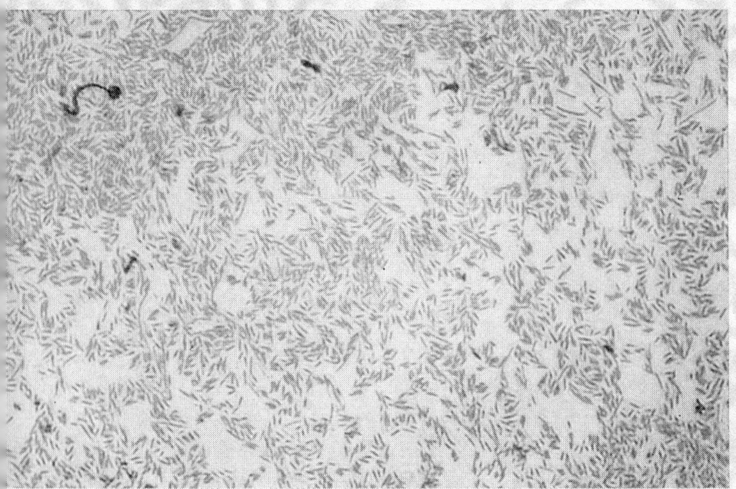

CAMPYLOBACTER JEJUNI

CHAPTER OUTLINE

VIBRIO
CAMPYLOBACTER
HELICOBACTER
AEROMONAS
PLESIOMONAS
LEGIONELLA
BORDETELLA
BRUCELLA
PASTEURELLA
FRANCISELLA
GARDNERELLA
STREPTOBACILLUS
CHROMOBACTERIUM AND *CARDIOBACTERIUM*
THIOSULFATE CITRATE BILE SALTS SUCROSE (TCBS) AGAR

KEY TERMS

BACTERIAL VAGINOSIS
CHOLERAGEN
CLUE CELL
FEBRILE AGGLUTININS
HALOPHILIC
LEGIONNAIRE'S DISEASE
PASTEURELLOSIS
PERTUSSIS
TULAREMIA
UNDULANT FEVER
ZOONOSES

Miscellaneous Gram-Negative Bacilli

CHAPTER THIRTEEN

LEARNING OBJECTIVES

1. Explain why the number of miscellaneous gram-negative bacilli associated with human infections has increased.
2. Name the agent of cholera, and explain how this organism is identified.
   a. Name the two biovars of cholera.
   b. Explain how cholera is transmitted.
3. Describe the unique characteristics of the genus *Campylobacter.*
   a. Explain how *Campylobacter* infections are transmitted.
   b. Differentiate *C. jejuni* subspecies *jejuni* from *C. coli.*
4. Explain the clinical significance of *Helicobacter pylori.*
5. Describe the clinical significance and differentiate *Aeromonas* from *Plesiomonas.*
6. Name the etiologic agent of legionnaires' disease.
   a. Describe and compare the types of legionellosis.
   b. List two other species of *Legionella* associated with human infection.
   c. Name the media used to isolate *Legionella.*
   d. Explain how *Legionella* is identified.
7. For each of the following bacteria:
   a. Name the media required for isolation.
   b. Name or describe the infectious process.
   c. Explain how the organism is identified.
      (1) Bordetella pertussis
      (2) Brucella
      (3) Pasteurella
      (4) Francisella
8. Name four species of Brucella, and list the animal source of each. Differentiate the species based on biochemical reactions and growth characteristics.
9. Describe the characteristics of bacterial vaginosis, and name the agent associated with this condition.
10. Identify and describe the gram-negative bacillus associated with rat-bite fever.

The miscellaneous or unusual gram-negative bacilli are a diverse group of gram-negative bacilli that are not easily placed into any specific category. Although these bacteria were once rarely associated with human infection, the infections have increased in recent years. This increase is a result of several factors, including the increase in the number of immunosuppressed hosts. In addition, methods of detection, including the use of highly selective media and immunological techniques, have been developed that facilitate the identification of these bacteria. Finally, changes in social factors, such as eating habits, also may have contributed to the increased incidence of the unusual gram-negative bacilli.

Many of these organisms are associated with **zoonoses,** infections in which the bacteria are transmitted from animals to humans. Transmission can follow a direct route through direct contact with an infected animal, ingestion of contaminated animal products, or an indirect route through tick or flea vectors.

Most of the bacteria in this group grow slowly on blood and chocolate agar and do not grow on MacConkey agar. Growth is usually enhanced with increased carbon dioxide (CO_2) and humidity.

VIBRIO

Vibrio organisms are natural habitants of sea water, and all species except *V. cholerae* and *V. mimicus* require increased sodium chloride (NaCl) for growth. **Halophilic** refers to this preference for increased salt and is attributed to the organism's need for increased chloride ions. Most species are associated with infections caused by contaminated water or seafood. *Vibrio* species have been isolated from the gastrointestinal tract as causes of gastritis and also have been found in blood and wound infections.

Vibrio organisms grow on blood agar, and selective media are also available to assist in their identification. The organisms grow on some differential media but may be overgrown by the normal flora coliforms. Thiosulfate citrate bile salts sucrose (TCBS) agar can be used to isolate most *Vibrio* species. TCBS agar contains sucrose, oxgall, sodium cholate, and bromthymol blue and thymol blue indicators. The medium is alkaline (pH of 8.6), which enhances the growth of *Vibrio.* The high pH of TCBS, oxgall, and cholate inhibit gram-positive bacteria and some lactose-fermenting gram-negative bacilli. The fermentation of sucrose TCBS can be used in the speciation of *Vibrio.* Sucrose fermentation is positive for *V. cholerae* but negative for *V. parahaemolyticus.*

Vibrio organisms are gram-negative straight or curved rods (Figure 13-1 [Color Plate 48]) and are motile with a single polar flagellum. They are facultative anaerobes or aerobic, and some prefer increased CO_2. *Vibrio* species are oxidase positive and fermentative in their metabolism of carbohydrates. There are more than 20 species, with 12 known to cause human infection. These 12 clinically significant *Vibrio* species are divided into six groups using differential biochemical tests.

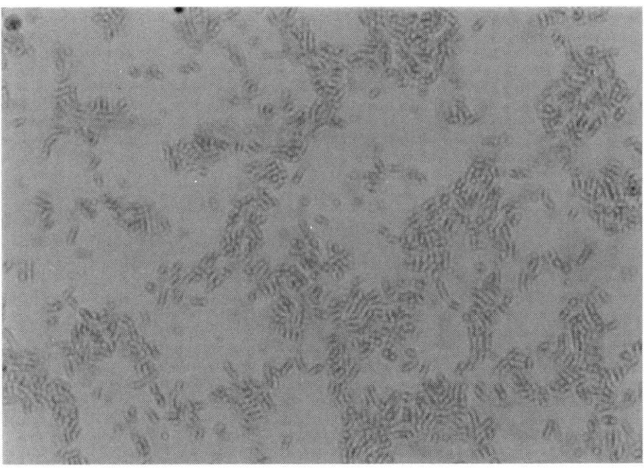

FIGURE 13–1

Photomicrograph of *Vibrio parahaemolyticus* showing gram-negative curved bacilli.

Vibrio infections have a low incidence in the United States and should be suspected if one has traveled to a foreign country, ingested shellfish, or has had contact with sea water. Certain species are seen more frequently near the Chesapeake Bay area.

Vibrio cholerae O1 is the cause of cholera. There are more than 60 different serogroups (known as serovars) of the organism based on typing for the "O" antigen, although all share a common "H" antigen. The cholera-producing strains belong to the "O1 type," which means that the organisms agglutinate with a single antisera against "serotype O, subgroup 1." The O1 strains are associated with pandemics and epidemics. *V. cholerae* is also serotyped into three serogroups: Ogawa, Inaba, and Hikojima. These serogroups are used to follow pandemics or epidemics.

There are two biotypes (biovars) of *V. cholerae:* classical and El Tor. The classical strain, responsible for pandemics in the past, is nonhemolytic on sheep blood agar, is Voges-Proskauer (VP) negative, and fails to agglutinate chicken red blood cells. The El Tor strain, which has been associated with more recent pandemics, is beta hemolytic, is more resistant to environmental changes, is VP positive, and agglutinates chicken red blood cells. In addition, the El Tor strain is resistant to polymyxin B, whereas the classical strain is susceptible to this antibiotic.

Recent cholera pandemics include an outbreak in Louisiana in 1978 and the January 1991 epidemic in South America. This South American pandemic began in Peru and spread to Chile, Brazil, and Mexico.

V. cholerae produces smooth, yellow colonies on TCBS agar because it is a sucrose fermenter. The organism produces a positive string test. In this procedure, 0.5% sodium desoxycholate is mixed with the suspected colony. Viscous *stringing* resulting in the production of a long, tenacious string occurs in a positive test.

Cholera is acquired through the ingestion of contaminated food or fecally contaminated water, including unpreserved meat, fish, seafood, and dairy products. It is a severe diarrheal disease due to the production of the potent "cholera enterotoxin" **(choleragen),** which attacks the bowel mucosa, leading to a tremendous outpouring of water and electrolytes. This is characteristically described as the "rice-water stool," which is watery and gray with mucin. Death may result from dehydration, extreme loss of fluid and electrolytes, hypovolemic shock, and acidosis. The infection may range from a mild form, lasting 3 to 5 days, to a more serious form. Mildly infected or asymptomatic individuals

Clinically Significant Vibrio Species

Vibrio cholerae **(serogroup O1)**

Nonhalophilic

Sucrose fermented

	Classical	El Tor
Red blood cell (RBC) hemolysis	Negative	Positive
Voges-Proskauer	Negative	Positive
Polymyxin B (50 U)	Susceptible	Resistant
Agglutination of chicken RBCs	Negative	Positive
Clinical significance (see text)	Cholera	Cholera

Vibrio parahaemolyticus

Halophilic

Lysine decarboxylase (LDC): positive

Arginine dehydrolase (ADH): negative

Fermentation of:

- Sucrose: negative
- Salicin: negative
- Cellobiose: negative

Clinical significance: gastroenteritis, usually associated with contaminated seafood

Vibrio vulnificus

Halophilic

LDC: positive

ADH: negative

Fermentation of:

- Sucrose: negative
- Salicin: positive
- Cellobiose: positive

Clinical significance: septicemia and wound infections involving marine environment

Vibrio mimicus

Nonhalophilic

Sucrose fermentation: negative

Voges-Proskauer: negative

Clinical significance: gastroenteritis and ear infections associated with marine environment

Vibrio anginolyticus

Halophilic

LDC: positive

ADH: negative

Voges-Proskauer: positive

Fermentation of:

- Sucrose: positive
- Arabinose: negative
- Salicin: negative
- Cellobiose: negative

Clinical significance: wound and ear infections associated with marine environment

Vibrio fluvialis **and** ***Vibrio furnissii***

Halophilic

ADH: positive

Voges-Proskauer: negative

Citrate: positive

Fermentation of sucrose: positive

Clinical significance: diarrhea associated with marine environment may excrete the organism and may serve as a source of transmission.

Replacement of fluids and electrolytes is essential therapy. Prevention of the infection is accomplished through proper sanitation, sewage disposal, and food handling.

Vibrio parahaemolyticus is a cause of wound and diarrheal infections. It is seen more frequently in the Far East and is associated with almost half of all causes of food poisoning in Japan. Infection is associated with contaminated or poorly cooked crab, shrimp, or lobster or with direct skin contact with contaminated water. It is now being found in the Chesapeake Bay area, mainly associated with contaminated crab. *V. parahaemolyticus* is a nonsucrose fermenter, producing green colonies on TCBS. It is halophilic and nonhemolytic on sheep blood agar.

Vibrio vulnificus has been isolated from marine sources and is mainly associated with wound infections and septicemia. Infections are most often seen in those handling seafood or working in the marine environment who have a preexisting liver condition. The production of a cytolysin by this species contributes to the high mortality rate associated with septicemia. Most strains produce green colonies on TCBS; the organism is a lactose fermenter and is positive for ONPG (*o*-nitrophenyl-beta-D-galactopyranoside).

V. mimicus, V. fluvialis, and *V. furnissii* are agents of gastroenteritis, and *V. alginolyticus* has been associated with ear, eye, and blood infections. The box on p. 241 summarizes some clinically important *Vibrio.*

CAMPYLOBACTER

Campylobacter species are microaerophilic and capnophilic, motile (via one polar flagellum), gram-negative, curved rods that are associated with gastroenteritis and diarrhea. The organisms are oxidase positive and nonfermentative. *Campylobacter* organisms are found as animal pathogens, causing abortion and sterility. Humans become infected through the fecal-oral route after contact with an infected animal, ingestion of contaminated animal products, or contact with another infected human. Animals known to harbor *Campylobacter* include farm animals, birds, cows, poultry, domestic pets, and water fowl. Infection is spread to humans who ingest raw milk, poorly cooked poultry, or contaminated water. The organism has also been isolated from environmental sources, such as soil and water.

The clinical signs of *Campylobacter* infection include fever, abdominal pain, and diarrhea. The stool characteristically contains segmented neutrophils and red blood cells. In its severe form the gastroenteritis may lead to intestinal bleeding that may mimic inflammatory bowel disease. The organism may invade the bloodstream and manifest as endocarditis, septic arthritis, or meningitis. Some individuals are asymptomatic carriers; they serve as a reservoir of infection.

Campylobacter infections have historically been seen more frequently in temperate climates but in recent years have surpassed *Salmonella* as agents in gastroenteritis in the United States.

Virulence factors for *Campylobacter* include the production of cytotoxin, cytotonic factor, and an enterotoxin.

Several species of *Campylobacter* have been described. The most frequently isolated species is *Campylobacter jejuni,* which is subdivided with two subspecies: *C. jejuni* subspecies *jejuni* and *C. jejuni* subspecies *doylei.* Following *C. jejuni* in frequency of human infection is *C. coli.*

Campylobacter species are isolated best on an agar selective for the organisms. One formulation is *Campylobacter* Blood Agar (Becton-Dickinson Microbiological Systems), which contains a blood agar base with the antibiotics vancomycin, polymyxin, cephalothin, trimethoprim, and amphotericin B added. Another example is Bacto *Campylobacter* Agar Skirrow (Difco Laboratories), which is a blood agar base with the antibiotics vancomycin, trimethoprim, and polymyxin B added. Several other media selective for *Campylobacter* are available commercially.

The enteric *Campylobacter* grow best at 42° to 43°C in a microaerophilic, capnophilic environment of 85% nitrogen, 5% oxygen, and 10% CO_2. The organisms also grow at 37°C. Currently, disposable plastic bags with generators providing this environment can be commercially purchased. An example is the Biobag Type Cf, available from Becton-Dickinson, which generates an environment of 5% to 10% oxygen and 8% to

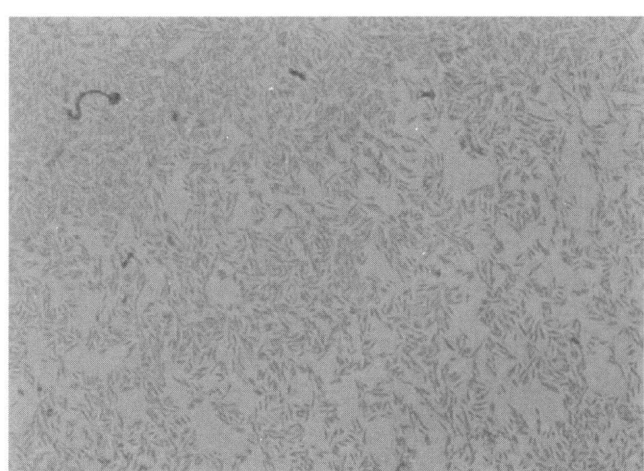

FIGURE 13–2
Campylobacter jejuni microscopic view showing curved gram-negative bacilli that may arrange to form a "sea gull" appearance in direct smears.

10% CO_2. The *Campylobactor* Microaerophilic System (Difco Laboratories) uses chemicals in envelopes and a standard anaerobe jar to generate a microaerophilic environment. Growth is usually present within 48 hours, and *Campylobacter* produces colonies that may be gray to pink or yellow to gray in color. Colonies are nonhemolytic and slightly mucoid.

A wet preparation should be prepared from any organism growing on *Campylobacter*-selective media at 42° to 43°C. The two species found most frequently in human infections, *C. coli* and *C. jejuni* subspecies *jejuni,* both grow at this temperature. Characteristic darting motility is observed in the wet preparation, as well as in a darkfield examination. Gram stains of *Campylobacter* are improved by substituting carbolfuchsin for safranin O in the final step. The organism appears as S-shaped or spiral forms and frequently is said to resemble the "wings of sea gulls" (Figure 13-2 [Color Plate 49]).

Another species of *Campylobacter* is *C. fetus* subspecies *fetus,* which is an agent of infective abortion in cattle and sheep. It has been known to cause extraintestinal infections in humans who are immunosuppressed. This species will not grow at 42°C and is susceptible to cephalothin.

Campylobacter can be differentiated by noting the reactions in Table 13-1.

HELICOBACTER

Helicobacter pylori was formerly known as *Campylobacter pylori.* The organism is differentiated from *Campylobacter* by the presence of four to six polar flagella and its very strong urease activity. The natural habitat for *H. pylori* is the human stomach, where the organism is found in the mucus-secreting cells. Current evidence may suggest a role between *H. pylori* and peptic and duodenal ulcers.

H. pylori is microaerophilic, preferring 85% nitrogen, 10% CO_2, and 5% oxygen. It grows optimally at 35° to 37°C and prefers increased humidity. The organism appears as a small, curved bacillus in Gram-stained smears and is positive for catalase, oxidase, and urease. Histological staining and culture of biopsies obtained from the stomach or duodenum are recommended for identification.

AEROMONAS

Aeromonas organisms are oxidase-positive, fermentative, gram-negative bacilli that are generally motile with polar monotrichous flagella. *Aeromonas* are naturally found in fresh water and sea water and are known to cause disease in cold-blooded animals. The organism is also found in drains, sink traps, distilled water, and tap water. The most common types of human infections include cellulitis and wound infections, acquired through contact with contaminated water or soil, as well as diarrheal disease. Miscellaneous types of infections associated with *Aeromonas* include septicemia, urinary tract infections, and ear infections.

Aeromonas organisms grow on MacConkey agar, eosin-methylene blue (EMB) agar, and *Salmonella-Shigella* agar but can be differentiated from Enterobacteriaceae by a positive oxidase reaction. *Aeromonas* also grow on cefsulodin-irgasan-novobiocin (CIN) medium used to isolate *Yersinia* species. They can be differentiated from *Pseudomonas aeruginosa* by their ability to ferment glucose and produce indole. *P. aeruginosa* oxidizes glucose and is indole negative. Most species of *Aeromonas* are motile.

The most common human isolate is *A. hydrophilia* ("water loving"), which is often associated with gastrointestinal disease. The organism produces a heat-labile enterotoxin and a heat-stable cytotoxic enterotoxin. A. hydrophila also produces a protease, lipase, and nuclease.

TABLE 13-1

Differentiation of *Campylobacter* Species

	C. JEJUNI SUBSP. *JEJUNI*	*C. COLI*	*C. FETUS* SUBSP. *FETUS*	*HELICOBACTER PYLORI*
Catalase	+	+	+	+
Nitrate	+	+	+	V
Urease	–	–	–	+
Hippurate hydrolysis	+	–	–	–
Growth at 42°C	+	+	–	V
Susceptible to:				
Nalidixic acid	S	S	R	R
Cephalothin	R	R	S	S

+, Most isolates give positive reaction; –, most isolates give negative reaction; V, variable reaction; S, susceptible; R, resistant.

PLESIOMONAS

Plesiomonas shigelloides is important in Japan and in the tropics and subtropics as a cause of gastritis. The organism is carried on various cold-blooded animals and is found in the water and soil. Infection is acquired through the ingestion of contaminated or unwashed foods. *P. shigelloides* grows on blood agar, MacConkey agar, and EMB. It can be differentiated from Enterobacteriaceae by a positive oxidase reaction.

Table 13-2 cites important biochemical reactions that can differentiate *A. hydrophila* from *P. shigelloides.*

LEGIONELLA

Legionella organisms are fastidious, narrow, gram-negative, non-spore-forming bacilli that are motile by one or more polar or subpolar flagella. Legionellae are the etiologic agents in **legionnaires' disease,** which was first documented in July 1976 as a pneumonia outbreak in Philadelphia at the American Legion Convention. The infectious agent was not known at that time. Legionellae are also associated with Pontiac fever, a milder form of legionnaires' disease.

In 1977, Dr. Joseph McDade of the Centers for Disease Control isolated the agent of legionnaires' disease. Two years later, the name *Legionella pneumophila* was proposed for this bacterium. Fourteen serotypes of *L. pneumophila* and 32 species of *Legionella* have been characterized. Many of the species are considered to be "potentially pathogenic" for humans, and most have been isolated from environmental sources. The most common type of infection involves sporadic cases or clusters of pneumonia.

Legionella organisms are naturally found in both natural and artificial water sources. The bacteria have been found in ponds, creeks and streams, wet soil, water-cooling towers for air-conditioning and heating systems, shower heads, and plumbing systems. It is believed that susceptible individuals inhale the organism from aerosols produced through these water sources. Many cases are nosocomial as patients contract the disease through inhalation of aerosols from contaminated water in showers, baths, humidifiers, and respiratory care equipment. It is important to note that person-to-person transmission does not seem to occur.

Legionellosis, which includes both legionnaires' disease and Pontiac fever, is more likely to attack middle-aged or geriatric male patients with an underlying medical disorder. Predisposing factors include, but are not limited to, diabetes, alcoholism, transplants, dialysis, cardiovascular illness, and pulmonary disease such as chronic obstructive pulmonary disease.

Legionnaires' disease is characterized by flulike symptoms, muscle aches, and fever. A dry cough, chest pain, and diarrhea may develop. Pneumonia and an accumulation of fluid in the lung occur next. Immunosuppressed patients may also have liver and renal involvement. Legionnaires' disease is a multisystemic condition that can affect almost any organ of the body. Common laboratory tests may reveal an elevated white blood cell count with an increase in immature forms. The serum sodium concentration is decreased, and protein may be found in the urine. Legionnaires' disease is fatal in up to 30% of all untreated patients.

The milder manifestation, Pontiac fever, is associated with mild symptoms such as low-grade fever and chills. Pneumonia and renal or liver impairments do not occur. Patients usually recover uneventfully.

Although most cases of legionellosis are attributed to *L. pneumophila,* other species have also been implicated in pneumonia. These species include *L. micdadei,* also known as Pittsburgh pneumonia agent, which has been isolated from respiratory care equipment and cooling towers. It has been associated with severe pulmonary infections in patients with leukemia, following renal transplants, and those undergoing corticosteroid therapy. "Wiga agent," or *L. bozemanii,* has also been isolated as an agent of pneumonia.

Legionella species do not grow on ordinary laboratory media and require an enriched media of buffered charcoal-yeast extract (BCYE) agar to grow. BCYE contains L-cysteine, activated charcoal, alpha-ketoglutarate, and other growth factors. Colonies of *Legionella* on BCYE are circular, glistening, and convex with an entire margin and may require up to 4 days to grow. Subcultures of suspected *Legionella* species growing on BCYE medium onto blood agar can be a useful tool to

TABLE 13–2

Differentiation of *Aeromonas hydrophila* from *Plesiomonas Shigelloides*

REACTION	*A. HYDROPHILIA*	*P. SHIGELLOIDES*
Hemolysis of blood agar	+	–
Oxidase	+	+
Indole	+	+
Glucose fermented	+	+
Gas from glucose	+	–
Motility	+	+
Deoxyribonuclease (DNase)	+	–
Esculin hydrolyzed	+	–
Ornithine decarboxylase (ODC)	–	+
Lysine decarboxylase (LDC)	+	+

identify *Legionella,* since *Legionella* will not grow on blood agar. Biochemical reactions for *Legionella* include a weakly positive catalase reaction, positive gelatinase, and positive motility. The organism Gram stains poorly, and Giemsa or basic fuchsin should be substituted for safranin O to improve the quality of the stain.

A direct fluorescent antibody (DFA) procedure is available for the rapid diagnosis of *Legionella* infection for respiratory tract specimens. The patient's specimen is fixed on a microscope slide and overlaid with *Legionella*-specific antisera labeled with conjugated fluorescein-isothiocyanate. The antigen, if present, binds to the globulin in the labeled antibody, forming an antigen-antibody complex that fluoresces as short rods under ultraviolet light. Serological diagnosis by immunofluorescent assay detects the patient's antibody for *Legionella.* In the assay, killed *Legionella* antigens and fluorescein-isothiocyanate-conjugated antihuman serum are used.

BORDETELLA

Bordetella organisms are aerobic, oxidative obligate parasites in animals and humans. The organisms bind to the ciliated epithelial cells in the mucous membranes of the respiratory tract. Of the following four species, *B. pertussis, B. parapertussis, B. bronchiseptica,* and *B. avium,* all can infect humans except *B. avium. B. bronchiseptica* is found in rabbits and dogs, whereas *B. avium* is found in turkeys. Human infection with *B. bronchiseptica* usually involves transmission from animals.

The most important human species, *B. pertussis,* the agent of **pertussis,** is only found in humans. It has been postulated that *B. parapertussis* is a nontoxigenic strain of *B. pertussis.* Pertussis, once a devastating childhood disease, has steadily declined in the United States since the advent of a vaccine in 1950. Today, the pertussis vaccine is given as a part of the DPT (diphtheria-pertussis-tetanus) vaccine to infants at 2, 4, and 6 months of age, with boosters at 12 to 15 months and 4 to 6 years. Pertussis showed an increase in the 1980s, presumably because children were not being immunized as a result of parental reaction to a small percentage of well-publicized adverse reactions to the vaccine. In addition, religious beliefs of some persons prohibit vaccination.

B. pertussis has a capsule and also produces pertussis toxin, which elicits several effects, including clinical symptoms, lymphocytosis, and impairment of neutrophil chemotaxis and phagocytosis. This absolute and relative lymphocytosis is unusual for a bacterial infection. Filamentous hemagglutinin is believed to allow the organism to attach to mucosal cells, while a cytotoxin damages the ciliated respiratory epithelial cells after the organism attaches. In addition, endotoxin is released on cell lysis, which has systemic effects such as fever.

Pertussis infection is extremely contagious and is directly spread through respiratory droplets. The incubation period ranges from 7 to 10 days. During this time, the patient may have flulike symptoms, such as a "runny nose," infrequent coughing, and a low-grade fever. During the catarrhal stage, bacteria multiply, spread to contiguous areas, and become concentrated in the ciliated epithelial cells and mucous membranes in the respiratory tract.

The paroxysmal coughing phase develops next. The severity of the cough increases, with some patients exhibiting the characteristic "whoop" that occurs as the patient inhales after a coughing spell. "Whooping cough" has been used in the past as a synonym for pertussis, although it is no longer considered to be accurate.

The convalescent phase, which may last for 4 to 8 weeks, may be accompanied by coughing. The cough eventually subsides, but secondary bacterial infections may occur.

Bordetella are tiny, gram-negative coccobacilli on primary isolation. The organisms are often pleomorphic on subculture. The bacteria are obligate aerobes and not very active metabolically. All species except *B. bronchiseptica* are nonmotile.

Primary isolation of *B. pertussis* requires a special medium known as Bordet-Gengou (B-G) agar, which contains potato, glycerol, and blood. In the past, patients suspected of pertussis simply coughed onto a B-G plate. This technique was referred to as a "cough plate." Today the specimen of choice is a nasopharyngeal swab or washings that are plated onto B-G agar or Regan-Lowe medium. B-G medium with methicillin or cephalexin, which inhibits normal flora, is preferable to traditional B-G agar. Regan-Lowe medium contains horse blood, charcoal agar, cephalexin, and amphotericin B and is preferred by many microbiologists. Ideally, two specimens are collected from the nasopharynx to increase the chances of isolation.

B. pertussis produces small, smooth colonies in 7 days on B-G or Regan-Lowe medium in increased CO_2 at 35° to 37°C. The colonies are shiny and are said to resemble mercury droplets or pearls. The organism appears as a tiny, gram-negative coccobacillus on Gram stain. Once isolated, identification can be confirmed by reacting the isolate with a fluorescent *B. pertussis* antibody. Important biochemical reactions for *B. pertussis* include:

Motility: nonmotile
Sheep blood agar: no growth
MacConkey agar: no growth
Bordet-Gengou agar: convex, shiny, silver, "mercury-like" droplets in 7 days
Catalase: positive
Citrate: negative
Indole: negative

TABLE 13-3

Differentiation of *Bordetella* Species

	UREASE	NITRATE	MOTILITY	OXIDASE
B. pertussis	−	−	−	+
B. parapertussis	+ (18 hours)	−	−	−
B. bronchiseptica	Strong + (4 hours)	+	+	+

The organism can be directly identified from nasopharyngeal specimens by using the DFA stain, which is the preferred method. In this technique, a smear is made from a nasopharyngeal specimen (swab or aspirate). Next, fluorescein-isothiocyanate-conjugated *B. pertussis* antibodies are added. After incubation, the slide is washed and examined under the fluorescent microscope. Some recommend that identification of *B. pertussis* include both culture and DFA.

B. parapertussis produces a brown pigment on B-G agar. It is nonmotile and has been associated with a pertussis-like syndrome that is a milder infection than seen with *B. pertussis.*

B. bronchiseptica is motile with peritrichous flagella and has been found to be a cause of a variety of infections, including septicemia and meningitis in immunosuppressed hosts. It is a rapid urease producer.

Some common biochemical reactions used to speciate *Bordetella* are found in Table 13-3.

BRUCELLA

Brucella organisms are catalase-positive, oxidase-positive, nonsaccharolytic, strictly aerobic gram-negative bacilli. The organisms are normal flora of the urinary and gastrointestinal tracts of goats, pigs, cows, and dogs. The organisms are agents of brucellosis in animals. Humans acquire *Brucella* infections through the ingestion of contaminated animal products, including meats and milk. Farmers can directly acquire *Brucella* infections through direct animal contact.

Brucella species are obligate parasites and can survive intracellularly in the reticuloendothelial system, bone, liver, and central nervous system of humans. The organism causes **undulant fever (brucellosis),** which is a chronic and recurring fever. The infection is characterized by weight loss and anorexia. Granulomatous infections occur in the reticuloendothelial system and in the bone. The infections become chronic because the organism resides intracellularly, protected from cell-mediated immunity.

Brucella can be isolated from blood cultures, which are positive the first 2 weeks of febrile illness. Blood cultures will become negative after the acute symptoms subside, since antibody production will begin. Although *Brucella* grows on blood and chocolate agar, *Brucella* agar plus 5% horse or rabbit serum is the recommended medium for isolation. *Brucella* agar contains a pancreatic digest of casein, a peptic digest of animal tissue, yeast, and sodium bisulfite. Plates are incubated in 5% to 10% CO_2 and are held for 3 weeks. Castañeda bottles are a biphasic system containing both agar and broth that can also be used to culture *Brucella.* In Gram-stained smears, *Brucella* organisms are tiny, gram-negative coccobacilli that may appear intracellular in tissue specimens. Carbolfuchsin should be substituted for safranin O to improve the quality of the Gram stain.

The "gold standard" for *Brucella* identification is **febrile agglutinins,** which is a serological test for antibodies in the patient's serum that react with antigen of killed *Brucella.* A fourfold increase between the acute and convalescent titer is considered significant.

Brucella is a type 3 biohazard that involves common and unusual pathogens. A biological safety cabinet must be used to prevent the generation of aerosols. All positive results should be sent to the state or another reference laboratory for confirmation. Most identifications are made in reference laboratories.

The species of *Brucella* can be identified using the biochemical reactions in Table 13-4.

PASTEURELLA

Pasteurella are nonmotile, oxidase-positive, fermentative, facultative, anaerobic gram-negative bacilli. The most important human species is *P. multocida,* which is the etiologic agent of pasteurellosis. *Pasteurella* is encapsulated, which enables it to resist phagocytosis. The organism is carried in the oral cavity and respiratory and gastrointestinal tracts of healthy domestic cats and dogs and also is normally found in many other animals, including rodents, rabbits, and birds. It is the agent of "shipping fever" in cattle, a hemorrhagic septicemia. Humans may acquire the infection following contact with domestic animals that harbor the bacterium. Most frequently the route of infection is from the bite or scratch of an infected animal, usually a cat. Local wound infections are the most common type of *Pasteurella* infection or **pasteurellosis,** which is characterized by pain, redness, swelling, cellulitis, and a purulent discharge. There is a rapid onset of inflammation, with a fever developing 3 to 5 days after the infection is acquired. Complications of pasteurellosis include osteomyelitis, meningitis, and joint infections. Bacteremia can result from the primary bite infection. A second route of infection is inhalation of the bacterium, which can lead to pneumonia, bronchitis, or sinusitis. Those at

TABLE 13–4

Speciation of *Brucella*

	B. ABORTUS	*B. MELITENSIS*	*B. SUIS*	*B. CANIS*
Animal source	Cattle	Sheep and goats	Pigs	Dogs
Urease (positive in)	1-2 hr	1-2 hr	0-30 min	0-30 min
Hydrogen sulfide (H_2S)	+	−	−	−
Growth on media containing:				
Thionin (20 μg)	−	+	+	+
Basic fuchsin (20 μg)	+	+	−	−
Thionin blue (2 mg/ml)	+	+	−	−

occupational risk for acquiring the infection via the respiratory route include those who handle or raise animals and those with a prior respiratory disorder. Other types of infections attributed to *Pasteurella* include endocarditis, peritonitis, and postoperative wound infections.

To identify *P. multocida,* the Gram stain reveals a small, gram-negative rod with bipolar staining. The bacterium grows on both blood agar and chocolate agar, but growth is not enhanced under increased CO_2. On sheep blood agar the colonies are small, smooth, gray or translucent, and nonhemolytic. The organism cannot grow on MacConkey or EMB agar. *P. multocida* produces a musty odor, which is said to resemble the smell of mushrooms. Important biochemical reactions to *P. multocida* are:

Oxidase: positive
Catalase: positive
Nitrate: positive
Indole: positive
Urease: negative
Acid but no gas produced from glucose, sucrose, and mannose
Acid not produced from maltose and lactose
Starch hydrolysis: negative

FRANCISELLA

Francisella tularensis, a small, nonmotile, pleomorphic gram-negative bacillus, is the agent of **tularemia,** a disease of rodents, primarily rabbits. The organism is carried on many wild animals, including rodents, rabbits, and beavers. Those individuals who handle infected animals, such as hunters, acquire this zoonosis through direct contact with blood or through an animal bite or scratch. The bacterium can also be inhaled or acquired indirectly through insect vectors, primarily ticks, which harbor *F. tularensis. F. tularensis* possesses a capsule and also has invasive properties that allow it to penetrate the intact skin. Once skin entry has occurred, the organism can cause bacteremia, living as an intracellular parasite within the recticulendothelial system and lymph nodes of the host. When acquired through inhalation, the most common type of infection is pneumonia.

F. tularensis requires a special medium, blood-cystine-glucose agar with thiamine, to grow. It also grows on modified charcoal-yeast agar and chocolate agar with IsoVitaleX. It requires 2 to 4 days to grow and is a strict aerobe. Colonies are smooth, bluish gray, and slightly mucoid with a narrow alpha-hemolytic zone. Biochemical reactions used to identify *Francisella* include catalase-positive, oxidase-negative, and positive fermentation of glucose, maltose, and mannose.

Serological techniques are the recommended method for identification. The DFA stain is used to detect antibodies to *F. tularensis* in the patient's serum. Enzyme-linked immunoassay techniques are also available.

Extreme caution should be exhibited when *F. tularensis* is suspected, since it is an easily acquired laboratory infection.

GARDNERELLA

Gardnerella vaginalis is a pleomorphic, gram-variable to gram-negative, nonmotile bacillus. This organism was previously known as *Corynebacterium vaginalis* and *Haemophilus vaginalis.* The organism is associated with **bacterial vaginosis,** which is characterized by a foul-smelling, grayish vaginal discharge. Characteristics of bacterial vaginosis include an excessive vaginal discharge, the presence of clue cells, a fishy aminelike odor on the potassium hydroxide (KOH) test, and a vaginal pH greater than 4.5. Although *G. vaginalis* is normally found in many healthy females, it is found in high numbers in patients with bacterial vaginosis. In addition, the normal vaginal flora may be decreased or lacking in this condition. Thus the isolation of *Gardnerella* is not always diagnostic for bacterial vaginosis.

Direct examination of vaginal secretions is an important diagnostic tool for bacterial vaginosis. The **clue cell** is a vaginal epithelial cell to which organisms are attached, obscuring the border of the epithelial cell. In addition, the vaginal secretions reveal a mixed flora with many small gram-negative and gram-variable rods. There are few or no lactobacilli, which are large gram-positive bacilli that constitute a part of the normal flora of the vaginal tract.

In the KOH test, commonly known as the "whiff test," vaginal secretions are mixed with KOH. A positive test is indicated by the fishy aminelike odor.

G. vaginalis is fastidious and will not grow on blood agar. It can be isolated on Columbia agar, which contains biotin, folic acid, niacin, and thiamine. It may also be isolated on human blood bilayer Tween (HBT) agar medium, on which the organism grows as small, opaque, beta-hemolytic colonies. Plates should be incubated in a candle jar, which provides increased CO_2. Significant biochemical reactions include:

HBT agar: beta hemolysis
Oxidase: negative
Catalase: negative
Hippurate hydrolysis: positive
Starch hydrolysis: positive

STREPTOBACILLUS

Streptobacillus moniliformis is a fastidious, gram-negative, pleomorphic bacillus normally found in the oropharynx of rodents, primarily wild and laboratory rats. Humans most frequently acquire the infection, **rat-bite fever,** through the bite of an infected animal. Other routes of inoculation include scratches or direct contact with rodents. Rat-bite fever is associated with a relapsing fever, chills, muscle aches, vomiting, a skin rash on the palms of the hands and soles of the feet, and lymphadenitis. The bite usually heals, but complications include arthritis, hepatic and splenic disorders, endocarditis, and meningitis. The disease is often difficult to diagnose because it resembles several other infections. Another type of *Streptobacillus* infection, known as Haverhill fever, is acquired by ingesting milk contaminated with *S. moniliformis.* It resembles rat-bite fever, but gastrointestinal signs are more pronounced.

The organism is difficult to identify and is rarely isolated. It is fastidious and requires media enriched with whole blood or serum for growth. It is biochemically inactive, and most reactions, including indole, catalase, oxidase, urease, and nitrates, are all negative. Serological identification for serum agglutinins against *S. moniliformis,* in which a fourfold increase between the acute and convalescent titers occur, is an important tool for diagnosis.

CHROMOBACTERIUM AND *CARDIOBACTERIUM*

Chromobacterium violaceum, a motile, facultative anaerobe that is oxidase positive, is a rare cause of human infection. It is found in soil and water and is unique in its ability to produce violacein, a purple pigment.

Cardiobacterium hominis is normally found in the upper respiratory tract and is isolated as a rare cause of endocarditis. It is nonmotile, oxidase positive, catalase negative, and indole positive. *C. hominis* grows on blood agar, with growth enhanced at increased CO_2. The organism ferments glucose and maltose but is negative for lactose.

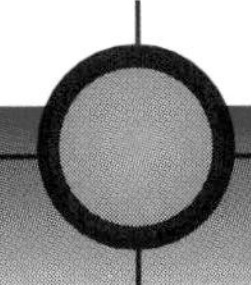

PROCEDURE

THIOSULFATE CITRATE BILE SALTS SUCROSE (TCBS) AGAR

PURPOSE

TCBS medium selectively isolates *Vibrio* from specimens, such as stools, that contain mixed flora.

PRINCIPLE

The medium contains sucrose, bile in the forms of oxgall and sodium cholate, sodium citrate, proteins, yeast, and pH indicators. *Vibrio* species prefer a high salt concentration and a high pH and thus grow well on TCBS, whereas other flora, such as *Proteus* and other members of the Enterobacteriaceae, are inhibited.

Fermentation of sucrose is indicated by a yellow color and is characteristic of certain *Vibrio* species, such as *V. cholerae* and *V. alginolyticus. V. parahaemolyticus* and *V. vulnificus* cannot ferment sucrose and appear as blue-green colonies.

METHOD

1. Inoculate plate and streak for isolation using stool culture suspected of containing *Vibrio.*
2. Incubate at 35° to 37°C for 24 to 48 hours.

INTERPRETATION

Growth usually indicates a *Vibrio* species. Occasionally, *Aeromonas* or *Pseudomonas* may grow on the medium.

Yellow colonies indicate a sucrose-fermenting *Vibrio.*

Blue-green colonies usually indicate a non-sucrose-fermenting *Vibrio.*

QUALITY CONTROL

Growth and fermentation of sucrose: *V. alginolyticus*—yellow colonies.

Growth and lack of fermentation of sucrose: *Vibrio parahaemolyticus*—blue-green colonies.

REVIEW QUESTIONS

MATCHING

Match the medium with the bacterium that the agar primarily is used to isolate:

_____ **1. Thiosulfate citrate bile salts sucrose agar.**
_____ **2. Bordet-Gengou agar**
_____ **3. Buffered charcoal-yeast extract**
_____ **4. Blood-cystine-glucose agar**

a. *Bordetella pertussis*
b. *Francisella tularensis*
c. *Pasteurella multocida*
d. *Legionella pneumophila*
e. *Vibrio cholerae*

Match the organism with its associated infection:

_____ **5. Whooping cough**
_____ **6. Undulant fever**
_____ **7. Cholera**
_____ **8. Rat-bite fever**

a. *Pasteurella multocida*
b. *Streptobacillus moniliformis*
c. *Vibrio cholerae*
d. *Bordetella pertussis*
e. *Brucella abortus*
f. *Francisella tularensis*

MULTIPLE CHOICE

9. Halophilic means that the organism requires:
a. Increased oxygen
b. Increased carbon dioxide
c. Decreased oxygen
d. Increased sodium chloride

10. Which is *not* a characteristic of *Vibrio cholerae?*
a. Motile with single polar flagellum
b. Oxidase negative
c. Ferments glucose and sucrose
d. Positive string test

11. The presence of clue cells may be diagnostic for:
a. *Gardnerella vaginalis*
b. *Campylobacter jejuni*
c. *Tularemia*
d. *Pertussis*

12. Which description is correct for *Campylobacter jejuni* subspecies *jejuni?*
a. Motile curved rod, halophilic, catalase negative
b. Nonmotile curved rod, grows at 42°C, catalase negative
c. Motile curved rod, grows at 42°C, catalase positive
d. Motile curved rod, cannot grow at 42°C, capnophilic

13. The population with increased susceptibility to *Legionella* infection is:
a. Newborns
b. Middle-aged females with autoimmune illness
c. Infants between ages 6 months and 4 years
d. Middle-aged males with an underlying medical problem

14. Legionnaires' disease is spread through:
a. Inhalation of contaminated aerosols
b. Ingestion of contaminated water
c. Direct contact with respiratory secretions of an infected individual
d. Direct contact with an infected animal or animal products

15. On Bordet-Gengou medium, *B. pertussis* appears:
a. Dry, heaped, serrated
b. Iridescent brown
c. Smooth, shiny, resembling mercury droplets
d. White, raised, rough

16. A *Vibrio* yielded the following biochemical reactions:
Growth in nutrient broth: –
Growth in nutrient broth with 1% NaCl: +
Oxidase: +
Nitrates reduced to nitrites
ADH: –
LDC: +
Fermentation of:
Sucrose: –
Salicin: –
Cellobiose: –

REVIEW QUESTIONS
(Continued)

This *Vibrio* species can most likely be identified as:
a. *V. cholerae*
b. *V. mimicus*
c. *V. parahaemolyticus*
d. *V. fluvialis*

17. A *Brucella* species gave the following reactions:
Urease positive in 1½ hours
H_2S negative
Growth in presence of:
20 μg thionin: +
2 μg thionin blue: +
20 μg basic fuchsin: +

This *Brucella* species is most likely:
a. *B. abortus*
b. *B. melitensis*
c. *B. suis*
d. *B. canis*

18. Which set of reactions is correct for *Pasteurella multocida?*

	Oxidase	Catalase	Growth on Blood Agar	Glucose Fermented	Acid from Glucose
a.	+	+	−	−	−
b.	−	+	+	+	−
c.	−	−	+	+	+
d.	+	+	+	+	−

BIBLIOGRAPHY

Beaser MJ et al: *Campylobacter enteritis:* clinical and epidemiologic features, *Ann Intern Med* 91:179, 1991.

Buck GE: *Campylobacter pylori* and gastrointestinal disease, *Clin Microbiol Rev* 3:1, 1990.

Buesching, WJ, Brust RA, Ayers, LW: Enhanced primary isolation of *Legionella pneumophila* from clinical specimens by low pH treatment, *J Clin Microbiol* 17:1153, 1983.

Campbell HW, Carnes L: *Pasturella meningitis, Lab Med* 13:175, 1982.

Carter GR: The epidemiology and pathogenesis of pasteurellosis in man, *J Med Tech* 1:718, 1984.

Catlin BW: *Gardnerella vaginalis:* characteristics, clinical considerations, and controversies, *Clin Microbiol Rev* 5:213, 1992.

Cholera-Peru, 1991, *MMWR* 40:108, 1991.

Edelstein PH: Improved semi-selective medium for isolation of *Legionella pneumophila* from contaminated clinical and environmental specimens, *J Clin Microbiol* 14:298, 1981.

Friedman RL: Pertussis: The disease and new diagnostic methods, *Clin Microbiol Rev* 1:365, 1988.

Hollis DG et al: Halophilic *Vibrio* species isolated from blood cultures, *J Clin Microbiol* 3:425, 1976.

Hughes JM et al: Non-cholera *Vibrio* infections in the United States, *Ann Intern Med* 88:602, 1978.

Kelly MT, Hickman-Brenner FW, Farmer JJ III: *Vibrio.* In Balows A, editor: *Manual of clinical microbiology,* ed 5, Washington, DC, 1991, American Society of Clinical Microbiology, pp 384-395.

Kirby BD et al: Legionnaires' disease: Report of 65 nosocomial acquired cases and review of the literature, *Medicine* 59:188, 1980.

Larsen HS: *Vibrio vulnificus:* more than a coastal pathogen, *Clin Lab Sci* 6:83, 1993.

McDade JE et al: Legionnaires' disease: isolation of a bacterium and demonstration of its role in other respiratory diseases, *N Engl J Med* 297:1197, 1977.

Pasculli AW, Rogers FG: *Legionella.* In Balows A, editor: *Manual of clinical microbiology,* ed 5, Washington, DC, 1991, American Society for Microbiology, pp 442-453.

Penner JL: *Campylobacter* and *Helicobacter* and related species. In Balows A, editor: *Manual of clinical microbiology,* ed 5, Washington, DC, 1991, American Society for Microbiology, pp 402-406.

Ramsay MK, Roberts GH: *Legionella pneumophila:* the organism and its implications, *Lab Med* 23:244, 1992.

Walker RI et al: Pathophysiology of *Campylobacter* enteritis, *Microbiol Rev* 50:81, 1986.

Winn WC Jr: Legionnaires' disease: a historical perspective, *Clin Microbiol Rev* 1:60, 1988.

Zeimis RT, Hanley OQ: Endocarditis caused by *Kingella kingae:* case report and review, *J Med Tech* 16:547, 1985.

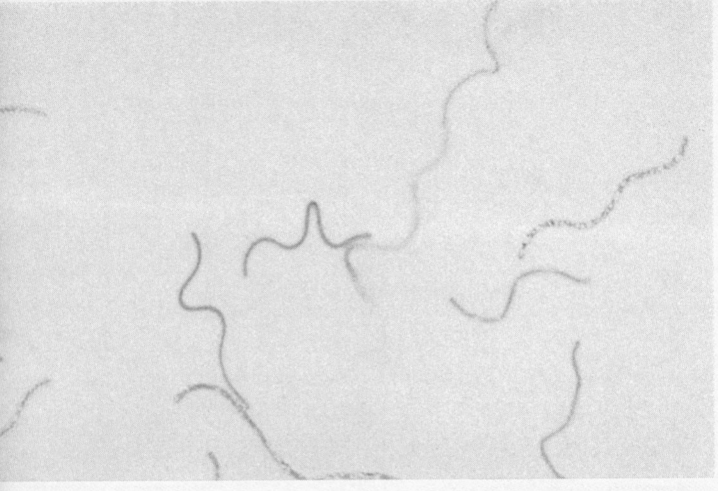

BORRELIA

CHAPTER OUTLINE

BORRELIA
- Relapsing Fever
- Lyme Disease

TREPONEMA

LEPTOSPIRA

KEY TERMS

BIOLOGICAL FALSE POSITIVES (BFPs)
ENDEMIC SYPHILIS
ERYTHEMA CHRONICUM MIGRANS
LEPTOSPIROSIS
LYME DISEASE
NONTREPONEMAL TESTS
PINTA
RELAPSING FEVER
TREPONEMAL TESTS
VENEREAL SYPHILIS
YAWS

Spirochetes

LEARNING OBJECTIVES

1. State the etiologic agent for the following diseases:
   a. Syphilis (venereal)
   b. Yaws
   c. Pinta
   d. Endemic syphilis (nonvenereal)
2. List and describe the stages of syphilis. Discuss laboratory methods to identify primary, secondary, and tertiary syphilis.
3. Compare and contrast the treponemal and nontreponemal tests for syphilis.
   a. State the principle for each of the following tests:
      (1) RPR
      (2) VDRL
      (3) FTA—absorbed
      (4) TPI
      (5) MHA
   b. Discuss biological false positives (BFPs) and explain how to differentiate a BFP from a true positive.
4. Name the etiologic agent and tick or louse vector for the following borrelioses:
   a. Relapsing fever
   b. Lyme disease
5. Explain how Lyme disease is acquired and diagnosed.
   a. List and describe the laboratory methods used to diagnose Lyme disease.
   b. Discuss the stages of Lyme disease.
6. Explain how relapsing fever is acquired and diagnosed.
7. Name the etiologic agent of leptospirosis and describe its significant characteristics.

Spirochetes are members of the family Spirochaetaceae. The bacteria are helically coiled and motile through periplasmic flagella. Periplasmic flagella are enclosed within the outer membrane of the bacterial cell. The outer membrane surrounds the protoplasmic cylinder, which contains both cytoplasmic and nuclear regions. One end of each flagellum is inserted near one pole of the protoplasmic cylinder, and the other end is not attached. Because of this unique flagellar arrangement, spirochetes can propel through the liquid environment using locomotion, rotation, and flexion. These organisms are motile even in viscous solutions.

Although spirochetes have the characteristics of a gram-negative cell wall, they typically do not Gram stain very well. Thus staining procedures have limited usefulness in the characterization of spirochetes.

The pathogenic spirochetes include the following genera: *Borrelia, Treponema,* and *Leptospira.*

BORRELIA

Borrelia organisms are microaerophilic, helically coiled bacteria that stain well with Giemsa dyes. Human pathogenic species are transmitted through arthropod vectors, including lice and ticks. *Borrelia* bacteria enter the host through the bite of a tick or through lice, which gain entrance through a damaged skin barrier.

Relapsing Fever

Borrelia recurrentis is the agent of louse-borne **relapsing fever,** which is found in South America, Europe, Asia, and Africa. Tick-borne relapsing fever occurs worldwide, and the infection can be attributed to several *Borrelia* species, including *B. hermsii* and *B. parkeri.* The vector in relapsing fever is the human body louse, *Pediculus humanus* subspecies *humanus,* and the infection is seen most often in impoverished areas with substandard sanitation in the Middle East and Asia. Since the body louse feeds only on humans, humans are the only vertebrate reservoir. Ticks of the genus *Ornithodoros,* including *O. hermsii* and *O. parkeri,* are the vectors in tick-borne relapsing fever. These ticks can also feed on rodents, prairie dogs, and squirrels and have been found to inhabit animal dwellings, caves, and decaying vegetation.

Relapsing fever has a dramatic onset with a high fever, muscle and bone pain, and confusion. The organism enters the blood, and multiple lesions may form in the spleen, liver, or kidneys. Hepatosplenomegaly and jaundice are possible clinical signs of infection. The fever persists for 2 to 6 days, and then the patient appears to "recover" spontaneously, only to "relapse" days or weeks later. Patients may enter several relapsing phases before recovery. These relapses are attributed to the ability of *Borrelia* to alter its antigenicity and thus require the host to develop "new" immunity to each altered strain.

Borrelia are difficult to culture in vitro and require modified Kelly's medium, also known as Barbour-Stoenner-Kelly medium (BSK-II), to grow. *B. recurrentis* is microaerophilic and will grow on the medium in 7 to 14 days at 30° to 35°C.

The preferred diagnostic tool is detection of the organism in peripheral blood smears. Thick blood films are recommended because the number of organisms is low. Also, the yield is enhanced in the blood when the specimen is collected during a febrile episode. Giemsa or Wright's stain can be used as suitable aniline dyes. *Borrelia* stains a blue color using either stain.

Lyme Disease

The first reported case of **Lyme disease** occurred in 1975. An increased incidence of rheumatoid arthritis in children in Lyme and Old Lyme, Conn., was brought to the attention of the state health department. It was also noted that several of the children had developed a unique red skin rash before the arthritis. This rash resembled a rash first noted by Arvid Afzelius of Sweden in 1909, who discovered a red papule that spread into a larger lesion. The rash typically appeared after the bite of a tick. He named the rash **erythema chronicum migrans.** Finally, most of the cases in Lyme were seen in the summer months. Based on these findings, an arthropod vector was suspected. Because of its minute size, many patients with Lyme disease did not recall a tick bite before the development of the rash. Finally, a tick was isolated from a patient's rash and identified as *Ixodes dammini.* This particular tick was present in abundant amounts in the wooded areas of Lyme and Old Lyme.

Soon after, Dr. W. Burgdorferi isolated a unicellular, loosely coiled spirochete from the gut of the *Ixodes* tick, and thus the organism was named *Borrelia burgdorferi.* It is now known that *B. burgdorferi* is found in the tissues of several mammals, including field mice and deer.

Several species of the *Ixodes* tick carry *B. burgdorferi:*

Ixodes dammini, found in the northeastern, eastern, and north central areas of the United States
Ixodes pacificus, found in the northwestern area of the United States
Ixodes ricinus, found in Europe

Today, Lyme disease is the most common arthropod-borne disease in the United States. More than 40,000 cases have been reported from 1982 to 1991. The disease has also been found in North and South America, Europe, Asia, Africa, and Australia.

The life cycle of the *Ixodes* tick spans 2 years (see the box on p. 255).

Life Cycle of *Ixodes* Tick

First spring: eggs are deposited and hatch into free-living larvae 1 month later.

First summer: larvae feed once on a host's blood.

First winter: larvae enter a resting stage.

Second spring: larvae molt and enter a second immature stage known as the nymphal stage, attach to an animal host, and feed. Hosts include many vertebrates, including humans and white-footed mice.

Second summer: nymphal stage molts into adult stage; ticks are found in brush approximately 1 yard above the ground. Ticks now can attach to larger animals, particularly the white-tailed deer. The adult ticks mate on the host soon after the female attaches and deposit eggs. The life cycle continues.

Because of its varied presentation, the diagnosis of Lyme disease may be missed or confused with other disease syndromes. Lyme disease has been divided into three stages:

Stage one: this follows the tick bite, with appearance of the lesion erythema chronicum migrans. Rash is present in some but not all patients with Lyme disease. Lymphadenopathy may also be present.

Stage two: dissemination occurs through the blood, and areas affected may include the bones (arthritis), central nervous system (meningitis and other neurological symptoms, such as dizziness and paralysis), heart (palpitations), and liver.

Stage three: also known as the chronic stage, this includes chronic neurological abnormalities, arthritis, and skin lesions.

General symptoms that may be present throughout the disease include headache, low-grade fever, fatigue, and abdominal pain. The symptoms of Lyme disease may vary and can be mistaken for several other diseases, including rheumatoid arthritis, systemic lupus erythematosus, and viral meningitis.

Although *B. burgdorferi* can be cultured in modified Kelly's medium, the yield of growth is usually low. Biopsy of the primary lesion or the erythema and subsequent silver impregnation can be used to demonstrate the spirochete in the lesion. This method is also considered to be quite insensitive. Therefore the patient history and serological methods are most often used to diagnose Lyme disease.

Serological methods demonstrate the presence of antibody to *B. burgdorferi* and include fluorescent immunoassay, indirect immunofluorescence, and enzyme-linked immunoassay. A Western blot method offers increased specificity; single cross-reacting antibodies have been identified as a concern in the other serological methods.

In fluorescent immunoassays, such as the Lyme FIAX (Whittaker Bioproducts), *B. burgdorferi* antigen is adsorbed onto an inanimate surface, such as a plastic stick. The antigen is incubated with the patient's serum and fluorescein-labeled antihuman conjugate. The reaction is read for fluorescence using a fluorometer.

In enzyme-linked immunoassay methods, such as the ImmunoCLONE (Medical Diagnostic Technologies) and LYME STAT (Whittaker Bioproducts), *B. burgdorferi* antigen is attached to a solid phase, such as the surface of microtiter wells. When present, the patient's antibody to *B. burgdorferi* will bind to the antigen. Unbound antibodies are washed away, and enzyme-conjugated antihuman immunoglobulin G (IgG) and IgM is added. The enzyme conjugate binds to the antigen-antibody complex. Excess enzyme conjugate is washed away, and substrate is added. Bound enzyme conjugate initiates a hydrolytic reaction. The color intensity is read spectrophotometrically and is proportional to the amount of *B. burgdorferi* antigen present in the specimen.

The Western blot test may be considered the "gold standard" in Lyme disease testing because of its high specificity and sensitivity. The Western blot method of Whittaker Bioproducts (AccuBlot) detects both IgG and IgM antibodies specific to *B. burgdorferi*. Specific *B. burgdorferi* proteins are separated according to molecular weight by sodium dodecyl sulfate (SDS) polyacrylamide electrophoresis. The separated proteins are transblotted to a microcellulose membrane that is washed, cut, and packaged. The strip is incubated with the patient's serum, enzyme conjugate (IgG or IgM), and substrate. A hydrolytic reaction enables the visualization of antibodies that specifically bind to various *B. burgdorferi* proteins. The antigen-antibody bands are compared with known positive and negative controls to determine the patient's status.

TREPONEMA

Treponemes are helically shaped bacteria that either fail to stain or stain very poorly with Gram and Giemsa stains. The organisms characteristically have tight, regular or irregular coils. There are thirteen species of *Treponema,* and most are anaerobic. However, the human pathogenic species are microaerophilic. In addition, these species have not been cultured in artificial media,

REVIEW QUESTIONS

MATCHING

Match the spirochete with its associated disease:

_____ **1.** ***Borrelia recurrentis***
_____ **2.** ***Treponema pallidum* subspecies *pertenue***
_____ **3.** ***Treponema pallidum* subspecies *endemicum***
_____ **4.** ***Treponema pallidum* subspecies *pallidum***
_____ **5.** ***Borrelia burgdorferi***

a. Syphilis
b. Lyme disease
c. Yaws
d. Relapsing fever
e. Pinta
f. Bejel

MULTIPLE CHOICE

6. Which statement is *incorrect* for the pathogenic spirochetes?
a. Stain well with Gram stain reagent
b. Cultured only in vivo
c. Fail to grow on solid culture media
d. Anaerobic

7. The stage of syphilis characterized by granulomatous lesions in various organs of the body, including cardiovascular and neurological disorders, is:
a. Primary
b. Secondary
c. Tertiary
d. Latent
e. Congenital

8. Primary syphilis is best diagnosed by:
a. Clinical signs and serological testing
b. Clinical signs and darkfield examination
c. Darkfield examination and serological examination
d. Growth on culture media and Gram stain

9. Secondary syphilis is best diagnosed by:
a. Clinical signs and serological testing
b. Clinical signs and darkfield examination
c. Darkfield examination and serological examination
d. Growth on culture media and Gram stain

10. A patient's serum yields a positive RPR and a negative FTA. These results most likely indicate:
a. Reactive for syphilis
b. False-negative FTA due to low sensitivity of the test
c. Biological false-positive RPR due to cross-reacting antibodies
d. Patient in remission for syphilis

11. The most common arthropod-borne disease in the United States is:
a. Pinta
b. Relapsing fever
c. Plague
d. Lyme disease

12. The diagnosis of Lyme disease can be made by:
a. Silver impregnation techniques to demonstrate spirochete in tissue
b. Serological demonstration of antibody in patient's serum using enzyme immunoassay
c. Growth on blood and chocolate agar
d. Both a and b
e. All the above

13. *Ixodes dammini* is the:
a. Name of the person who first isolated the agent of Lyme disease
b. Agent of leptospirosis
c. Species of one of the tick vectors of Lyme disease
d. Agent of rat-bite fever

REVIEW QUESTIONS
(Continued)

14. All the following are categorized as specific treponemal tests *except:*
a. RPR
b. TPI
c. FTA—absorbed
d. MHA

15. The preferred diagnostic method for relapsing fever is:
a. Biochemical identification
b. Giemsa stain of peripheral blood smears
c. Serological techniques
d. All the above

16. The stage of Lyme disease characterized by the appearance of erythema chronicum migrans is:
a. Primary
b. Secondary
c. Tertiary
d. Latent

17. During the second spring of the life cycle of the *Ixodes* tick:
a. Eggs are deposited and hatch into free-living larvae.
b. Larvae feed once on the host's blood.
c. Larvae molt and attach to the animal host and feed.
d. Lymphs molt into adult stage, and ticks attach to larger animals.

18. Which of the following methods is used most frequently to diagnose Lyme disease?
a. Culture on modified Kelly's medium
b. Silver impregnation of biopsy from erythema chronicum migrans
c. Serological demonstration of the patient's antibody
d. Darkfield examination of erythema chronicum migrans

19. Which statement is *incorrect* for *Leptospira interrogans?*
a. Tightly coiled spiral with one or both ends hooked
b. Primarily pathogenic on vertebrates other than humans
c. Stain well with aniline dyes
d. Infection may involve liver, kidney, or central nervous system.

BIBLIOGRAPHY

Burgdorfer W et al: Lyme disease: a tick-borne spirochetosis, *Science* 216:1317, 1982.

Centers for Disease Control: Lyme disease surveillance—United States 1989-1990, *MMWR* 40:417, 1991.

Chang YW: A guideline to serologic tests for syphilis, *Diagn Med,* March/April 1991, pp 51-67.

Craft JE, Grodzick RL, Steer AC: Antibody response in Lyme disease: evaluation of diagnostic tests, *J Infect Dis* 149:780, 1984.

Fitzgerald TJ: Treponema. In Lennette EH, editor: *Manual of clinical microbiology,* ed 4, Washington, DC, 1985, American Society for Microbiology, pp. 485-489.

Harlow RD, Stephenson S: Laboratory testing for Lyme disease, *Am Clin Lab,* May 1991, p 30.

Hook EW III, Marra CM: Acquired syphilis in adults, *N Engl J Med* 326:1060, 1992.

Keifer CR: Diagnosis of Lyme disease: evaluation of an enzyme linked immunobinding assay, *Am Clin Lab,* May 1991, pp 14-16.

Steere AC: Lyme disease, *N Engl J Med* 321:586, 1989.

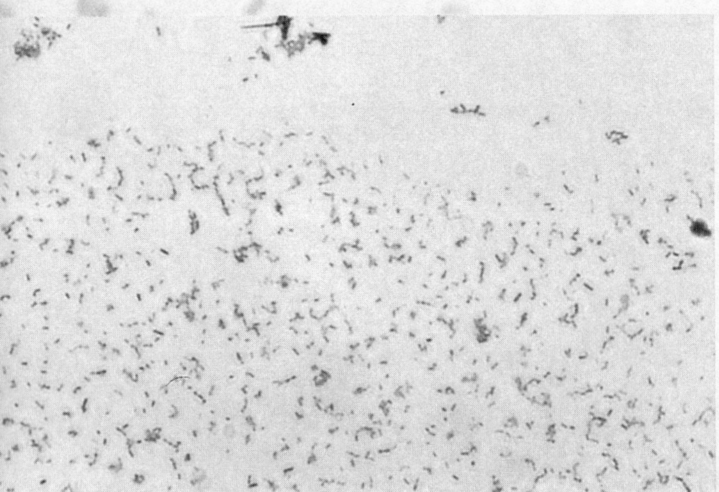

LISTERIA MONOCYTOGENES

CHAPTER OUTLINE

SPORE FORMERS

NON–SPORE FORMERS

- *Corynebacterium*
- Aerobic Actinomycetes
- *Listeria*
- *Erysipelothrix rhusiopathiae*
- *Lactobacillus*
- *Kurthia*
- *Rothia*

KEY TERMS

ANTHRAX

DIPHTHEROID

LISTERIOSIS

METACHROMATIC GRANULES

MYCETOMA

PARTIALLY ACID FAST

Gram-Positive Bacilli

CHAPTER FIFTEEN

LEARNING OBJECTIVES

1. **Describe and recognize the following:**
   a. Diphtheroid
   b. Metachromatic granules
   c. Pleomorphic
2. **State the purpose of the following media:**
   a. Tellurite medium
   b. Loeffler serum medium
3. **Discuss the identification and infectious process of *Corynebacterium diphtheriae.* Describe the significance and technique used to identify its exotoxin.**
4. **Describe the identification and clinical significance of *C. jeikeium* (group JK).**
5. **Explain the relevance of isolating:**
   a. *Corynebacterium ulcerans*
   b. *Corynebacterium pseudodiphtheriticum*
6. **Describe the identification and clinical significance of *Listeria monocytogenes.***
   a. List the outstanding characteristics of this organism.
   b. Describe the types of infections and how they are transmitted.
7. **Discuss the homeostatic mechanism of *Lactobacillus acidophilus.***
8. **Describe the infections attributed to *Erysipelothrix rhusiopathiae.***
9. **Based on colonical morphology and biochemical reactions, differentiate *Lactobacillus, Erysipelothrix,* and *Listeria.***
10. **Describe the significant morphological and microscopic characteristics of the genus *Bacillus.***
11. **List and describe the types of anthrax.**
12. **Compare and contrast *Bacillus anthracis* and *Bacillus cereus,* including biochemical reactions, morphological characteristics, and diseases.**
13. **Discuss the clinical significance of the nocardioforms and aerobic actinomycetes.**
    a. Relate epidemiological, clinical, and pathological aspects of *Nocardia.*
    b. Differentiate *Nocardia* from other aerobic actinomycetes.

SPORE FORMERS

Bacillus organisms are large, gram-positive, aerobic or facultatively anaerobic bacilli. The spores may be either small and contained within the cell or large and swollen beyond the width of the cell. Figure 15-1 illustrates a photomicrograph of *Bacillus subtilis.* Although more than 40 species of *Bacillus* are known, most are saprophytic, contaminants, or considered to be normal flora of the gastrointestinal tract of animals. *Bacillus* species are catalase positive and sporulate aerobically. These are important characteristics in differentiating *Bacillus* from *Clostridium,* which are anaerobic, spore-forming, gram-positive bacilli. *Clostridium* species are usually catalase negative.

Almost all species of *Bacillus* are motile, except for the most virulent, which is ***Bacillus anthracis,*** the agent of anthrax. Anthrax is associated with cattle hides, goat hairs, and other herbivorous animals. Humans acquire the infection through direct contact with infected animal products, wool, or hair. Anthrax is an occupational hazard for those who handle livestock. Although rarely found in the United States in Texas, Louisiana, and Nebraska, the infection has a worldwide distribution and occurs in Europe, Asia, and Africa.

Once the disease is established in an area, bacterial spores from dead infected animals can contaminate the soil. The resistant spore form can remain dormant indefinitely in the soil, and the area can remain infected for years.

There are three types of anthrax. **Cutaneous anthrax** is the most common but least severe form of the disease. Infection occurs as the organism enters the body through a small cut. A lesion occurs at the site of entry and develops into a black necrotic area. If left untreated, invasion of the regional lymph nodes and blood may occur. **Woolsorters' disease,** or **pulmonary (inhalational) anthrax,** results from the inhalation of spores during shearing or sorting of animal hair or hides. Although this form occurs less frequently than cutaneous anthrax, the mortality rate is higher. **Gastrointestinal anthrax,** the most severe form, results from ingestion of the bacilli or spores in contaminated food. Although no cases have been documented in the United States, cases have been reported in other parts of the world. Extreme safety precautions are required when working with a suspected case of anthrax. Level 3 precautions, with the avoidance of aerosols, a biosafety hood, and protective laboratory gowns, gloves, and masks are all necessary.

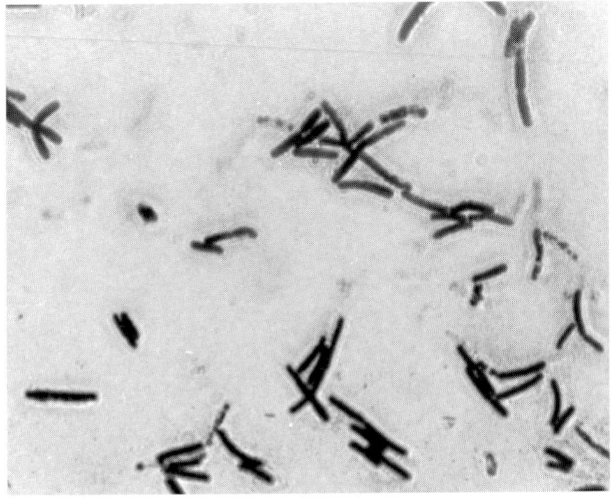

FIGURE 15–1
Bacillus subtilis photomicrograph showing large bacilli, which are gram positive.

B. anthracis is a large gram-positive bacillus. The cells typically occur in long chains, which give the organism a "bamboo rod" appearance. Virulent strains may be encapsulated. The spores are oval, located centrally to subterminally, and usually not swollen.

The specimen collected for diagnosis may be blood or skin vesicles. The organism grows well on blood agar but is somewhat inhibited on colistin-nalidixic acid (CNA) by nalidixic acid. Colonies are large (4 to 6 mm), white to gray, and raised, with an irregular curled margin and whirling projections. This has been described as a "Medusa head" appearance when seen under the dissecting microscope. When the colony is lifted with an inoculating loop, it has the consistency of a "beaten egg white." *B. anthracis* is nonhemolytic on blood agar, an important reaction in differentiating it from other *Bacillus* species.

Important biochemical reactions include:

- Nonmotile
- Produces acid from glucose, sucrose, and maltose
- Fails to produce acid from xylose, mannitol, lactose, or salicin
- Lecithinase: most strains positive
- Starch hydrolysis: positive

The organism also produces a "string of pearls" when it is streaked on Mueller-Hinton agar and a 10 U penicillin disk is added and a coverslip applied. The plate is incubated 3 to 6 hours at 37°C, and the growth beneath the coverslip is viewed microscopically.

Bacillus cereus is associated with food poisoning isolated from several foods. The organism is found in the environment in the soil, water, and vegetation. Foods implicated in *B. cereus* food poisoning include rice and other cereals, vegetables, and milk. The food poisoning is associated with vomiting resulting from the release of an emetic toxin by the organism. This emetic toxin is heat stable, with vomiting occurring within 6 hours after ingestion of the contaminated food. Most patients recover without medical intervention. The emetic toxin has been isolated primarily from boiled rice allowed to remain at room temperature or held warm. The spores are not killed during cooking and germinate when left unrefrigerated. A diarrheal syndrome associated with *B. cereus* food poisoning results from a heat-labile enterotoxin. The diarrheal effects are seen within one-half day after ingestion of the contaminated food. Implicated foods include poultry and desserts; the toxin is produced while the foods are left at room temperature. Refrigeration of foods decreases the likelihood of toxin production.

In addition to food poisoning, *B. cereus* has also been isolated from a variety of opportunistic infections, including septicemia, pneumonia, meningitis, and peritonitis.

B. cereus produces various colonial types on blood agar, ranging from small, shiny colonies to large, spreading ones. The organism may produce a grayish to lavender color on blood agar and produces a wide zone of beta hemolysis.

Important biochemical reactions for *B. cereus* include:

Motility: positive
Hemolysis: wide-zone beta
Produces acid from glucose, maltose, and salicin
Fails to produce acid from xylose, mannitol, or lactose
Lecithinase: positive

NON–SPORE FORMERS

The gram-positive, non-spore-forming bacilli that are clinically important include the following:

Corynebacterium
Listeria
Erysipelothrix
Lactobacillus
Kurthia
Rothia
Nocardioforms and aerobic actinomycetes

Many of the bacteria in this chapter have a **diphtheroid** microscopic appearance. Diphtheroid cells have variable shapes and sizes and have been described as "Chinese letters" or "picket fences" (Figure 15-2). This pleomorphic appearance is believed to result from irregular snapping during cell division. Bacteria in the genus *Corynebacterium* exhibit a diphtheroid appearance. In addition, *Lactobacillus, Listeria, Erysipelothrix, Rothia,* and *Nocardia* may also appear as diphtheroids.

Corynebacterium

Corynebacterium organisms are slender, pleomorphic, gram-positive bacilli that are aerobes or facultative anaerobes. Klebs first isolated the *Corynebacterium* in 1883, and the identification of diphtheria was attributed to Loeffler. Thus a common name for *Corynebacterium* has been "Klebs-Loeffler" bacillus. The bacteria are non-spore formers and are positive for both the catalase and the oxidase reactions. The diphtheroid appearance in Gram-stained smears is evident.

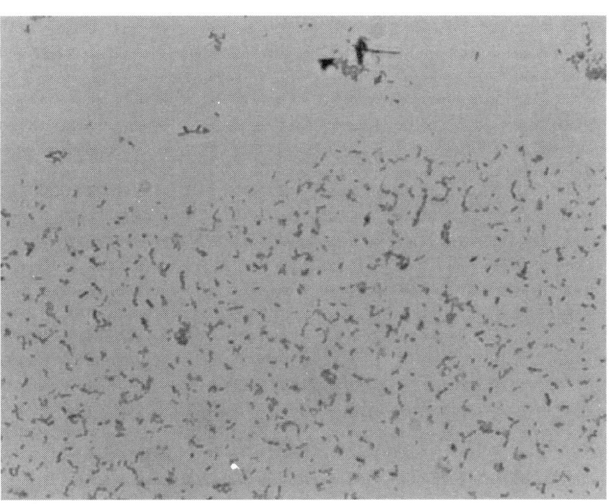

FIGURE 15–2
Listeria monocytogenes species showing characteristic diphtheroid appearance. The organism is gram positive.

The *Corynebacterium* can be divided into three groups:

Group I: human and animal pathogens
Group II: plant pathogens
Group III: nonpathogenic

The bacteria are widely distributed in nature and can be found in the soil and water. Some species are found as normal flora of the mucous membranes of humans and other animals. Unless isolated from the blood or spinal fluid, species other than *C. diphtheriae* are considered to be commensal.

The most virulent species is ***Corynebacterium diphtheriae***, the etiologic agent of **diphtheria**, a severe and acute infection. The organism produces a very powerful exotoxin that first attacks the mucous membranes of the respiratory tract. This results in an inflammation and "pseudomembrane" formation of the oropharynx, leading to respiratory obstruction. As the bacteria grow, more exotoxin is produced. The exotoxin can then be absorbed, resulting in damage to the heart and peripheral nerves. The organism can be carried in the nasopharynx of infected individuals or healthy carriers, which leads to the spread of the infection. As a result of childhood immunizations through the DPT (diphtheria-pertussis-tetanus), the incidence of diphtheria is very low in the United States.

A cutaneous form of diphtheria characterized by necrotic lesions occurs in the tropics and subtropics.

Nasopharyngeal swabs of the inflamed areas or a vigorously swabbed culture of the pseudomembrane are collected to diagnose diphtheria. Wound or skin cultures can be used to diagnose cutaneous diphtheria. A direct smear using both Gram stain and Loeffler–methylene blue should be performed. The "Chinese letters" typical of *Corynebacterium* are better visualized with the methylene blue smear, as are **metachromatic granules** (or **Babès-Ernst bodies**). Metachromatic granules are irregularly staining granules that appear as beads. It is believed that these areas serve as storage depots for materials needed by the bacterial cell. These staining characteristics are typical for most *Corynebacterium,* including those species that are normal flora of the throat. Thus a diagnosis of diphtheria cannot be made from the smear alone.

C. diphtheriae is isolated using blood agar, Loeffler serum medium, and potassium tellurite medium. The organism produces a narrow zone of beta hemolysis on blood agar. Loeffler medium enhances metachromatic granule formation. *C. diphtheriae* produces gray to black colonies on potassium tellurite medium. This is an important medium for primary isolation, since it inhibits most of the normal flora of the upper respiratory tract. Isolates from Loeffler medium should be subcultured onto Tindale's medium, which also contains tellurite. *C. diphtheriae* produces black colonies with a brown halo that are distinct from the normal flora *Corynebacterium.*

There are three colonial types of *C. diphtheriae:*

Gravis type: 1 to 2 mm colonies on blood agar; largest colonial type

Mitis type: "fried egg" appearance on blood agar (clear colonies with white centers); bleachlike odor on tellurite medium

Intermedius type: small colonies (0.5 mm) on blood agar; black colonies with gray borders on tellurite medium

Since nontoxigenic strains of *C. diphtheriae* may exist, it is necessary to demonstrate the exotoxin. In vivo toxigenicity tests include direct animal inoculation into guinea pigs. More often an in vitro toxigenicity test known as the **modified Elek test** can be used. In this procedure a filter paper strip impregnated with diphtheria antitoxin is placed in a medium containing rabbit serum, potassium tellurite, and prepared agar. The medium is allowed to solidify, and the antitoxin diffuses through the medium. The plate is inoculated with a toxigenic strain of *C. diphtheriae.* The streak is made at a right angle to the strip of antitoxin. A negative control is streaked in the same manner. The unknown culture is streaked parallel to the positive and negative controls. After incubation at 35°C for 24 to 48 hours, the plate is observed for lines of precipitation, which form where the toxigenic strain reacts with the antitoxin.

Corynebacterium jeikeium (formerly **group JK**) were first recognized in 1976 when the Centers for Disease Control characterized 95 diphtheroid bacilli. The bacteria were isolated from a number of sites, including blood, spinal fluid, and wounds. All held one unique characteristic: they were resistant to a number of antibiotics. Today it is known that the group JK bacteria are also associated with endocarditis, pneumonia, and peritonitis. This bacterial group consists of pleomorphic, non-spore-forming, gram-positive bacilli that produce pinpoint white colonies on sheep blood agar after incubation at increased carbon dioxide (CO_2) at 30°C for 24 hours.

Corynebacterium ulcerans produces a diphtheria-like toxin and causes a diphtheria-like infection in humans and mastitis in cattle. Infections in humans frequently follow exposure to cattle or ingestion of contaminated milk.

Corynebacterium pseudotuberculosis, formerly known as *C. ovix,* is a rare cause of lymphadenitis in humans, frequently following contact with infected livestock through direct contact or ingestion of contaminated milk.

Corynebacterium xerosis is part of the normal flora of human skin, the nasopharynx, and the conjunctival sac and is a rare cause of endocarditis.

Corynebacterium pseudodiphtheriticum is found in the normal flora of the human oropharynx and is a rare cause of endocarditis.

Aerobic Actinomycetes

Members of the aerobic actinomycetes include ***Nocardia, Nocardiopsis, Streptomyces, Actinomadura,*** and ***Dermatophilus.***

Nocardia is found in the soil and water, and humans can become infected through inhalation of the organism. The species most frequently found in human infections is *Nocardia asteroides.* Other species include *N. brasiliensis* and *N. caviae.* Infections are usually chronic in nature and most frequently involve the respiratory tract and central nervous system. The organism typically infects immunosuppressed hosts, and the infection is characterized by necrosis and abscesses. Because the organism can resist phagocytosis, it can remain within the host indefinitely.

Nocardia species are unique in their ability to retain carbolfuchsin after decolorization with mild acid. They are thus termed "**partially acid fast.**" A specimen of a lesion of sputum will yield long, thin, branching gram-positive bacilli. The organism grows well on Sabouraud dextrose agar but is inhibited by chloramphenicol. Growth is enhanced in 10% CO_2 and appears in 3 days to 4 weeks as waxy, bumpy, velvety, yellow-orange colonies. This growth may resemble that of the mycobacteria, which are acid fast.

Actinomadura, Dermatophilus, Nocardiopsis, and *Streptomyces* are associated with chronic granulomas of the skin and subcutaneous tissue. **Mycetoma,** a swelling, draining lesion of the extremities, can be caused by fungi and the aerobic actinomycetes. The infection, termed **actinomycetoma,** is acquired through inoculation (because the organisms normally reside in the soil) and is usually an opportunistic infection.

Listeria

Listeria is found in the environment in soil, water, sewage, and decaying vegetation and in the feces of humans, swine, and poultry. Animals, soils, and plants can become contaminated through contact with animal products. Although primarily an animal pathogen, human infections may be initiated through contact with infected animals or animal products. An increased frequency of isolation of *Listeria* from human sources may indicate that *Listeria* infections have gone undetected in the past.

There are six species of *Listeria,* and ***Listeria monocytogenes*** is the most significant human isolate. The major source of infection is contaminated food, and those at highest risk include pregnant females, their fetuses, and newborns. Foods contaminated with *Listeria* include cabbage, raw fruit, and pasteurized and unpasteurized dairy products. In 1988 an outbreak of **listeriosis** was attributed to contaminated Mexican cheese. The most common manifestation of listeriosis is meningitis. In early-onset listeriosis the fetus becomes infected either in utero or during the first days following birth. A common manifestation is pneumonia, as well as meningoencephalitis and brain abscess. Often the infection may result in spontaneous abortion or stillbirth when acquired in utero. Infants who survive are critically ill during the first days following birth. In late-onset listeriosis the infection is acquired 1 to 4 weeks after birth. Meningitis is typically associated with late-onset listeriosis, as is conjunctivitis and septicemia.

In immunosuppressed adults, particularly those who have undergone transplants or treatment for malignancies, *Listeria* may cause meningitis, endocarditis, conjunctivitis, and urethritis.

L. monocytogenes is a classical intracellular parasite that can resist phagocytosis. It is taken up by the cells of the host's reticuloendothelial system.

L. monocytogenes is a tiny, gram-positive, motile diphtheroid and a facultative anaerobe. The organism is most frequently isolated from blood cultures or cerebrospinal fluid. It grows on blood agar, producing smooth, clear to gray colonies 1 to 2 mm in diameter with a narrow band of beta hemoloysis. The organism grows best at 25° to 35°C, slowly at 4°C, and poorly at 42°C.

The organism possesses unique motility characteristics. First, *L. monocytogenes* produce a characteristic **tumbling motility** when observed in a wet mount or through a hanging-drop technique. The bacillus flips "end over end." Also, when a semisolid agar is used to demonstrate motility, the organisms produce an **umbrella-like growth** 2 to 5 mm below the agar surface. Others have described this pattern as an "inverted Christmas tree." The organism has optimal motility at 25°C, and these unique characteristics are best observed at this temperature when compared with those observed at 35°C.

Important reactions to identify *L. monocytogenes* include:

Catalase: positive
Oxidase: negative
Indole: negative
Hydrogen sulfide (H_2S): negative
CAMP reaction: positive rectangle observed
Bile-esculin hydrolysis: positive
Ferments glucose, trehalose, and salicin

The **ocular test of Anton** is performed to determine the pathogenicity of an isolate suspected of being *L. monocytogenes.* The isolate is suspended in sterile water, and two or three drops of the suspension are inoculated into the conjunctival sac of a rabbit's eye. A positive test is indicated by the development of purulent conjunctivitis. The other eye serves as a negative control.

Erysipelothrix rhusiopathiae

Erysipelothrix (red skin, thread) *rhusiopathiae* (red disease) is a veterinary infection and an occupational hazard for those handling meat, poultry, fish, and rabbits. The organism is carried asymptomatically or causes infection in fish, cattle, horses, turkeys, and pigs. Infections most frequently occur as a cutaneous inflammation of the hands or fingers. The infection is known as erysipeloid, which describes its red, spreading nature. Most infections remain localized, but rarely they may disseminate to the blood, resulting in bacteremia and arthritis.

The organism is nonmotile and gram positive but decolorizes easily and grows as alpha-hemolytic or nonhemolytic colonies on blood agar. Specimens collected for diagnosis include skin biopsies, tissue aspirates, and blood cultures. Important biochemical reactions for *E. rhusiopathiae* include:

Catalase: negative
Indole: negative
Nitrate: negative
H_2S: positive

Lactobacillus

Lactobacillus acidophilus is normal flora of the mouth, gastrointestinal tract, and vaginal canal. It is usually nonpathogenic and has little clinical significance. The organism is a rare cause of bacteremia and pneumonia.

The organism helps to maintain the normal homeostatic environment by producing large quantities of lactic acid. This acidic environment is intolerable to many pathogenic bacteria. *Lactobacillus* tolerates this highly acidic environment and can grow at a pH of 3 to 4.

Lactobacillus is a gram-positive, catalase-negative, pleomorphic bacillus. It is nonmotile and unable to

TABLE 15–1

Biochemical Reactions to Differentiate Gram-Positive Non–Spore-Forming Bacilli

	LISTERIA MONOCYTOGENES	*ERYSIPELOTHRIX RHUSIOPATHIAE*	*LACTOBACILLUS* SPECIES	*CORYNEBACTERIUM*	
				DIPHTHERIAE	*JEIKEIUM*
Beta hemolysis	+	−	−	V	−
Catalase	+	−	−	+	+
Motility	+*	−	−	−	−
H_2S	−	+	−	−	−
Esculin hydrolysis	+	−	−	−	−
Fermentation of:					
Glucose	+	+	+	+	+
Mannitol	−	−	V	+	−
Salicin	+	−	V	−	−

+, Most isolates give positive reaction; −, most isolates give negative reaction; V, variable reaction.

*Umbrella growth in semisolid media. Motile at 25°C.

produce H_2S or hydrolyze esculin. It is an ingredient in many natural yogurts.

Kurthia

Kurthia bessonnii is found in the soil and is an opportunistic pathogen. It is motile by peritrichous flagella, is an obligate aerobe, and is catalase positive and oxidase negative.

Rothia

Rothia is normal flora of the human mouth and a rare cause of abscesses and endocarditis.

• • •

Table 15-1 outlines important reactions to identify the gram-positive bacilli.

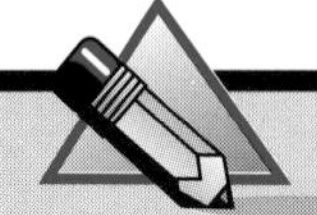

REVIEW QUESTIONS

MATCHING

1. **Which of the following is *not* a characteristic of *Corynebacterium diphtheriae?***
   a. Pleomorphic morphology
   b. Gram-positive bacillus
   c. Spore former
   d. Nonmotile
2. **To differentiatfe *Bacillus anthracis* from *Bacillus cereus:***
   a. B. anthracis is beta hemolytic on blood agar and nonmotile; B. cereus is nonhemolytic and motile.
   b. B. cereus is beta hemolytic on blood agar and motile; B. anthracis is nonhemolytic on blood agar and nonmotile.
   c. B. anthracis produces acid from glucose and maltose; B. cereus does not.
   d. B. anthracis is lecithinase positive; B. cereus is lecithinase negative.
3. ***Bacillus cereus* has been implicated in which of the following diseases?**
   a. Anthrax
   b. Pseudomembranous colitis
   c. Gastroenteritis
   d. Meningitis
4. **On potassium tellurite medium, *Corynebacterium diphtheriae* produces:**
   a. Beta-hemolytic colonies
   b. Enhanced pleomorphic properties

REVIEW QUESTIONS

(Continued)

c. Black colonies
d. Pink to red colonies

5. **Which species of *Corynebacterium* was characterized in 1976 as a multidrug-resistant agent in a variety of clinical infections?**
   a. *C. diphtheriae*
   b. *C. ulcerans*
   c. *C. pseudotuberculosis*
   d. *C. jeikeium*

6. **"Partial acid fastness" is a characteristic of:**
   a. *Listeria monocytogenes*
   b. *Nocardia*
   c. *Lactobacillus acidophilus*
   d. *Bacillus anthracis*

7. **A gram-positive bacillus isolated from the spinal fluid of a 1-month-old infant is catalase positive, beta hemolytic, and bile-esculin positive and exhibits tumbling motility in a wet preparation. This organism is most likely:**
   a. *Lactobacillus acidophilus*
   b. *Listeria monocytogenes*
   c. *Erysipelothrix rhusiopathiae*
   d. *Corynebacterium jeikeium*

8. **Which statement correctly describes *Lactobacillus acidophilus?***
   a. Prefers alkaline pH range
   b. Strict pathogen
   c. Produces large quantities of lactic acid
   d. Characteristic tumbling motility

BIBLIOGRAPHY

Clarridge JE: When, why, and how far should coryneforms be identified, *Clin Microbiol Newsletter* 8:32, 1985.

Coyle MB, Lipsky BA: Coryneform bacteria in infectious disease: clinical and laboratory aspects, *Clin Microbiol Rev* 3:227, 1990.

Coyle MB, Hollis DG, Groman NB: *Corynebacterium* species and other coryneform organisms. In Lennette EH, editor: *Manual of clinical microbiology,* ed 4, Washington, DC, 1985, American Society for Microbiology, p. 193.

Doyle RJ, Keller KF, Ezzell JW: Bacillus. In Lennette EH, editor: *Manual of clinical microbiology,* ed 4, Washington, DC, 1985, American Society for Microbiology, p. 211.

Gellin BG, Broome CV: Listeriosis, *JAMA* 261:1313, 1989.

Gorby GL, Peacock JE Jr: *Erysipelothrix rhusiopathiae* endocarditis: microbiologic, epidemiologic, and clinical features of an occupational disease, *Rev Infect Dis* 10:31, 1988.

Hollis DG, Weaver RE: *Gram positive organisms: a guide to identification,* Atlanta, 1981, Centers for Disease Control.

Holt JG et al: *Bergey's manual of determinative bacteriology,* ed 9, Baltimore, 1994, Williams & Wilkins.

Matthews EK, Gullberg RM, Warren JR: A diagnostic protocol for bacteremia due to aerobic coryneforms, *Lab Med* 17:217, 1986.

Riley PS et al: Characterization and identification of 95 diphtheroid (group JK) cultures from clinical specimens, *J Clin Microbiol* 9:418, 1979.

Schlech WF III et al: Epidemic listeriosis: evidence for transmission by food, *N Engl J Med* 308:203, 1983.

Skalka B, Smola J, Elischerova K: Routine test for *in vitro* differentiation of pathogenic and apathogenic *Listeria monocytogenes* strains, *J Clin Microbiol* 15:503, 1982.

Tuazon CU et al: Serious infection from *Bacillus* species, *JAMA* 241:1137, 1979.

Turnbull PCB, Kramer JM: Nongastrointestinal *Bacillus cereus* infections: an analysis of exotoxin production by strains isolated over a two year period, *J Clin Pathol* 36:1091, 1983.

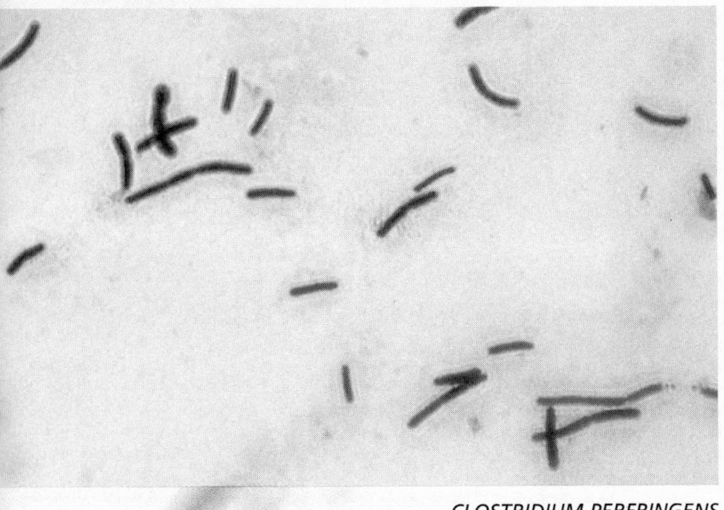

CLOSTRIDIUM PERFRINGENS

CHAPTER OUTLINE

SPECIMEN COLLECTION AND TRANSPORT
ANAEROBIC MEDIA AND INCUBATION
IDENTIFICATION
ANAEROBIC GRAM-NEGATIVE BACILLI
ANAEROBIC GRAM-POSITIVE SPORE-FORMING BACILLI: *CLOSTRIDIUM*
- *Clostridium botulinum*
- *Clostridium perfringens*
- Miscellaneous Clostridia

ANAEROBIC GRAM-POSITIVE NON–SPORE-FORMING BACILLI
ANAEROBIC COCCI
ANAEROBIC BLOOD AGAR
ANAEROBIC BLOOD AGAR WITH KANAMYCIN AND VANCOMYCIN
MISCELLANEOUS TESTS TO IDENTIFY ANAEROBES
ANAEROBIC BLOOD AGAR WITH PHENYLETHYL ALCOHOL
PRELIMINARY IDENTIFICATION OF ANAEROBES
ANTIBIOTIC DISK TESTS

KEY TERMS

ACTINOMYCOSES
AEROTOLERANCE
BOTULISM
FACULTATIVE ANAEROBE
GAS-LIQUID CHROMATOGRAPHY
MICROAEROPHILIC
MODERATELY OBLIGATE ANAEROBE
MYONECROSIS
OBLIGATE ANAEROBE
POLYMICROBIC
STRICT OBLIGATE ANAEROBE
TETANOSPASMIN
TETANUS

Anaerobes

LEARNING OBJECTIVES

1. **Define and differentiate among obligate anaerobes, facultative anaerobes, and obligate aerobes.**
2. **List at least 10 types of infections in which anaerobes may be found.**
3. **Identify three anaerobes that are normal flora of the body and identify the site(s) of each.**
4. **When given types of specimens submitted for anaerobic culture, indicate if each specimen is acceptable or not. Explain why needle aspiration is preferred over collection by swab for anaerobes.**
5. **State the purpose of each of the following anaerobic media:**
   a. Anaerobic blood agar
   b. Phenylethyl alcohol blood agar
   c. Kanamycin-vancomycin blood agar
   d. Paromomycin-vancomycin laked blood
   e. Thioglycollate
   f. *Bacteroides* bile-esculin agar
6. **Explain how an anaerobic environment may be achieved through the anaerobic jar, evacuation-replacement, glove box, or other methods.**
7. **List and briefly explain how anaerobes are identified.**
8. **Perform and interpret Gram stains on at least four anaerobes.**
9. **Recite the important characteristics (Gram stain, colonial morphology, biochemical reactions) to identify each of the following gram-negative bacilli:**
   a. *Bacteroides fragilis*
   b. *Prevotella intermedius*
   c. *Porphyromonas asaccharolyticus*
   d. *Fusobacterium nucleatum*
   e. *Fusobacterium necrophorum*
   f. *Fusobacterium mortiforum*
10. **Discuss the clinical relevance of isolation of the gram-negative anaerobic bacilli.**
11. **For each of the following *Clostridium*, discuss the disease process and explain how each is identified:**
   a. *C. botulinum*
   b. *C. tetani*
   c. *C. perfringens*
   d. *C. difficile*

Continued.

12. **List and describe the five *Clostridium* groups.**

13. **Describe the clinical relevance of isolation of the following gram-positive non–spore-forming bacilli:**
   a. *Actinomyces israelii*
   b. *Propionibacterium acnes*

14. **List the clinically important gram-negative anaerobic cocci.**

15. **Explain how the following gram-positive anaerobic cocci are identified, and relate the clinical significance of each.**
   a. *Peptostreptococcus anaerobius*
   b. *Peptococcus niger*

16. **Perform and interpret at least four of each of the following anaerobic procedures:**
   a. Lombard-Dowell medium
   b. Antibiotic disk testing

17. **When given an unknown anaerobe, identify without error.**

Anaerobes are those bacteria that require a reduced oxygen tension for growth and fail to grow on solid media in the presence of oxygen. This is a simple definition, but in reality the oxygen requirements of bacteria are not so clear-cut. **Obligate aerobes** require oxygen as the final electron acceptor, whereas **obligate anaerobes** do not use oxygen and are inhibited by its presence. Bacteria classified as **facultative anaerobes** can grow in both the presence and the absence of oxygen. **Microaerophilic** bacteria prefer reduced oxygen tension but can grow on solid media in 10% carbon dioxide (CO_2) in air.

When considering the obligate anaerobes, a further differentiation can be made. There are varying degrees of tolerance to oxygen and peroxides as well as differing limits of oxidation-reduction potentials. It is believed that the varying oxygen tolerance depends on the organism's ability to produce superoxide dismutase, catalases, and peroxidases that protect against toxic oxygen products. These toxic oxygen products include the superoxide radical and hydrogen peroxide, which are believed to react to form free hydroxyl radicals, which are very powerful oxidants. Superoxide dismutase catalyzes the conversion of superoxide radicals to less toxic hydrogen peroxide and molecular oxygen. Catalase converts hydrogen peroxide to water and oxygen. Anaerobes that produce some superoxide dismutase are more resistant to the toxic effects of oxygen. An example is *Clostridium perfringens,* which is classified as a **moderately obligate anaerobe,** since it can grow at oxygen levels of 2% to 8%. Most anaerobes associated with human infection belong to this category. Other anaerobes are classified as **strict obligate anaerobes** and cannot grow on the agar surface when it is exposed to as little as 0.5% oxygen.

Anaerobes are frequently involved in **polymicrobic** infections, those involving more than one bacterial species. Often, both aerobes and anaerobes can be isolated from the same site. Anaerobes can cause almost every type of infection known, and these infections are often fulminating and devastating. They follow trauma, vascular stasis, or tissue necrosis, which makes the environment of the tissue favorable for anaerobic growth. Infections in which anaerobes are found or are the predominant pathogen are:

Brain abscess
Chronic otitis media
Dental infection
Aspiration pneumonia
Lung abscess
Liver abscess
Peritonitis
Appendicitis
Intraabdominal abscess
Wound infections following surgery or trauma
Postabortion sepsis
Gynecological infections
Cellulitis
Myonecrosis

Although some anaerobic infections are **exogenous** (from an outside source) in nature, most are **endogenous** and arise from sources within the mouth, intestinal tract, or female genital tract. Examples of exogenous anaerobic infections include food-borne botulism, myonecrosis, tetanus, infant botulism, and *Clostridium difficile* nosocomial diarrhea. Anaerobes are the predominant normal flora in the lower intestine, where they outnumber aerobes by as much as 1000:1 and are a constant source of endogenous infection when removed to other sites through surgery, disease, or trauma. For example, a major normal flora of the bowel, the anaerobe *Bacteroides fragilis,* is a significant cause of intraabdominal abscesses. The upper respiratory tract, including the mouth, nasopharynx, oropharynx, and nasal passages, are inhabited by *Fusobacterium* and other anaerobic cocci and bacilli associated with aspiration pneumonia and lung abscesses. *Actinomyces* species may be normally found in the upper respiratory and gastrointestinal tracts and may cause actinomycoses of the mouth, chest, and abdomen. Anaerobes, including *Propionibacterium acnes* and the anaerobic gram-positive cocci, are members of the normal flora of the skin, while anaerobic gram-positive non-spore-forming bacteria, such as *Lactobacillus,* are found as normal flora in the female genital tract.

SPECIMEN COLLECTION AND TRANSPORT

Whenever possible, it is preferred to collect a specimen for anaerobic examination by needle aspiration instead of by a swab. Collection using a swab has several drawbacks, including contamination with normal flora, collection of a small volume of specimen, the danger of the swab drying out, and exposure of the swab to toxic oxygen. Although often difficult when culturing mucous membranes near a site of infection, the area should be properly disinfected with a surgical soap scrub, alcohol, and iodine to avoid normal flora contamination.

Blood cultures should allow the growth of obligate anaerobes, aerobes, and facultative anaerobes. The skin over the venipuncture site must be cleansed using alcohol and povidone-iodine to avoid contamination from the normal flora of the skin, especially *Staphylococcus epidermidis* and the anaerobic *P. acnes.* All cultures should be checked twice daily for growth for the first 3 days, as evidenced through hemolysis, gas production, or turbidity when using a manual method. Cultures should then be checked once daily and held for a total of 5 to 7 days until reported as negative. The box at right lists general guidelines for the collection of anaerobic specimens.

It is also important to maintain the specimen in an anaerobic state after collection until transport to the laboratory. Several systems are commercially available that provide an agar surface and anaerobic environment once a specimen is inserted. The PRAS (prereduced and anaerobically sterilized) system of Remel provides a semisolid agar and an anaerobic atmosphere. It is suitable for use with swabs and aspirates. "Gassed-out collection" tubes also provide an anaerobic environment for transport. A nonsupportive medium with cystine as a reducing agent and the redox indicator resazurin are parts of the system. The tube is flushed with oxygen-free CO_2. The specimen is then injected through a rubber stopper. In the Port-A-Cul (Becton-Dickinson Microbiology Systems), prereduced transport media maintain the anaerobe's viability while an indicator monitors the anaerobiosis of the system.

GENERAL GUIDELINES FOR COLLECTION OF ANAEROBIC SPECIMENS

Preferable Specimens

Abscesses of the liver, lung, brain and abdomen

Necrotic tissue associated with poor vascular perfusion, trauma, or malignancy

Wound infections proximal to mucous membranes

Exudates from deep wounds or abscesses, especially when associated with the production of gas, necrosis, or a foul smell

Gram stain that indicates anaerobes

Serous fluid exudates from normally sterile sites, such as amniotic, pleural, peritoneal, and synovial fluids

Infected human or animal bites

Food suspected of causing botulism

Specimen containing sulfur granules

Specimens to Avoid or Reject

Nasal, pharyngeal, vaginal, cervical, and rectal swabs

Voided urine

Swabs of surface skin ulcers and abscesses

Sputum

Feces, gastric contents, and small bowel contents

ANAEROBIC MEDIA AND INCUBATION

Anaerobic media contain supplements, such as hemin, blood, and vitamin K, as well as sodium bicarbonate, which provides a source of CO_2. Reducing agents, such as thioglycolic acid, sodium thioglycollate,

TABLE 16–1

Anaerobic Media

MEDIUM	PURPOSE
Anaerobic blood agar	Trypticase soy agar with 5% sheep blood; supplements: yeast, hemin, vitamin K–reducing agent: L-cystine Isolation of all anaerobes, including obligate and facultative
Anaerobic phenylethyl alcohol (PEA) blood agar	Anaerobic blood agar plus phenylethyl alcohol Inhibits swarming of *Proteus* and growth of facultative anaerobes, such as the Enterobacteriaceae Isolation of gram-positive and gram-negative obligate anaerobes. Gram-positive facultative anaerobes such as *Staphylococcus, Streptococcus,* and *Corynebacterium* also grow on PEA.
Anaerobic kanamycin-vancomycin blood agar (KV)	Anaerobic blood agar plus the antibiotics kanamycin and vancomycin Vancomycin inhibits facultative and obligate gram-positive anaerobes while kanamycin inhibits facultative gram-negative rods. Isolation of gram negative anaerobes, especially *Bacteroides, Prevotella,* and some *Fusobacterium*
Anaerobic paromomycin-vancomycin laked blood (PVLB) agar	Similar to KV and can be used instead; medium is "laked:" blood is frozen and thawed. Isolation of gram-negative anaerobes, especially *Bacteroides, Prevotella,* and some *Fusobacterium;* pigment production of *Prevotella* detected earlier because of "laked" blood
Thioglycollate	Enriched broth with hemin and vitamin K Supplement to plating media for slower-growing bacteria; supports growth of most anaerobes found in clinical specimens
Bacteroides bile-esculin (BBE)	Detects organism's ability to grow in 20% bile and to hydrolyze esculin; interpret plate for growth and hydrolysis of esculin, which is indicated by a brown-black color.

and cystine, can be added to the media to absorb oxygen.

For primary isolation of anaerobes, a nonselective blood agar plate, anaerobic-selective media, and an enriched broth should be used. The enriched broth, such as thioglycollate, is used as a supplement, which may be needed if the anaerobic system fails. Also, if the agar plates do not grow, growth may occur in the thioglycollate, from which a second set of plates can be inoculated. Table 16-1 describes frequently used anaerobic plating media.

Although anaerobic media do not need to be stored anaerobically, they should be held in a reduced form 8 to 16 hours before inoculation.

Anaerobic systems for incubation include the anaerobic jar method, evacuation-replacement systems, the glove box, and disposable anaerobic bags. In the **anaerobic jar method** (Figure 16-1), oxygen is removed from the system through reaction with hydrogen, which has been added externally to the system. The reaction takes place in the presence of a palladium catalyst. In the GasPak System (Becton Dickinson Microbiology Systems), a generator envelope is opened and activated by adding water. This activates the generation of hydrogen and CO_2. In the presence of the palladium catalyst, the following reaction occurs:

$$2H_2 + O_2 \rightarrow 2H_2O$$

The palladium must be replaced or reactivated each time the jar is used, since it can be inactivated by the production of metabolic products of the bacteria. Reactivation is accomplished through heating the pellets in a dry-heat oven for 2 hours at 160° to 170°C. The pellets must be stored in a desiccator until use.

To determine the effectiveness of the system, methylene blue strips should be used. When minimal anaerobic conditions are achieved, the strip becomes white. If the strip remains blue or reverts back to blue, the system is failing and an anaerobic environment has not been achieved.

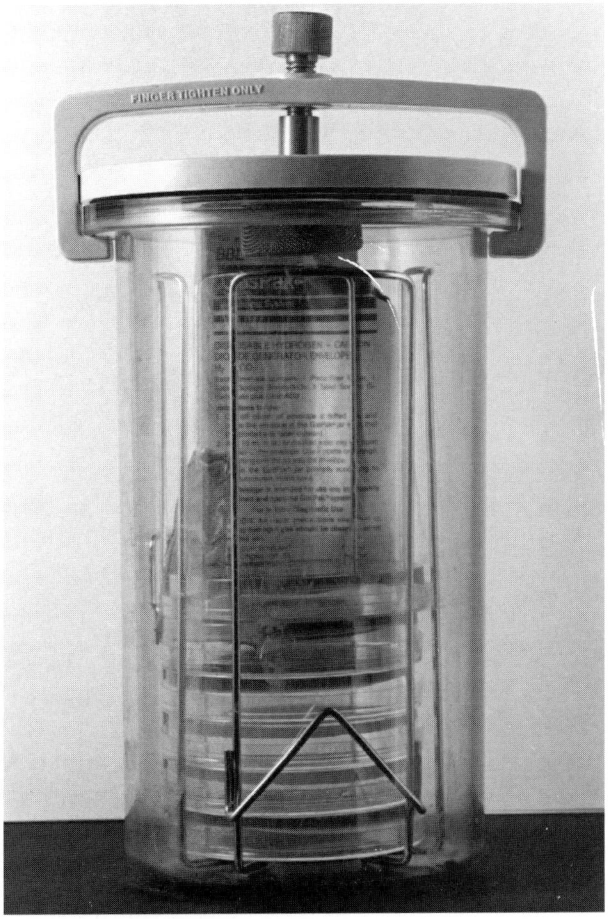

FIGURE 16–1
Anaerobic jar showing plates, generator envelope, indicator, and palladium catalyst. *(Becton Dickinson Microbiology Systems.)*

In the **evacuation-replacement system,** an airtight container, such as a Brewer jar or GasPak jar (Becton Dickinson Microbiology Systems), is used. The air in the jar is removed and replaced with a mixture of gas containing 85% N_2, 10% H_2, and 5% CO_2. An anaerobic environment is quickly established using this method. A redox indicator system, such as the methylene blue strips, should be used to monitor the effectiveness of this system. This method has largely been replaced by more modern techniques.

In the **glove-box method,** a self-contained anaerobic environment of 85% N_2, 10% H_2, and 5% CO_2 is provided through external gas sources. Specimens and other materials are passed into the chamber through an entry lock system. Cultures can be incubated in an incubator within the glove box. The system also permits one to perform most techniques necessary to isolate and identify anaerobes within the glove box. The glove box is useful for large laboratories that handle a great volume of anaerobic cultures.

Disposable anaerobic bags provide a convenient anaerobic incubation system. The BioBag System (type

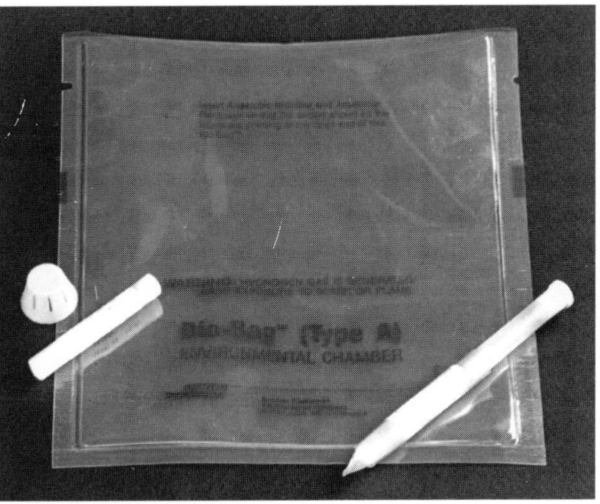

FIGURE 16–2
BioBag (Type A) for incubation of anaerobic agar plates. Bag contains ampule for generation of hydrogen, palladium catalyst, and indicator for anaerobiosis. *(Available from Becton Dickinson Microbiology Systems.)*

A) of Becton Dickinson (Figure 16-2) consists of a plastic bag with a H_2CO_2 gas generator that is released on addition of water. Palladium pellets act as catalysts while a resazurin indicator monitors the system's effectiveness. The bag is sealed after activation of the gases. The bags can hold from one to three Petri plates. The BBL GasPak Pouch (Becton Dickinson) operates without a catalyst. In this self-contained system, a liquid activating agent is added to citric acid, releasing CO_2 and H_2. Oxygen is removed by reacting with iron powder to form iron oxides. The pouches used in this system can hold one or two Petri plates.

An anaerobic holding jar can be used to hold media, recently inoculated plates, or plates to be subcultured. This is a three-jar system in which the first jar holds uninoculated plates, the second jar holds plates with colonies for subculture, and the third jar holds freshly inoculated plates. Nitrogen or CO_2 gas is piped into the system.

Anaerobic cultures are incubated at 35° to 37°C for at least 48 hours. After examination, plates should be reincubated for an additional 2 to 4 days to ensure that some of the slower-growing organisms, such as *Actinomyces,* are not missed. Broth cultures should be held for 7 days before reporting growth as negative. It is essential to limit exposure to air because this may be toxic to the organisms.

Aerotolerance tests can be performed on any colony type found growing anaerobically. The colony is subcultured onto an aerobic blood agar plate, which is incubated in increased CO_2 (using a CO_2 incubator or candle jar), and onto an anaerobic blood agar plate, which is incubated anaerobically. The growth can be interpreted as shown in Table 16-2.

TABLE 16–2

Aerotolerance Interpretation

COLONY TYPE	GROWTH ON AEROBIC BLOOD	GROWTH ON ANAEROBIC BLOOD
Obligate aerobe or microaerophile	Growth	No growth
Obligate anaerobe	No growth	Growth
Facultative anaerobe	Growth	Growth

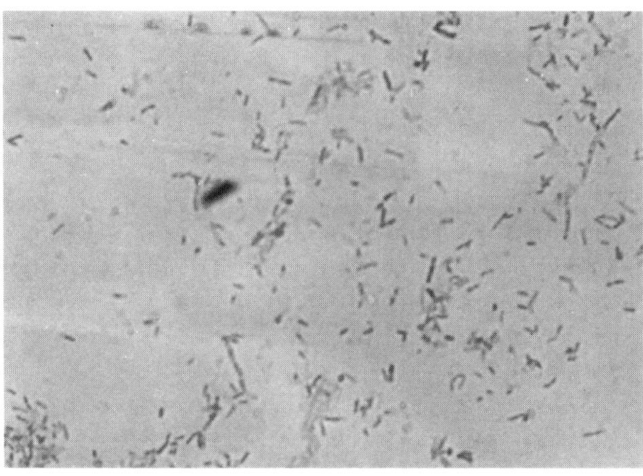

FIGURE 16–3
Photomicrograph of *Bacteroides fragilis* showing pale-staining pleomorphic bacillus. Appearance is also characteristic of *Prevotella.*

IDENTIFICATION

The Gram stain is very important in the identification of anaerobes. Methanol fixation provides better results than the traditional heat fixation. *Bacteroides* and *Prevotella* species typically appear as pale, pleomorphic, gram-negative coccobacilli with bipolar staining (Figure 16-3 [Color Plate 50]). *Fusobacterium* species are long, thin, filamentous gram-negative bacilli with tapered ends and often are arranged end to end (Figure 16-4 [Color Plate 51]). *Actinomyces* species appear as branching gram-positive bacilli. *Fusobacterium necrophorum* may appear as pale, irregularly staining, highly pleomorphic, gram-negative bacilli with swollen areas.

In addition, the presence or absence of spores as well as their location should be noted. This is particularly important for the genus *Clostridium.* **Terminal spores** appear at the end of organism, whereas **central spores** appear in the middle. **Subterminal spores** appear between the end and the middle of the organism.

Colonial morphology is also an important tool to identify anaerobes. For example, *Actinomyces israelii,* a gram-positive non-spore-forming bacillus, appears as rough, heaped, white colonies that are said to resemble a "molar tooth" on anaerobic blood agar. *Prevotella melaninogenica* (formerly *Bacteroides melaninogenicus*) develops a brown to black pigment on anaerobic blood agar after 7 days of incubation.

Gas-liquid chromatography (GLC) involves the analysis of metabolic end products released into broth during anaerobic growth. Fermentative products produced by bacteria from organic compounds, primarily glucose, can be used to identify anaerobes. Certain organisms characteristically produce one or a pattern of end products. Short-chain volatile fatty acids can be identified through a gas chromatograph. Typically, one can identify the following volatile acids: acetic, propionic, butyric, isobutyric, isovaleric, valeric, caproic, and isocaproic. Volatile acids are identified by comparing unknown results with known standards. Nonvolatile acids identified include pyruvic, lactic, succinic, and phenylacetic. The box on p. 275 lists metabolic end products of some common anaerobes.

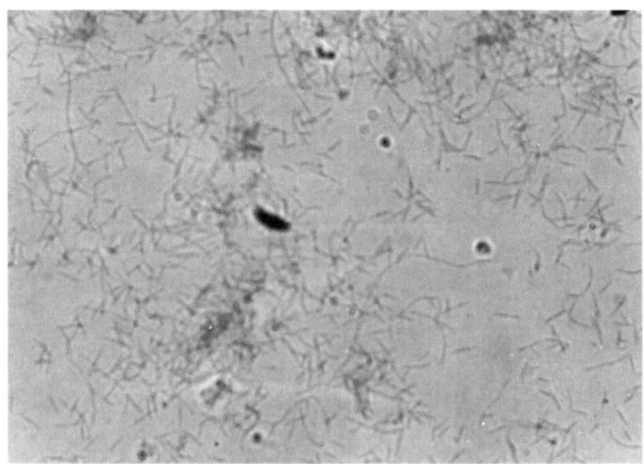

FIGURE 16–4
Fusobacterium Gram stain showing typical morphology of long, thin, filamentous gram-negative bacilli.

Biochemical reactions can also be used to identify anaerobes. Commercially, packaged kits are available and include the Minitek system (Becton Dickinson), the API 20A System (bioMérieux Vitek), and the RapID-ANA (Innovative Systems). The Lombard Dowell Presumpto Plate System offers a series of 12 biochemical reactions that can be used to identify anaerobes. In addition, the **catalase, nitrate, urease,** and **indole** reactions, which have been discussed in previous chapters, pro-

METABOLIC PRODUCTS OF SOME COMMON ANAEROBES: MAJOR END PRODUCTS FROM PEPTONE-YEAST EXTRACT-GLUCOSE BROTH

Gram-Negative Bacilli

Bacteroides fragilis: acetic, lactic, succinic, phenylacetic*

Porphyromonas asaccharolyticus: acetic, propionic, isobutyric, butyric, isovaleric, succinic

Prevotella intermedius: acetic, isovaleric, succinic

Fusobacterium nucleatum: acetic, propionic, butyric

Fusobacterium necrophorum: acetic, propionic, butyric

Fusobacterium mortiferum: acetic, propionic, butyric

Cocci

Peptococcus niger: acetic, isobutyric, butyric, isovaleric

Peptostreptococcus asaccharolyticus: acetic, butyric

Peptostreptococcus anaerobius: acetic, isocaproic

Veillonella spp: acetic, propionic

Gram-Positive Bacilli

Actinomyces israelii: acetic, lactic, succinic

Bifidobacterium spp: acetic, lactic

Propionibacterium acnes: acetic, propionic

Gram-Positive Spore-Forming Bacilli

Clostridium botulinum: acetic, isocaproic

Clostridium difficile: acetic, isobutyric, butyric, isovaleric

Clostridium perfringens: acetic, butyric

Clostridium ramosum: acetic

Clostridium septicum: acetic, butyric

Clostridium sordellii: acetic, isocaproic

*Refers to volatile and nonvolatile acids throughout (see text).

vide additional information for identification. The box on p. 276 lists the biochemical reactions of the Presumpto Plates.

Also, the **susceptibility** of anaerobes to high-level antibiotic disks, such as 1 mg kanamycin, can be used as a preliminary tool in identification. MicroRings AN and AC (Medical Wire and Equipment Company) are a commercially available system to determine the susceptibility pattern of the anaerobe (Figure 16-5).

ANAEROBIC GRAM-NEGATIVE BACILLI

The anaerobic gram-negative bacilli are the major normal flora in the colon, outnumbering aerobes by 1000:1. These organisms are also a major normal flora of the oral cavity. The gram-negative bacilli are the most common anaerobes isolated clinically. Infections usually involve the presence of anaerobes in normally sterile sites, such as after surgery, trauma, or disease, which disrupts the normal mucosal surface of the bowel. Identification is accomplished through grouping based on colonial morphology, Gram stain appearance, pigment production, antibiotic susceptibility, hemolysis, and biochemical testing. The "gold standard" for identification of anaerobic gram-negative bacilli is gas-liquid chromatography (GLC), although the procedure is not typically performed in clinical laboratories. See the box above for typical results of GLC.

The ***Bacteroides fragilis*** group is composed of nonmotile gram-negative bacilli. The bacilli have rounded ends and may be pleomorphic with vacuoles. On anaerobic blood agar, colonies are nonhemolytic

LOMBARD-DOWELL PRESUMPTO PLATES

Presumpto Plate 1

LD agar

LD esculin agar

LD egg-yolk agar

LD bile agar

Presumpto Plate 2

LD glucose agar

LD starch agar

LD milk agar

LD DNA agar

Presumpto Plate 3

LD mannitol agar

LD lactose agar

LD rhamnose agar

LD gelatin agar

and gray, with an entire margin and ringlike structures. Growth is enhanced in 20% bile, and the organisms are resistant to penicillin (2 U), kanamycin (1 mg), vancomycin (5 μg), and colistin (10 μg) but are susceptible to rifampin (15 μg). These bacteria are saccharolytic, and the specific carbohydrates fermented depend on the species.

B. fragilis is extremely virulent and can cause widespread tissue destruction. The organism has a capsule and also produces several enzymes, including deoxyribonuclease (DNase), heparinase, fibrinolysin, and superoxide dismutase. Important reactions for *B. fragilis* are summarized as follows:

Growth in 20% bile (resistant to bile)
Bile-esculin hydrolysis: positive
Catalase: positive
Lipase: negative
Lecithinase: negative
Gelatinase: positive
No pigment or spore production

The **pigmented saccharolytic gram-negative bacilli** include the pigmented *Bacteroides* that have been renamed ***Prevotella.*** These organisms ferment glucose and other carbohydrates. Species included in this group include *Prevotella melaninogenica, P. corporis, P. denticola, P. loescheii,* and *P. intermedius.* The organisms are normal flora of the oropharynx, nose, gastrointestinal (GI) tract, and

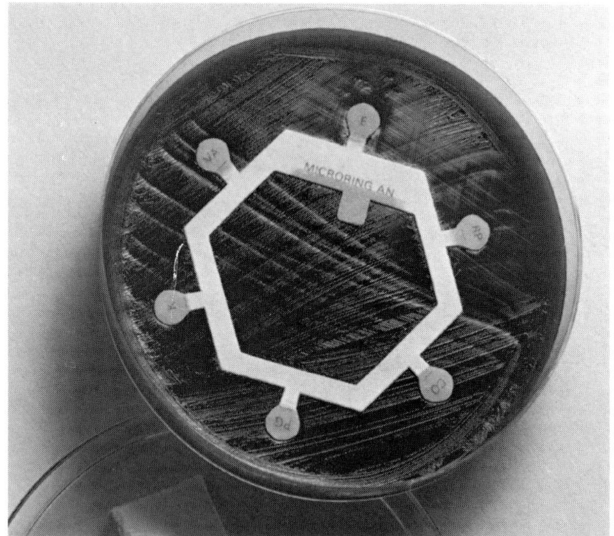

FIGURE 16–5

MicroRings showing anaerobic bacteria's susceptibility or resistance to various antibiotics. The antibiotic pattern can be used in the identification of the microorganism. *(Medical Wire and Equipment Company.)*

urogenital tract and cause infections in the head and neck and lower respiratory tract. The bacteria are typically slow growing, requiring up to 3 weeks to grow. Young colonies are tan to buff in color. An important characteristic is brick-red fluorescence when viewed under ultraviolet light at 365 nm. Older colonies develop a brown to black pigment. Some of these bacteria (*P. denticola, P. loescheii, P. melaninogenica*) ferment lactose, while others (*P. intermedia, P. corporis*) are lactose negative. Other important reactions include:

Inhibition by 20% bile
Susceptible to rifampin (15 μg)
Resistant to kanamycin (1 mg)

P. intermedia produces black colonies in 2 to 3 weeks and ferments sucrose but not lactose. It is indole and lipase positive. *P. corporis* (formerly *B. intermedius*) is indole and lipase negative and cannot ferment sucrose. *P. denticola* is a slow pigment producer, ferments ribose, and is esculin positive, whereas *P. melaninogenica* cannot ferment ribose and is esculin negative.

The **asaccharolytic pigmented gram-negative bacilli** include the genus *Porphyromonas,* which are normal flora of the oropharynx, nose, urogenital tract, and GI tract. The bacteria are associated with infections of the head, neck, oral cavity, and urogenital tract and with pleuropulmonary infections. Important species include *Porphyromonas asaccharolyticus, P. endodontalis,* and *P. gingivalis.*

Similar to *Prevotella,* the bacteria are typically slow growing, requiring 48 hours to as long as 2 weeks to grow. Colonies characteristically show a brick-red

TABLE 16–3

Identification of Anaerobic Gram-Negative Bacilli

	BACTEROIDES FRAGILIS	PORPHYROMONAS ASACCHAROLYTICUS	PREVOTELLA INTERMEDIA	FUSOBACTERIUM		
				NECROPHORUM	NUCLEATUM	MORTIFERUM
PRESUMPTO PLATE 1						
Indole	–	+	+	+	+	–
Esculin hydrolysis	+	–	–	–	–	+
H_2S	–	–	–	V	V	–
Catalase	+	–	–	–	–	–
Lecithinase	–	–	–	–	–	–
Lipase	–	–	+	+	–	–
Growth on 20% Bile	E	I	I	I	I	E
PRESUMPTO PLATE 2						
Glucose fermented	+	–	+	+	–	+
Starch hydrolysis	–	–	+	–	–	–
Milk digested	–	+	+	V	–	–
DNase	–	–	+	–	–	–
PRESUMPTO PLATE 3						
Gelatin hydrolysis	–	+	+	V	–	–
Fermentation of						
Mannitol	–	–	–	–	–	–
Lactose	+	–	–	–	–	+
Rhamnose	–	–	–	–	–	–

+, Most strains positive; –, most strains negative; V, variable reaction; E, growth on 20% bile equal to that without bile; I, growth on 20% bile inhibited.

fluorescence when viewed under ultraviolet light (365 nm). Older colonies develop a black to brown pigment. The asaccharolytic pigmented gram-negative bacilli do not grow on kanamycin-vancomycin anaerobic media, since the organisms are inhibited by vancomycin. These bacteria are also inhibited by 20% bile. The organisms are inhibited by penicillin (2 U) and rifampin (15 μg) and are susceptible to kanamycin (1 mg). Finally, these bacteria are indole positive and do not ferment carbohydrates.

The *Fusobacterium,* another group of gram-negative anaerobic bacilli, are found as normal flora of the upper respiratory tract, GI tract, and urinary tract. Infections include serious pulmonary and blood infections, brain abscesses, and sinus and dental infections. These infections often are associated with metastatic conditions. The species isolated most frequently is *Fusobacterium nucleatum,* which is associated with pleuropulmonary infections, including lung abscesses and pneumonia. The organism appears as spindle-shaped cells in long filaments with tapered or pointed ends. An important characteristic is the colonial morphology, which is opalescent with speckles when viewed under a stereoscope. *F. nucleatum* is quite inactive biochemically, yielding a positive indole reaction but negative reactions for catalase, esculin hydrolysis, growth in 20% bile, gelatin, lipase, and lecithinase. It cannot ferment glucose.

Another important species is *Fusobacterium necrophorum,* which is associated with particularly virulent infections, including septicemia and metastatic infections such as lung and liver abscesses, arthritis, and osteomyelitis. The organism is indole and lipase positive. Negative reactions are seen for catalase, esculin hydrolysis, growth in 20% bile, gelatin, and lecithinase. The organism can ferment glucose.

Table 16-3 outlines reactions used to identify some of the more important gram-negative anaerobes.

after ingestion and include foul-smelling stools and diarrhea, but usually no vomiting occurs. The organism is also known to cause a necrotizing bowel disease characterized by abdominal cramps, vomiting, bloody diarrhea, and acute inflammation. Death may occur from fluid and electrolyte loss. These effects are caused by the production of beta toxin. The condition is rare in the United States but occurs in other parts of the world.

C. perfringens is identified through the clinical picture and its typical **double zone of hemolysis** on anaerobic blood agar. The inner zone is completely lysed due to **theta toxin,** while the outer zone is incompletely hemolyzed due to **alpha toxin** and **lecithinase** activity. It is lecithinase positive and ferments glucose, lactose, maltose, and fructose. Lecithinase produces an opaque yellow halo on egg yolk agar. Spores are round and subterminal but are usually impossible to demonstrate. The organism is nonmotile.

If *C. perfringens* is suspected, a **Nagler plate** can be inoculated. One-half the surface of the plate is streaked with a few drops of *C. perfringens* type A antitoxin. Then the suspected culture is streaked across the plate at a right angle to the antitoxin. A zone of precipitation around the colonies on the side without antitoxin, with little or no precipitation around colonies on the side with antitoxin, indicates a positive lecithinase test. A limited number of *Clostridium* species, including *C. perfringens, C. sordellii,* and *C. bifermentans,* give a positive Nagler reaction. Because the antisera is difficult to obtain commercially, the Nagler reaction is not usually performed in clinical laboratories.

The **reverse CAMP** procedure can be performed to confirm the presence of *C. perfringens.* In this technique the suspected clostridial species is streaked on a blood agar plate. Group B streptococcus *(Streptococcus agalactiae)* is streaked at a right angle to the first streak. After incubation, a positive reaction is indicated by the formation of an arrowhead at the intersection of the two streaks.

Miscellaneous Clostridia

Clostridium ramosum is normal flora of the large bowel and is an important agent in intraabdominal infections following trauma. It usually stains gram negative, which can lead to erroneous results. To differentiate from *Fusobacterium, C. ramosum* is indole negative, whereas *Fusobacterium* species are indole positive. *C. ramosum* grows well on 20% bile agar, hydrolyzes esculin, and does not produce lecithinase, catalase, or lipase. It produces round to oval terminal spores that are difficult to demonstrate. The organism is highly fermentative and can utilize glucose, lactose, maltose, fructose, and mannitol.

Clostridium septicum is a cause of bacteremia associated with malignancies, such as colon and breast cancer, and leukemia. The organism produces oval, subterminal spores and is gelatinase positive. *C. septicum* does not produce lecithinase, lipase, or indole but ferments glucose, lactose, maltose, and fructose. The organism does not ferment mannitol.

Clostridium difficile was first isolated in 1975 and was considered nonpathogenic until a few years later, when it was isolated as an important cause of antibiotic-associated pseudomembranous colitis. The organism is carried as normal flora in the GI tract and urethra of a small percentage of healthy adults and up to one third of hospitalized adults. It is also found in the soil and water. As an important cause of hospital-acquired diarrhea and colitis, *C. difficile* is frequently found in patients who have received one or more broad-spectrum antibiotics, including the aminoglycosides, penicillins, second- and third-generation beta-lactams, cephalosporins, erythromycin, clindamycin, and rifampin. It has also been associated as a cause of pseudomembranous colitis and diarrhea in patients who have not undergone antibiotic therapy.

C. difficile produces toxin A, an enterotoxin, and toxin B, a cytotoxin. Several commercial products are available that demonstrate the cytotoxin. Identification of *C. difficile* is usually accomplished through demonstration of the cytotoxin. Methods include enzyme immunoassay, tissue culture, and latex agglutination. Enzyme immunoassay procedures currently available include the *C. difficile* toxin A procedure (Meridian Diagnostics) and the Culturette Brand Toxin CD (Becton Dickinson Microbiology Systems). The Culturette Brand CDT, also available from Becton Dickinson, uses latex agglutination and is a useful screening procedure. Tissue culture remains the "gold standard" for toxin identification. Although more cumbersome to perform, some recommend that tissue culture be used as a confirming test. Although it can be isolated from stool culture, this generally is no longer performed.

C. difficile produces gelatinase but is negative for lecithinase, lipase, and indole. It ferments glucose and fructose but not lactose, maltose, or xylose. Spores are oval and subterminal. The organism is motile and fluoresces under ultraviolet light.

Table 16-4 outlines biochemical reactions to identify *Clostridium* species.

ANAEROBIC GRAM-POSITIVE NON–SPORE-FORMING BACILLI

The anaerobic gram-positive non–spore-forming bacilli are predominantly normal flora. The organisms, which include ***Bifidobacterium, Eubacterium, Lactobacillus, Actinomyces,*** and ***Propionibacterium,*** are normal flora of the human urinary tract, oral cavity, bowel, and vagina.

Actinomyces may be normal flora of the mouth and urogenital tract. It is associated with opportunistic in-

TABLE 16–4

Identification of *Clostridium* Species Using Lombard-Dowell Medium

	DIFFICILE	*PERFRINGENS*	*RAMOSUM*	*SEPTICUM*	*SORDELLII*	*TETANI*
PRESUMPTO PLATE 1						
Indole	–	–	–	–	+	+
Esculin hydrolysis	+	V	+	+	–	–
H_2S	–	N/A	N/A	N/A	V	V
Catalase	–	–	–	–	–	–
Lecithinase	–	+	–	–	+	–
Lipase	–	–	–	–	–	–
Growth on 20% Bile	E	E	E	E	E	E
PRESUMPTO PLATE 2						
Glucose fermented	+	+	+	+	+	–
Starch hydrolysis	–	V	–	–	–	–
Milk digested	–	–	–	V	+	–
DNase	V	+	–	+	–	+
PRESUMPTO PLATE 3						
Gelatin hydrolysis	V	+	–	+	+	+
Fermentation of mannitol	+	–	+	–	–	–
Lactose	–	+	+	+	–	–
Rhamnose	–	–	+	–	–	–

+, Most strains positive; –, most strains negative; V, variable reaction; E, growth on 20% bile equal to that without bile; I, growth on 20% bile inhibited; N/A, not applicable.

fections of endogenous origin. The most significant species is ***Actinomyces israelii,*** which is usually isolated in mixed anaerobic infections and as an agent of pelvic **actinomycoses.** Actinomycosis is characterized by the presence of "sulfur granules" in the exudate of the infection. Cells are branching and diphtheroid in appearance. On agar, the organism grows heaped, rough, and white, and the colonies are described as resembling a "molar tooth."

Bifidobacterium is normal flora of the GI tract and is a rare cause of pulmonary infections.

Propionibacterium acnes is the most frequent gram-positive non-spore-forming bacillus isolated from clinical cultures. It is normal flora of the skin, nasopharynx, oral cavity, and GI tract. A rare cause of endocarditis, *P. acnes* is more often found as a skin contaminant in blood cultures. Because it is a frequent contaminant, an emphasis must be placed on the proper disinfection of skin in preparation for blood cultures, lumbar puncture, or aspiration of abscesses. *P. acnes* produces propionic acid as the major end product of glucose metabolism. Sometimes referred to as "anaerobic diphtheroids," the organism resembles the corynebacteria as "Chinese letters" or "picket fences."

Eubacterium is rarely isolated from wounds and abscesses in mixed infections.

ANAEROBIC COCCI

The anaerobic cocci are normal flora of the bowel, female genital tract, oral cavity, skin, and respiratory tract. They are associated with abscesses of the liver and brain and with wound infections and infections of the female genital tract, abdominal cavity, and respiratory tract.

The anaerobic gram-positive cocci include:

Peptococcus niger
Peptostreptococcus anaerobius, P. productus, P. tetradius, P. micros, P. macros, P. magnus
Anaerobic *Streptococcus intermedius, S. constellatus*
Ruminococcus
Coprococcus

Peptococcus is commonly known as "anaerobic staphylococcus." It typically appears in clusters and is catalase positive. It is a rare cause of human infections.

There are seven species of *Peptostreptococcus,* which are commonly known as "anaerobic streptococci." *P. anaerobius* appears as large coccobacilli in chains on Gram-stained preparations, and *P. tetradius* appears as tetrads. *P. anaerobius* is unique in its resistance to sodium polyanethol sulfonate (SPS); it is also resistant to kanamycin and colistin.

The gram-negative anaerobic cocci include:

Veillonella
Megasphaera
Acidoaminococcus

Veillonella appears as gram-negative cocci arranged in pairs, short chains, or irregular clumps. It is a rare cause of human infection. Because of its high sensitivity to oxygen, *Veillonella* is not usually isolated unless a glove box is used.

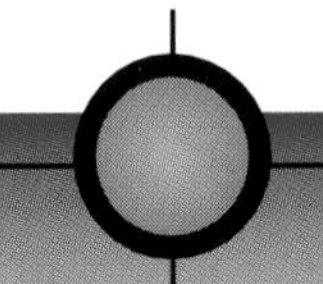

PROCEDURE
ANAEROBIC BLOOD AGAR

PURPOSE
Anaerobic blood agar (CDC) is an enriched medium to isolate all anaerobic bacteria, including obligate, facultative, and fastidious anaerobes.

PRINCIPLE
The medium contains 5% defibrinated sheep blood base, which is enriched with yeast, hemin, and vitamin K. The reducing agent L-cystine is also incorporated into the medium.

PROCEDURE
1. Streak plate for isolation.
2. Incubate anaerobically at 35°C for a minimum of 48 hours.
3. Interpret plate at 48 hours for growth, colonial morphology, and hemolysis.
4. Plates are generally incubated for an additional 2 to 4 days.

QUALITY CONTROL
Clostridium perfringens: growth with double zone of hemolysis around colonies
Bacteroides fragilis: growth

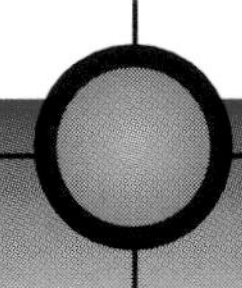

PROCEDURE

ANAEROBIC BLOOD AGAR WITH KANAMYCIN AND VANCOMYCIN

PURPOSE

Anaerobic blood agar with kanamycin and vancomycin is recommended for isolation of gram-negative anaerobes, particularly *Bacteroides, Prevotella,* and some *Fusobacterium.*

PRINCIPLE

The medium is the anaerobic blood agar base (CDC) with the antibiotics kanamycin and vancomycin. Kanamycin inhibits facultative gram-negative bacilli. Vancomycin inhibits facultative and obligate gram-positive bacteria.

PROCEDURE

1. Streak plate for isolation.
2. Incubate anaerobically for a minimum of 48 hours.
3. Interpret plate at 48 hours for growth.
4. Plates are generally incubated for an additional 2 to 4 days.

QUALITY CONTROL

Bacteroides fragilis: growth
Clostridium perfringens: no growth

NOTES

1. Laked blood agar with paromomycin or kanamycin and vancomycin is similar to anaerobic blood agar with kanamycin and vancomycin (CDC). Laked blood is prepared by freezing and then thawing whole blood.
2. Pigment production by *Prevotella melaninogenica* is enhanced on laked blood medium.

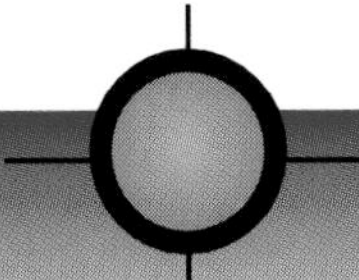

PROCEDURE

MISCELLANEOUS TESTS TO IDENTIFY ANAEROBES

1. Susceptibility to **sodium polyanethol sulfonate (SPS)** can be performed by placing a 1 mg SPS disk on the culture streaked on anaerobic blood agar. A zone of 12 mm or more is considered sensitive.
2. **Catalase** activity is determined by suspending the suspected colony in one drop of 10% to 15% hydrogen peroxide. A positive reaction is indicated by bubbling. Take care to avoid picking up the blood agar, since this can lead to a false-positive reaction.
3. **Nitrate** reduction can be determined by adding one drop of sulfanilic acid and one drop of alpha-naphthylamine to a nitrate disk that has been placed on the inoculum on anaerobic blood agar. A pink to red color is positive. Sprinkle zinc dust on all negative reactions to ensure that nitrates were not totally reduced to nitrogen gas. A pink-red color after zinc application indicates the presence of nitrate (a negative reaction).
4. **Indole** production is determined by rubbing growth from a pure culture grown on tryptophan medium onto a piece of filter paper. Add 1% paradimethylaminocinnamaldehyde reagent. The test can also be performed by placing a sterile blank disk on the heavy growth area of a pure culture plate for 5 minutes. Remove the filter paper and place it into a empty Petri dish. Add one drop of reagent. Positive reactions are indicated by a blue color.
5. Growth in **20% bile** is useful for classification of the anaerobic gram-negative bacilli. Thioglycollate medium containing 20% bile is inoculated with the test organism. A control tube without the bile is similarly inoculated. Growth is compared between the two tubes. Members of the *Bacteroides fragilis* group grow well in 20% bile, whereas other members of the genus *Bacteroides* are inhibited.

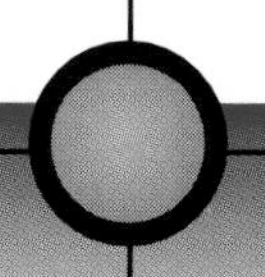

PROCEDURE

ANAEROBIC BLOOD AGAR WITH PHENYLETHYL ALCOHOL

PURPOSE

Anaerobic blood agar with phenylethyl alcohol (PEA) isolates gram-positive and gram-negative obligate anaerobes.

PRINCIPLE

The medium is an anaerobic blood agar base with PEA added. The medium inhibits the growth of gram-negative facultative anaerobes, such as the Enterobacteriaceae, and the swarming of *Proteus.* The medium permits the isolation of obligate anaerobes. Facultative gram-positive anaerobes, such as *Staphylococcus,* can also grow on PEA.

PROCEDURE

1. Streak PEA plate for isolation.
2. Incubate anaerobically for a minimum of 48 hours.
3. Interpret plate for growth.
4. Plates are generally incubated for an additional 2 to 4 days.

QUALITY CONTROL

Peptostreptococcus anaerobius: growth
Escherichia coli: no growth

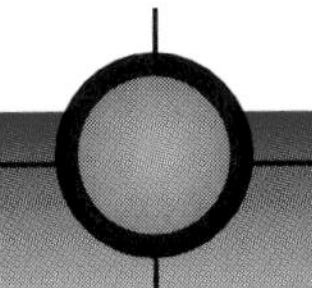

PROCEDURE

PRELIMINARY IDENTIFICATION OF ANAEROBES

Key factors in identification of anaerobes include colonial characterizations, pigment production, hemolysis, pitting of agar surface, Gram stain morphology, presence and location of spores, and susceptibility to high levels of antibiotics. Also, various biochemical reactions can be used to identify anaerobes. Packaged systems are available commercially.

PRINCIPLE

The **Presumpto Plates** developed by Dowell and Lombard provide 12 biochemical reactions (three plates with four quadrants each) that can be used in the preliminary identification of anaerobes. Presumpto Plates are available through Remel or Carr Scarborough. The basal medium of Lombard Dowell (LD) agar supports the growth of almost all anaerobes.

PROCEDURE

1. Prereduce plates in anaerobic jar or glove box for 2 to 4 hours at room temperature before use.
2. Prepare a no. 1 McFarland standard in LD broth for the organism to be tested.
3. Add one or two drops of broth culture to each quadrant, or saturate a swab in the broth and inoculate each quadrant with the swab. Streak three quarters of quadrant.
4. Place a sterile piece of filter paper over the LD agar to test for indole production.
5. Incubate anaerobically for 24 to 48 hours.

INTERPRETATION

PRESUMPTO PLATE 1

LD agar—growth on LD medium: note degree of growth—light, moderate, or heavy.

Indole: add two drops of paradimethylaminocinnamaldehyde reagent to the paper disk. A positive reaction is a blue or blue-green color within 30 seconds. The development of pink or red color or the lack of color development is considered negative.

Catalase: add two drops of 3% hydrogen peroxide to LD medium after exposing plates to air for at least 30 minutes. Sustained bubbling is considered a positive reaction. Reaction may take 1 minute to develop. Test can also be performed on LD esculin quadrant.

LD esculin agar—esculin hydrolysis: expose plate to air for 15 minutes. A positive reaction is given by a red-brown or dark-brown color in the agar surrounding the growth.

Hydrogen sulfide: blackening of medium is a positive reaction. It is best to observe H_2S production anaerobically or when first exposing plates to air, since it disappears when exposed to air.

PROCEDURE

PRELIMINARY IDENTIFICATION OF ANAEROBES

(Continued)

LD egg-yolk agar—lecithinase: positive reaction is a zone of insoluble precipitate in the area surrounding the growth.
Lipase: positive reaction is an "iridescent sheen" characterized by a pearly layer on the surface of the colonies and on the agar surrounding the bacteria. Add a few drops of water to questionable reactions; a thin film floating on the water is a positive reaction.
Proteolysis: positive reaction is a clearing of the medium in the area near the bacterial growth.
LD bile: compare amount of growth on LD bile with that observed on plain LD agar. Record "E" if growth is equal to or more than that observed on LD agar. Record "I" if growth is less inhibited on LD bile when compared with that on LD agar.

PRESUMPTO PLATE 2

LD glucose: fermentation of glucose is indicated by a yellow color. A blue color is negative. To determine if glucose enhances bacterial growth, compare the amount of growth on the LD glucose with that observed on LD agar.
LD starch: flood quadrant with Gram's iodine. Clearing around the colony indicates a positive reaction. Negative reactions show a brown color, which indicates nonhydrolyzed starch.
LD milk: casein hydrolysis is indicated by a clear zone around the growth and a positive reaction. A cloudy medium indicates that the milk proteins have not been hydrolyzed and a negative reaction.
LD DNA: positive DNase production is indicated by a pink-red zone surrounding the colony. A blue color is considered negative.

PRESUMPTO PLATE 3

LD mannitol—LD lactose—LD rhamnose: fermentation of the carbohydrates is indicated by a yellow color. A blue color is considered negative.
LD gelatin: add acidified mercuric chloride reagent, which binds to unhydrolyzed gelatin. A zone of complete clearing around the growth on the quadrant indicates positive gelatin hydrolysis.

LD Presumpto I, II, III, insert, Carr Scarborough Microbiologics, Inc, Stone Mountain, GA.

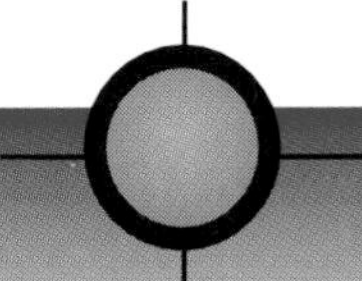

PROCEDURE
ANTIBIOTIC DISK TESTS

PURPOSE
The use of antibiotic disks to determine an anaerobe's inhibition can be a useful identification method. Most anaerobes have a characteristic susceptibility pattern to colistin (10 μg), vancomycin (5 μg), and kanamycin (1 mg).

PRINCIPLE
After streaking an anaerobic blood agar plate to obtain a lawn of growth, each antibiotic disk is placed over the area of the streak. After incubation, the plates are interpreted by measuring the zone of inhibition.

MEDIA AND MATERIAL
5 μg vancomycin disk (Va)
1 mg (1000 μg) kanamycin disk (K)
10 μg colistin disk (Co)
Anaerobic blood agar (ABA)

PROCEDURE
1. Transfer a portion of one colony to the ABA plate, and streak the first quadrant of the plate to produce a heavy lawn of growth.
2. Streak the other quadrants for isolation.
3. Place the Co, K, and Va disks in the first quadrant well separated from each other.
4. Incubate the plates anaerobically for 48 hours at 35°C.

INTERPRETATION
Observe for a zone of inhibition of growth. A zone of 10 mm or less indicates resistance, and a zone greater than 10 mm indicates susceptibility. Zone-size interpretation is not to be used as an indicator to predict clinical susceptibility.

PROCEDURE
ANTIBIOTIC DISK TESTS
(Continued)

QUALITY CONTROL

Fusobacterium necrophorum: susceptible to K and Co; resistant to Va
Bacteroides fragilis: resistant to K, Co, and Va
Clostridium perfringens: susceptible to Va and K; resistant to Co

NOTES

1. Gram-positive anaerobes are usually susceptible to Va and K and resistant to Co.
2. Kanamycin can be used to separate *Fusobacterium,* which are susceptible, from *Bacteroides,* which are usually resistant.

ORGANISM	KANAMYCIN (1000 µg)	COLISTIN (10 µg)	VANCOMYCIN (5 µg)
Bacteroides fragilis *group*	*R*	*R*	*R*
Other Bacteroides *species*	*R*	*V*	*R*
Pigmented Bacteroides *species*	*R*	*V*	*V*
Fusobacterium	S	S	R
Veillonella	S	S	R
Peptostreptococcus	V	R	S
Clostridium	S	R	S
Propionibacterium	*S*	*R*	*S*

R, Resistant; S, susceptible; V, variable.

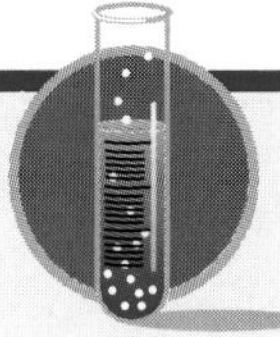

LABORATORY EXERCISES

1

Observe prepared Gram-stained smears of the following anaerobes and make a sketch of your findings.

Bacteroides fragilis

Clostridium perfringens

Peptostreptococcus anaerobius

Peptococcus niger

Fusobacterium nucleatum

LABORATORY EXERCISES

(Continued)

2

Plate the following stock organisms on phenylethyl alcohol (PEA) and kanamycin-vancomycin (KV), and inoculate a thioglycollate (Thio). Incubate under anaerobic atmosphere. Describe your findings and record your observations.

	PEA	KV	Thio
B. fragilis			
F. nucleatum			
P. niger			
C. perfringens			

3

Explain the principle of the anaerobic jar method. Properly prepare the activator, catalyst, and indicator for incubation of cultures.

Continued.

LABORATORY EXERCISES

(Continued)

4

Using the Lombard Dowell medium, inoculate one set for each of the following organisms and an unknown anaerobe. Interpret and record your results.

	B. fragilis	*F. nucleatum*	*C. perfringens*	*Unknown*
Unknown number: ______				
Indole				
Esculin hydrolysis				
H_2S				
Catalase				
Lecithinase				
Lipase				
Growth 20% bile				
Glucose fermented				
Starch hydrolysis				
Milk digested				
DNase				
Gelatin hydrolysis				
Mannitol fermented				
Lactose fermented				
Rhamnose fermented				
Gram stain				
Colonial morphology				
Identification:				

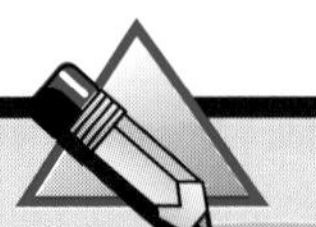

REVIEW QUESTIONS

MATCHING

Match each of the following anaerobic media with its purpose:

____ **1. Enriched broth to supplement plating media**
____ **2. Isolation of obligate and facultative anaerobes**
____ **3. Inhibition of gram-positive anaerobes and facultative gram-negative bacilli**
____ **4. Ability of organism to grow in 20% bile and hydrolyze esculin**
____ **5. Inhibition of Enterobacteriaceae and swarming of *Proteus;* allows for isolation of gram-positive and gram-negative obligate anaerobes.**

a. Thioglycollate
b. Anaerobic blood agar
c. Anaerobic PEA
d. Anaerobic KVBA
e. BBE

Match the *Clostridium* species with its associated infection:

____ **6. *C. tetani***
____ **7. *C. botulinum***
____ **8. *C. difficile***
____ **9. *C. perfringens***

a. Pseudomembranous colitis
b. Myonecrosis
c. Tetanus
d. Botulism

MULTIPLE CHOICE

10. An organism that cannot use oxygen as the final electron acceptor and is inhibited by its presence is a(an):
a. Obligate aerobe
b. Obligate anaerobe
c. Facultative anaerobe
d. Microaerophile

For each of the following, indicate if the specimen is acceptable (A) or unacceptable (U) for anaerobic culture.

11. ____ **Peritoneal fluid**
12. ____ **Vaginal swab**
13. ____ **Exudate from abscess**
14. ____ **Feces**
15. ____ **Necrotic tissue**
16. ____ **Sputum**
17. ____ **Tissue from liver abscess**
18. ____ **Swab of wound**

19. Which of the following is the environment achieved in the anaerobic glove box?
a. 85% hydrogen, 5% carbon dioxide, 5% nitrogen
b. 85% nitrogen, 10% hydrogen, 5% carbon dioxide
c. 85% oxygen, 10% hydrogen, 5% carbon dioxide
d. 75% nitrogen, 15% hydrogen, 10% carbon dioxide

20. After the incubation of cultures in an anaerobic jar, the methylene blue strip has reverted to its original blue color. This indicates.
a. Anaerobiosis has been achieved.
b. Oxygen may have entered the system.
c. The system has failed.
d. Both b and c are correct.
e. All are correct.

21. An organism isolated from anaerobic blood agar was subcultured onto both aerobic blood agar, which was incubated aerobically, and anaerobic blood agar, which was incubated anaerobically. After 48 hours, growth was evident only on the anaerobic blood agar plate. This organism is most likely:
a. An obligate aerobe
b. An obligate anaerobe
c. A facultative anaerobe
d. Capnophilic

Continued.

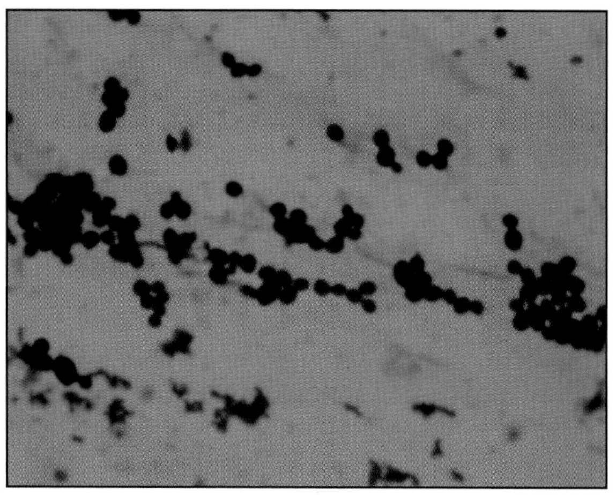

Plate 7 Gram stain of sputum, showing yeast—large, oval to round organisms that stain dark purple—with a few gram-negative bacilli, and gram-positive cocci.

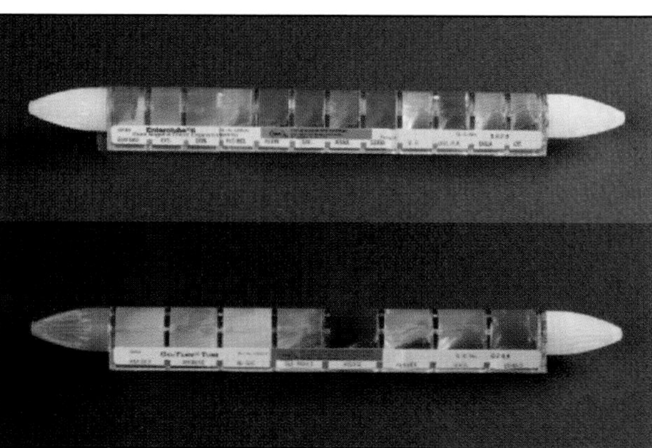

Plate 10 Enterotube and Oxi-Ferm multitest systems, which feature small pieces of agar substrates and an inoculation wire that is contained within the system.

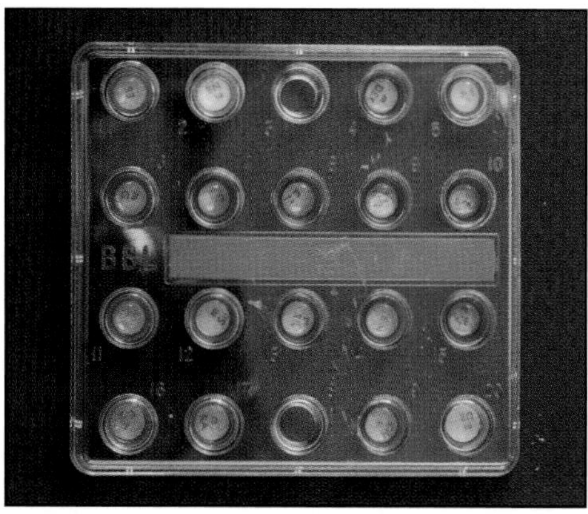

Plate 8 Minitek system is a miniaturized, multitest system for the identification of Enterobacteriaceae, anaerobes, and *Neisseria.* The system uses filter paper disks impregnated with various substrates.

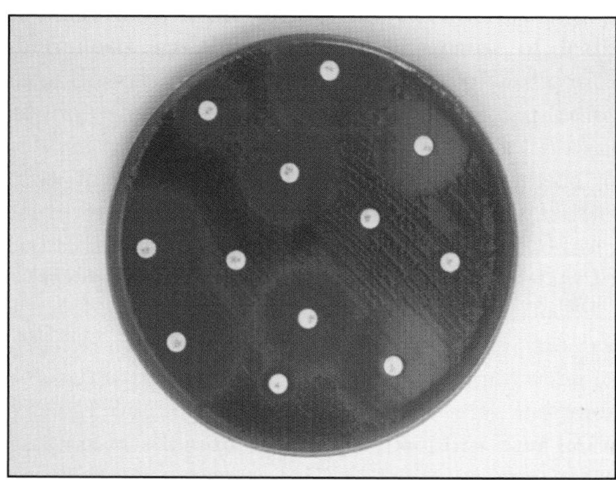

Plate 11 Kirby-Bauer susceptibility test showing Mueller-Hinton agar that has been supplemented with sheep blood. The organism is *Streptococcus pneumoniae,* which requires sheep blood for growth.

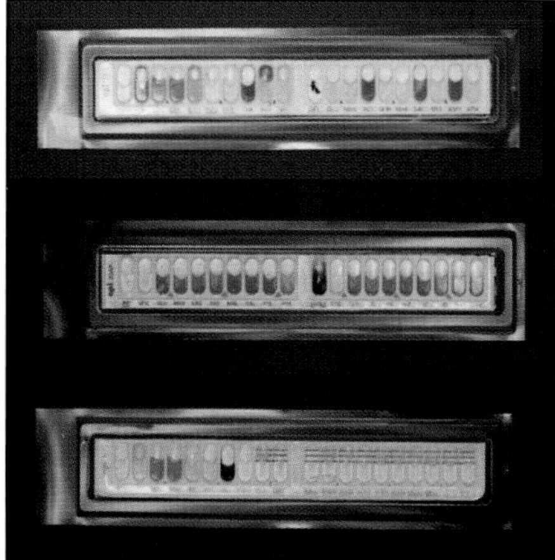

Plate 9 Miniaturized multitest systems. **A,** API 20E for identification of Enterobacteriaceae, **B,** API 20A for identification of anaerobes, and **C,** NFT for identification of nonfermentative gram-negative bacilli.

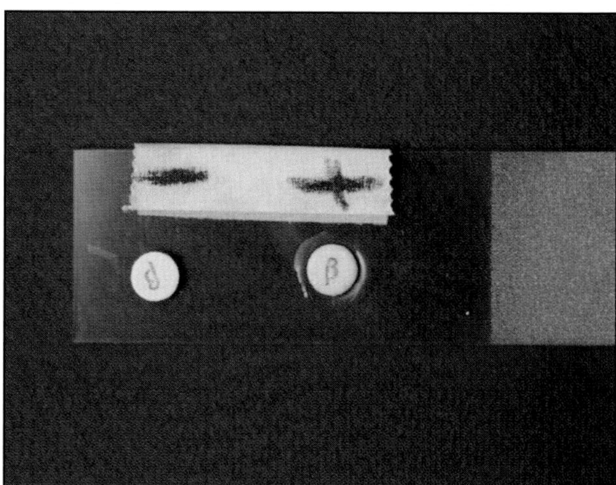

Plate 12 Cefinase procedure for determination of beta lactamase activity.

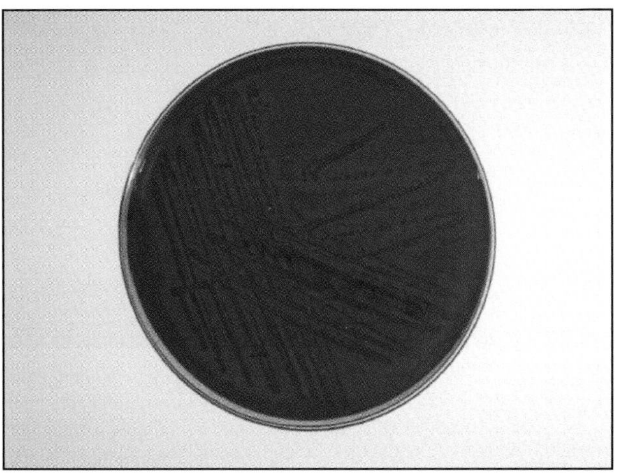

Plate 13 *Staphylococcus aureus* on sheep blood agar. Large, convex, creamy colonies of *S. aureus* may be pigmented white to golden yellow, with a narrow zone of beta hemolysis.

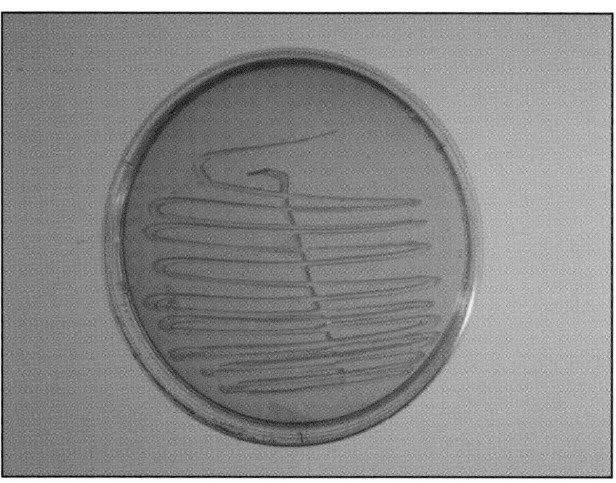

Plate 16 Mannitol salt agar showing positive fermentation of mannitol, as indicated by a yellow color. Reaction is typical of *Staphylococcus aureus.*

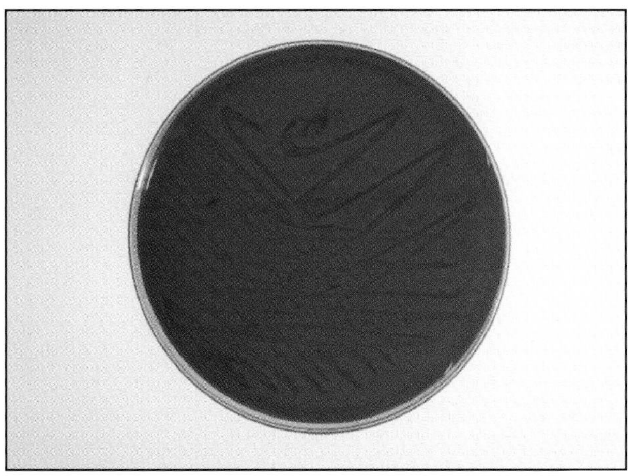

Plate 14 *Staphylococcus epidermidis* on sheep blood agar shows medium, white, creamy nonhemolytic colonies.

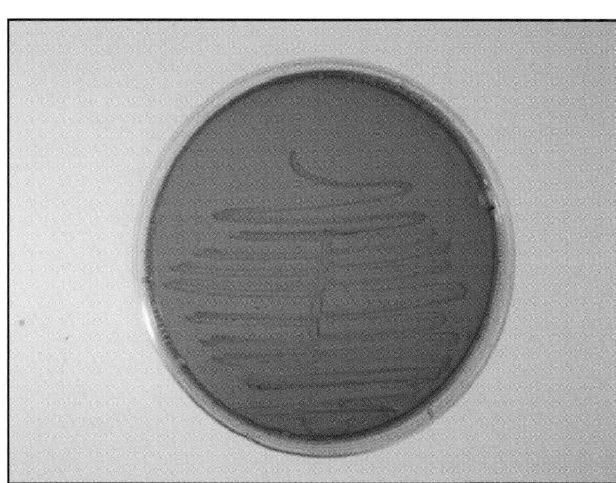

Plate 17 Mannitol salt agar showing negative fermentation of mannitol. Reaction is typical of *Staphylococcus epidermidis.*

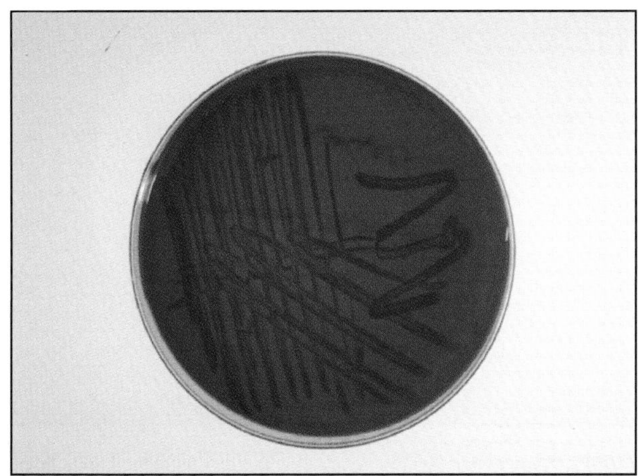

Plate 15 *Staphylococcus saprophyticus* on sheep blood agar shows medium, white, creamy, nonhemolytic colonies.

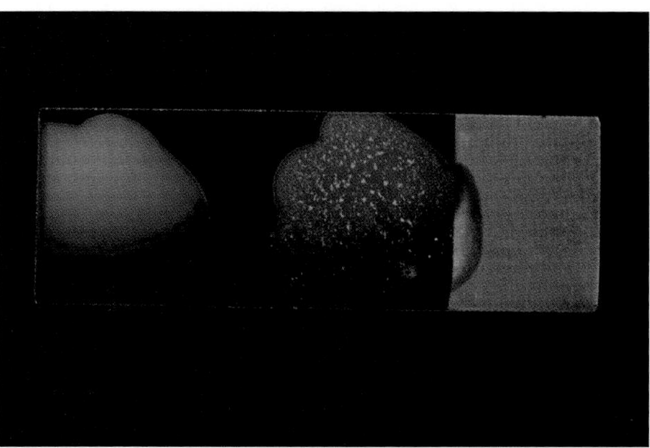

Plate 18 Bacto Staph Latex technique showing positive agglutination with yellow latex beads on the right with a negative smooth suspension on the left, indicating the presence of bound coagulase and/or protein A.

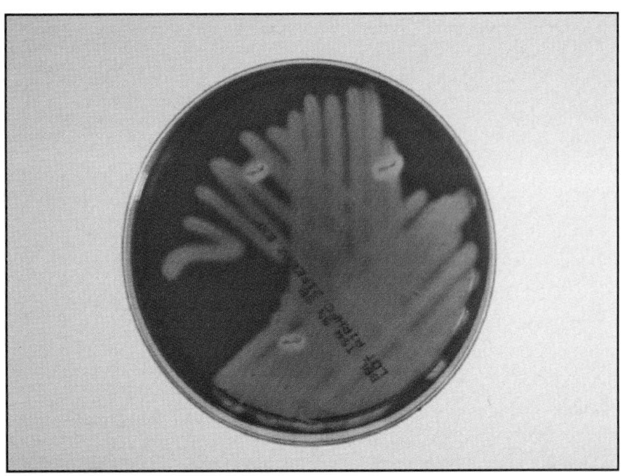

Plate 19 Group A beta-hemolytic *Streptococcus* on sheep blood agar showing small pinpoint colonies and wide zone of beta hemolysis.

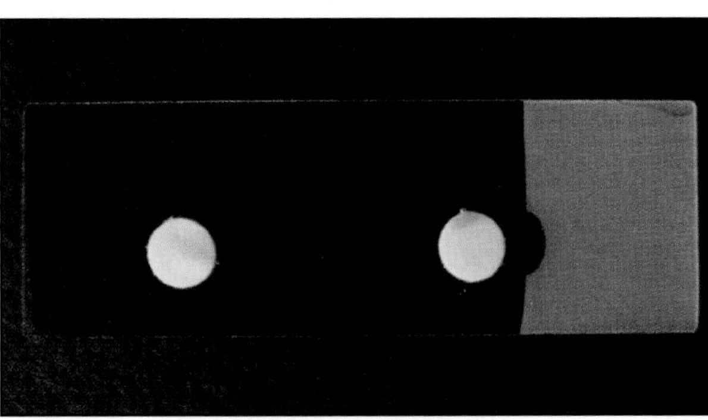

Plate 22 PYRase activity is positive for Group D *Enterococcus* and group A *Streptococcus*. The reaction can be used to differentiate *Enterococcus* (+) (*right*) from non-*Enterococcus* (−) (*left*) and as an additional test to aid in the identification of group A *Streptococcus*.

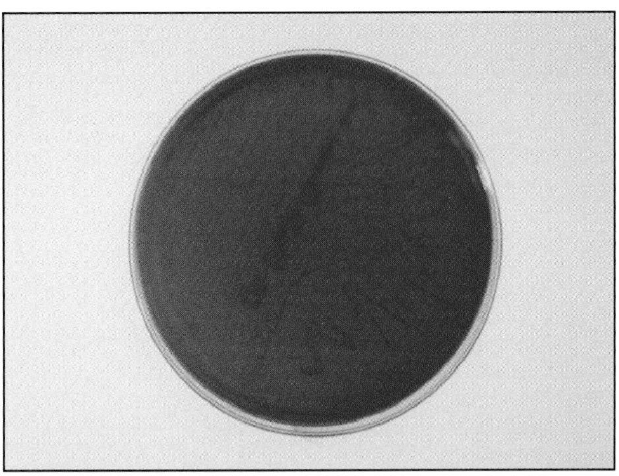

Plate 20 Group B *Streptococcus* on sheep blood agar. Colonies are pinpoint, clear, and either narrow-zone beta hemolytic or nonhemolytic.

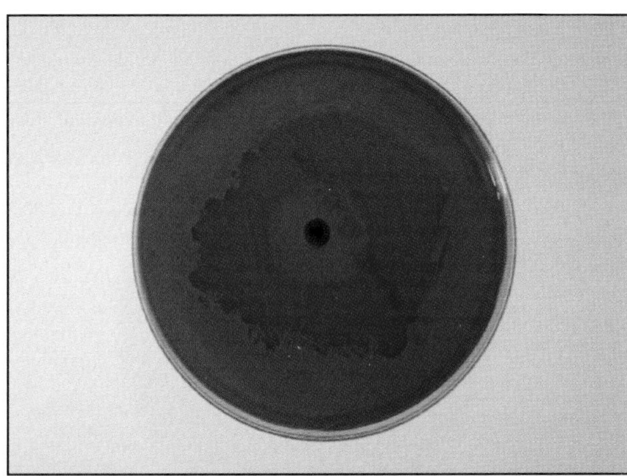

Plate 23 Optochin test for *Streptococcus pneumoniae* indicating susceptibility of the organism to 6 μg optochin. Organism is alpha hemolytic and mucoid at 24 hours.

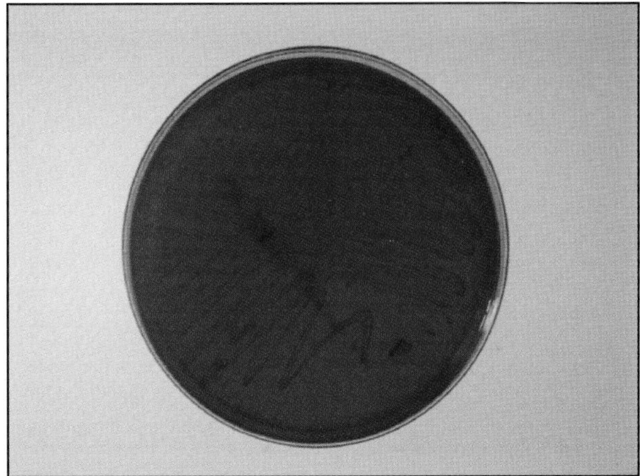

Plate 21 *Enterococcus* on sheep blood agar. Colonies are small, grayish, and may be alpha hemolytic, beta hemolytic, or nonhemolytic.

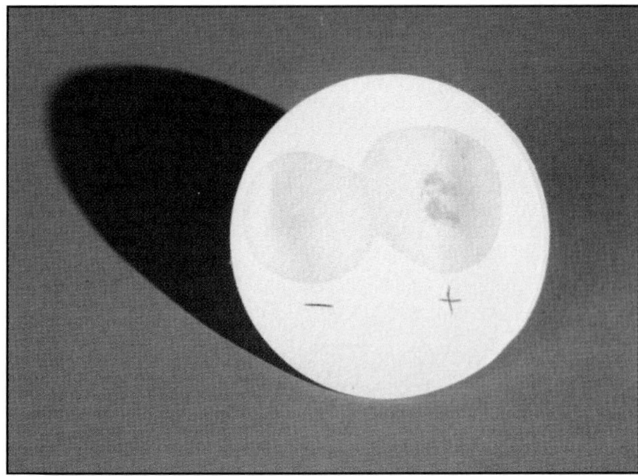

Plate 24 Cytochrome oxidase reaction illustrating positive violet color (*right*) when a *Neisseria* organism is mixed with oxidase reagent (1% tetra-methyl-para-phenylenediamine dihydrochloride). Negative reaction is shown on the left.

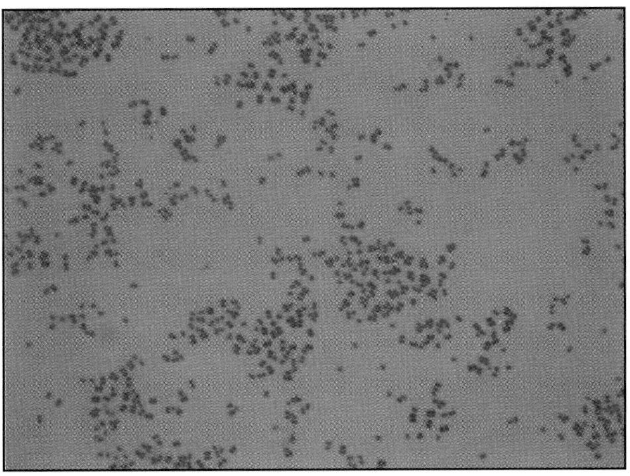

Plate 25 Gram stain smear of *Neisseria sicca* showing gram-negative diplococci.

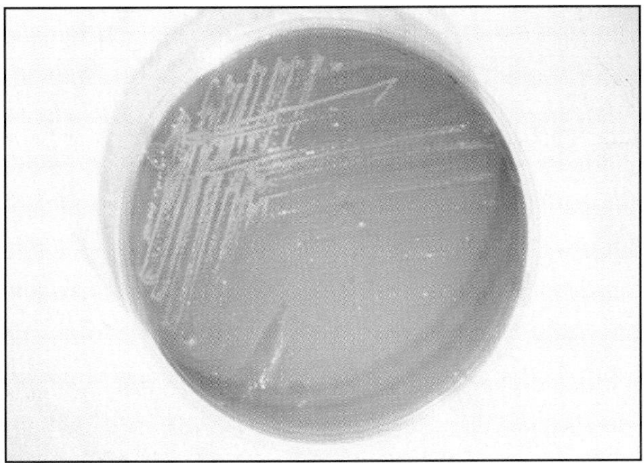

Plate 26 *Neissseria gonorrhoeae* on Martin-Lewis medium showing typical gray, translucent, shiny colonies.

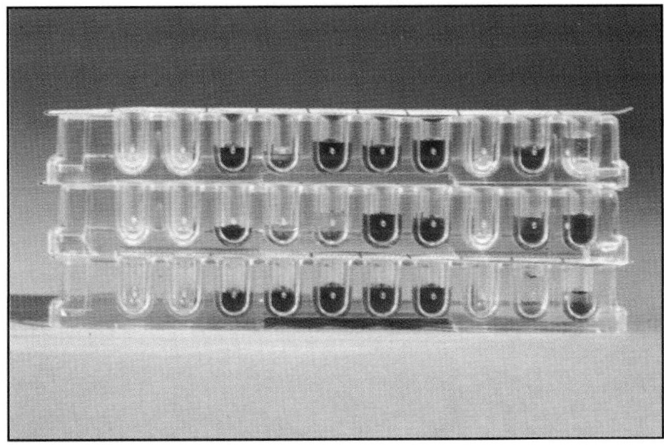

Plate 27 Quad FERM+ showing reactions typical of *Neisseria gonorrhoeae* (positive for glucose) (*top*), *N. lactamica* (positive for glucose, maltose, and lactose) (*center*), and *Moraxella catarrhalis* (negative for all carbohydrates and positive DNase activity) (*bottom*).

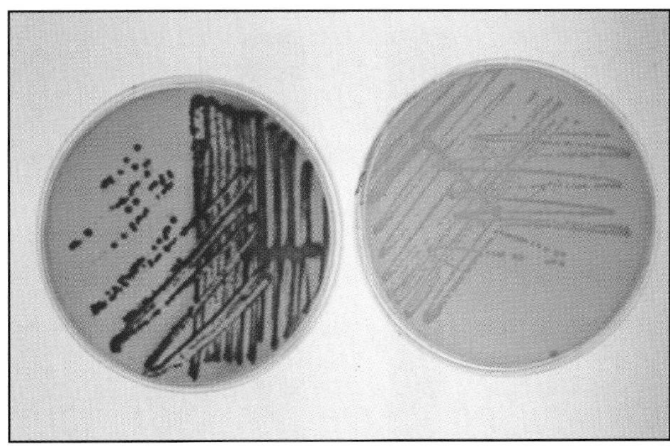

Plate 28 MacConkey agar showing pink colonies indicative of lactose fermentation and colorless colonies indicative of nonlactose fermenters.

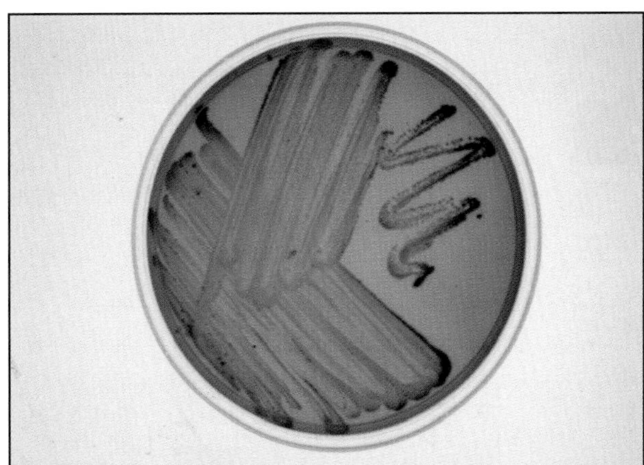

Plate 29 Hektoen-enteric agar, used to isolate and cultivate stool pathogens, showing *Salmonella* species, which grows as an H_2S positive nonferementer.

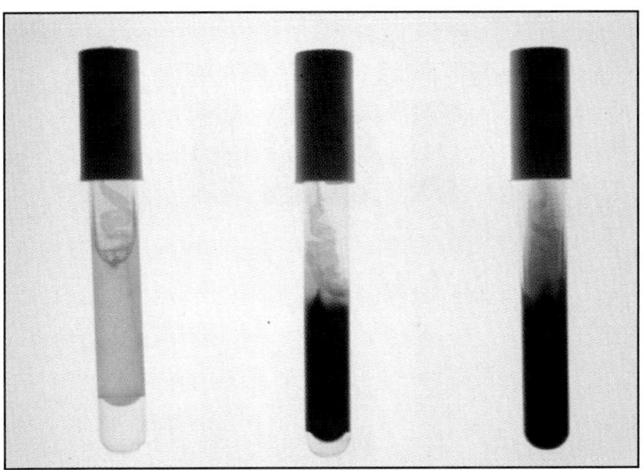

Plate 30 Triple sugar iron agar. A yellow deep indicates fermentation of glucose, whereas a yellow slant indicates fermentation of lactose and/or sucrose. Blackening indicates production of H_2S gas, and cracks in the medium indicate gas production.

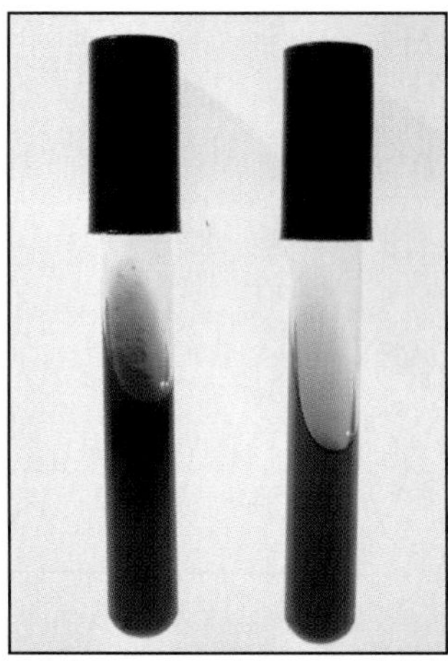

Plate 31 Citrate reaction. Positive reactions are indicated by growth and/or development of a blue color. Negative reactions are characterized by the inability of the organism to grow, with the medium remaining a green color.

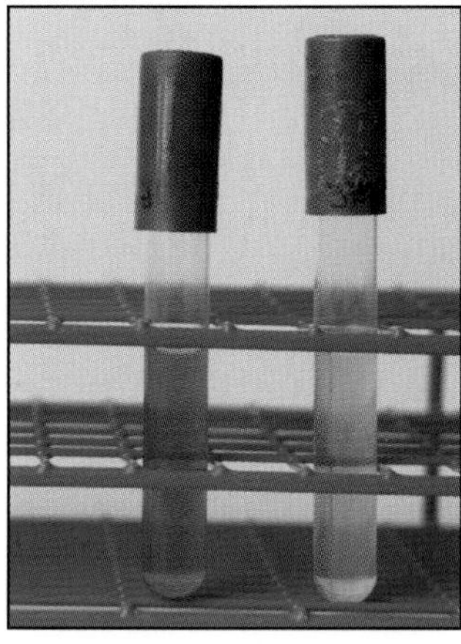

Plate 32 Ornithine decarboxylase and arginine dihydrolase reactions: a yellow color indicates the organism's ability to ferment glucose. Positive decarboxylation is illustrated by a reversion of the medium to its original purple color.

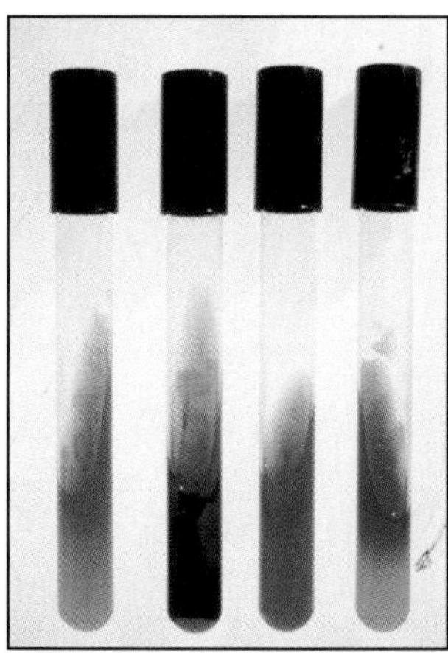

Plate 33 Lysine iron agar showing decarboxylation of lysine (purple slant/purple deep), and deamination of lysine (red slant); blackening of the medium indicates H_2S production.

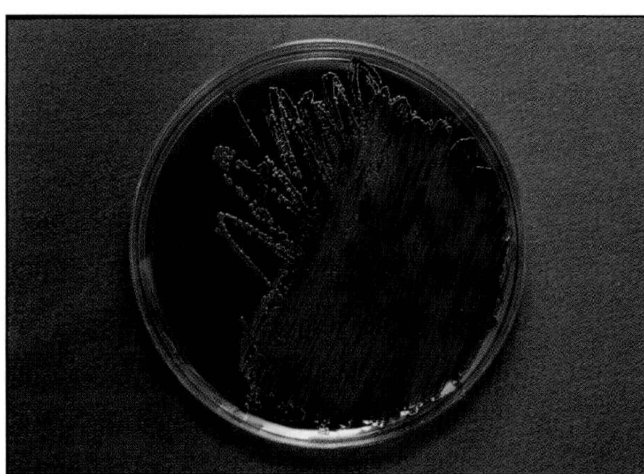

Plate 34 Eosin-methylene blue medium with *Escherichia coli,* showing the characteristic green metallic sheen of the organism on EMB, which occurs with strong lactose fermentation and precipitation of the dyes eosin and methylene blue.

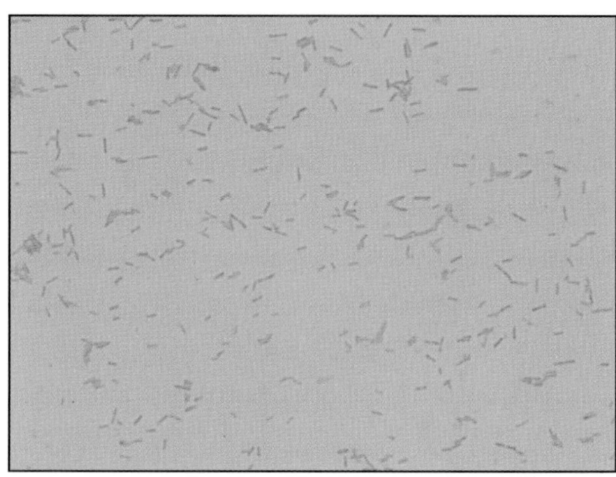

Plate 35 Gram stain of *Pseudomonas aeruginosa* illustrating long, narrow, non–spore-forming gram-negative bacillus.

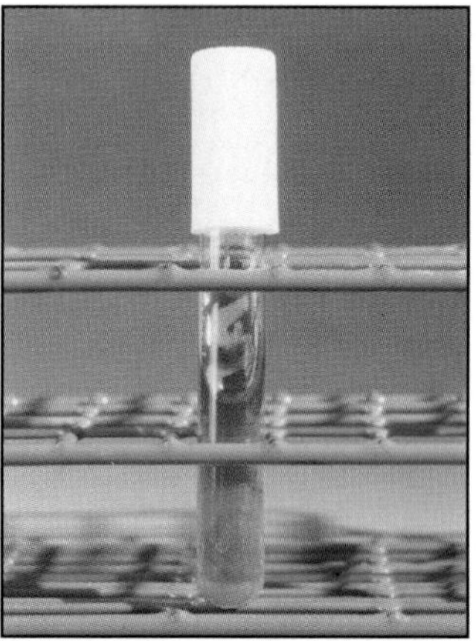

Plate 36 Triple sugar iron (TSI) agar, K/K indicates the organism's inability to ferment glucose or any carbohydrates in the TSI; this is the typical reaction of the nonfermenters. In addition, many nonfermenters are cytochrome oxidase positive.

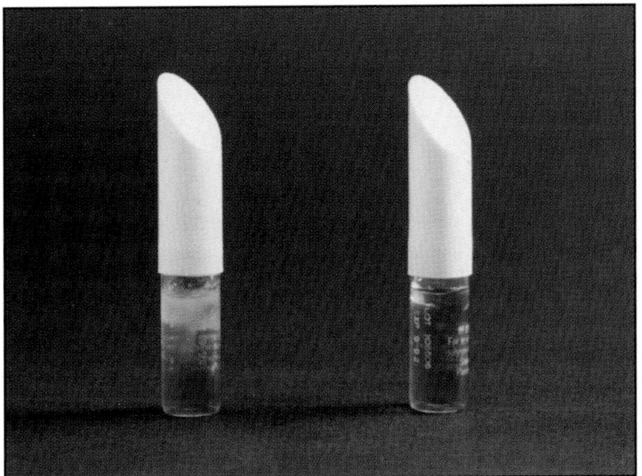

Plate 37 Oxidative-fermentative (OF) medium of Hugh and Leifson showing oxidation of glucose (yellow color), since the carbohydrate is utilized only in the open tube where oxygen is present.

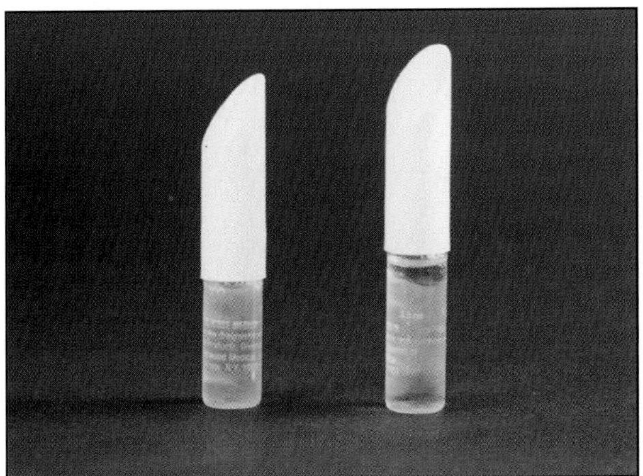

Plate 38 OF medium; fermentative. Fermentation of glucose is illustrated by utilization of the carbohydrate glucose (yellow color) in both the open and the closed tubes. Reaction is typical of members of the Enterobacteriaceae.

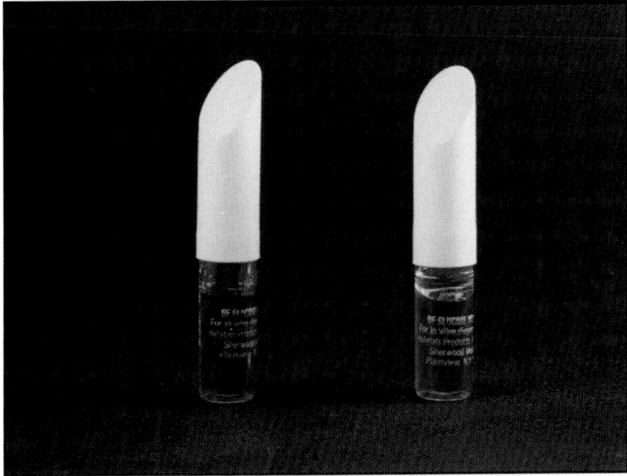

Plate 39 OF medium: nonsaccharolytic. Inability of organism to use carbohydrate either oxidatively or fermentatively is illustrated by negative (green to blue-green) reactions in both the open and closed tubes.

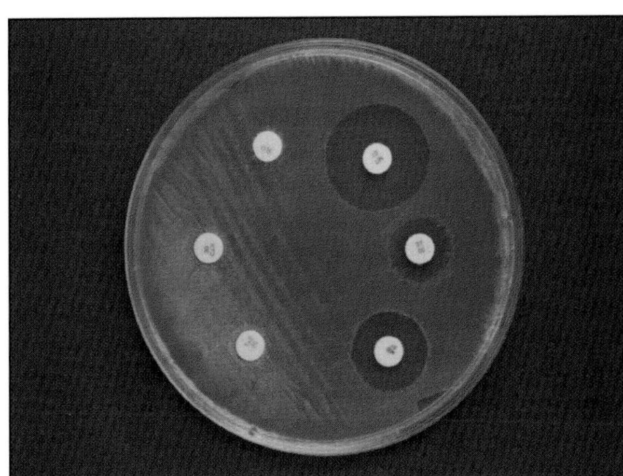

Plate 40 *Pseudomonas aeruginosa* on Mueller-Hinton medium illustrating its characteristic green to blue-green pigment.

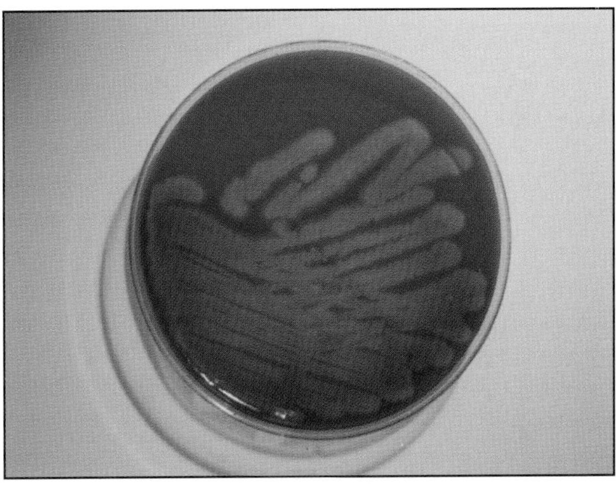

Plate 41 *Pseudomonas aeruginosa* on sheep blood agar with its typical large, dull, gray colonies that are beta hemolytic. Colonies typically have a "feathery edge" and may resemble ground glass.

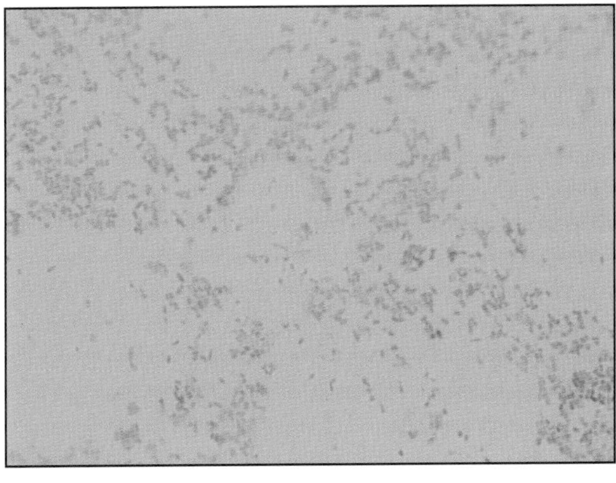

Plate 42 Gram stain of *Acinetobacter baumanni* illustrating typical morphology of the gram-negative coccobacillus.

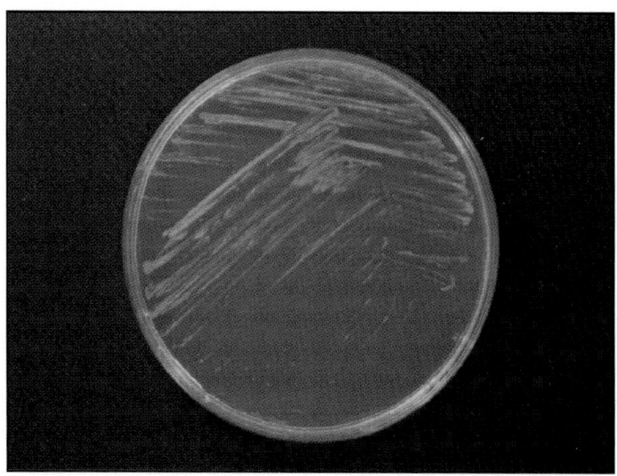

Plate 43 *Flavobacterium meningosepticum* showing its characteristic yellow pigment.

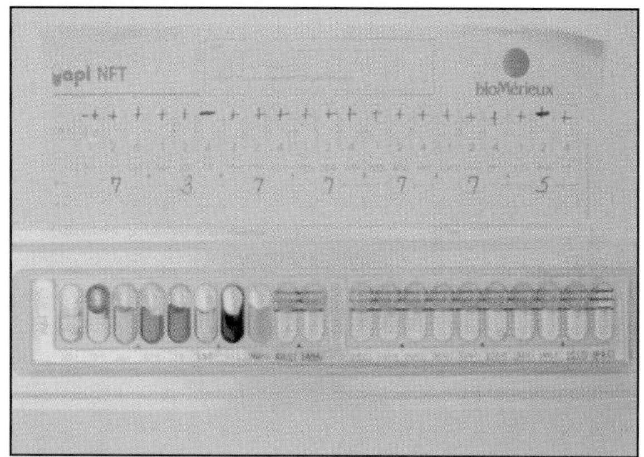

Plate 44 Rapid NFT test of *Pseudomonas aeruginosa* illustrating biochemical reactions as well as the organism's ability to assimilate various carbohydrates. A profile number is determined that can be matched to an identification number in the database.

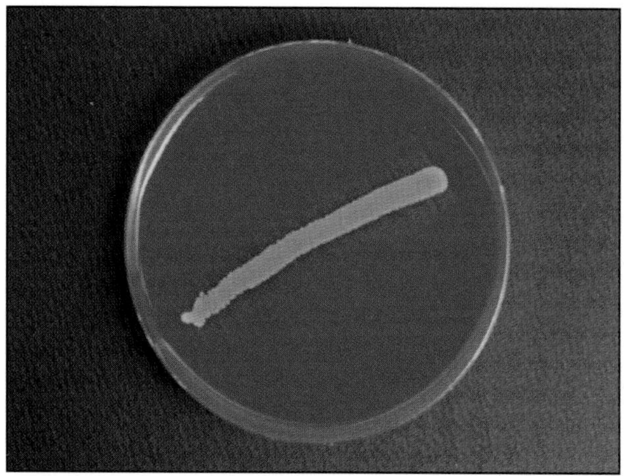

Plate 45 Satellitism on *Haemophilus influenzae* around beta-hemolytic *Staphylococcus aureus.*

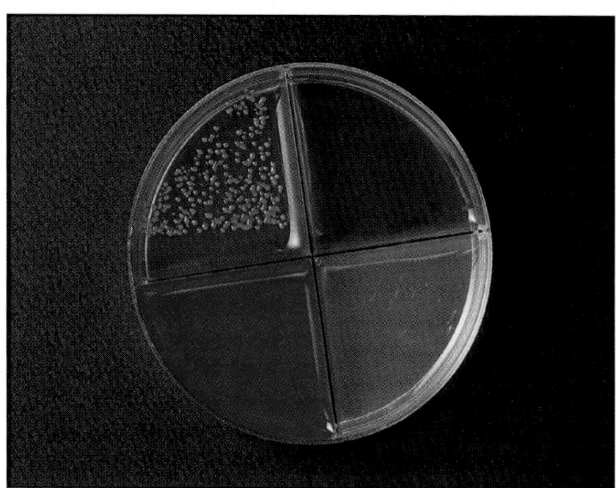

Plate 46 *Haemophilus influenzae* on *Haemophilus* ID plate showing requirement of both X and V factors and lack of hemolysis on horse blood agar.

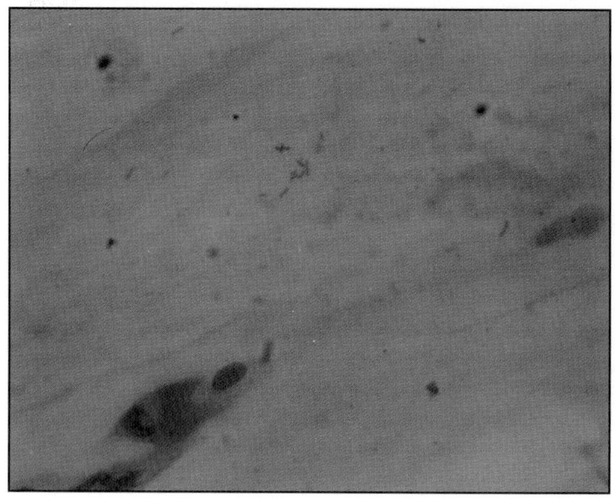

Plate 47 Gram stain of *Haemophilus influenzae* in a sputum specimen showing small, gram-negative coccobacilli.

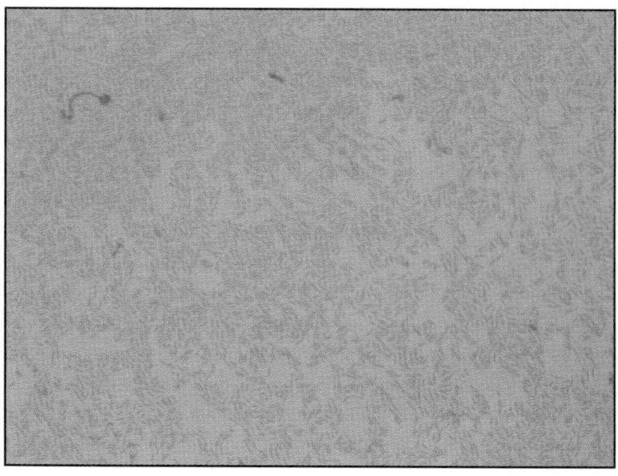

Plate 48 Gram stain of *Vibrio parahaemolyticus* showing gram-negative curved bacilli.

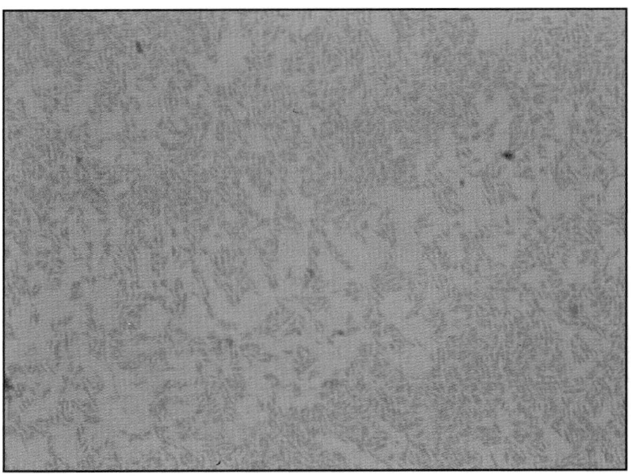

Plate 49 *Campylobacter jejuni* Gram stain showing curved gram-negative bacilli that may arrange to form a "sea gull" appearance in direct smears.

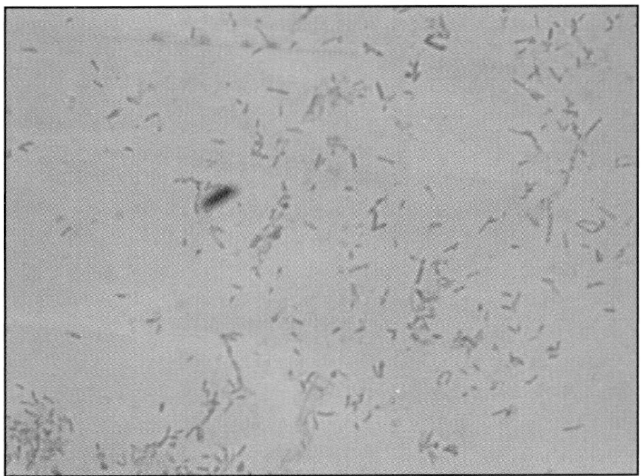

Plate 50 *Bacteroides fragilis* Gram stain showing pleomorphic, gram-negative coccobacilli that may stain bipolar.

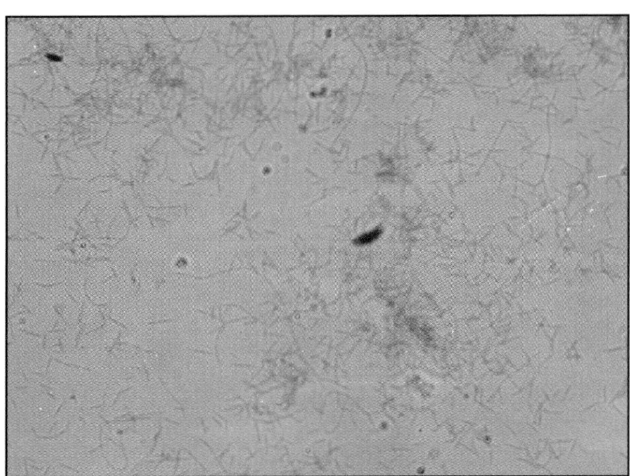

Plate 51 *Fusobacterium* Gram stain showing typical morphology of long, thin, filamentous gram-negative bacilli.

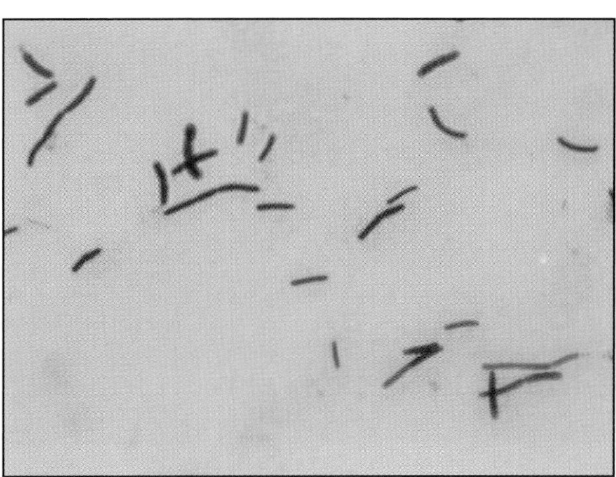

Plate 52 *Clostridium perfringens* Gram stain showing gram-positive bacilli; spores are rarely observed.

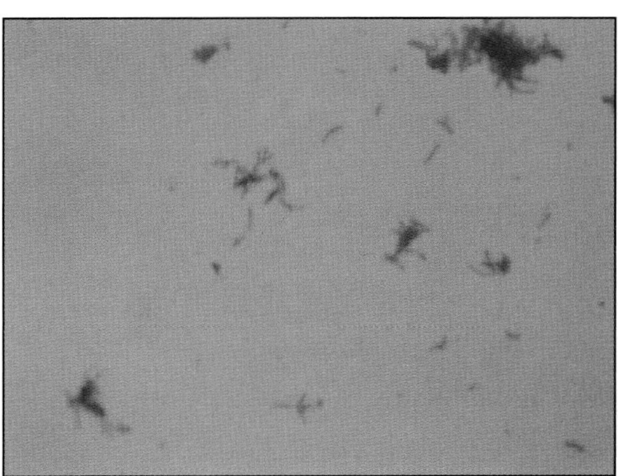

Plate 53 Carbolfuchsin stain showing red-staining acid-fast bacilli.

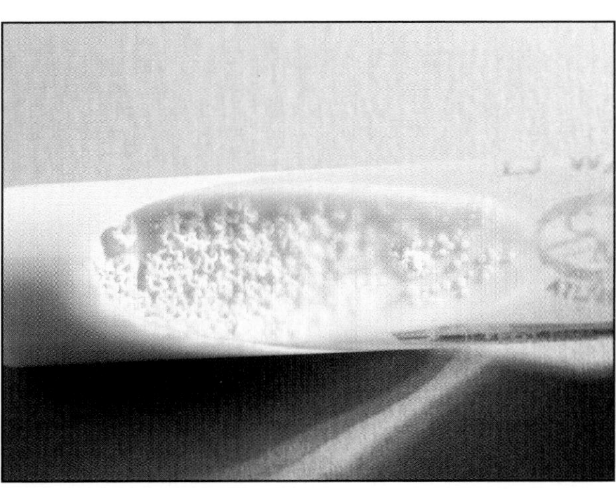

Plate 54 *Mycobacterium tuberculosis* on Löwenstein-Jensen (LJ) slant showing characteristic nonpigmented, dry, granular colonies.

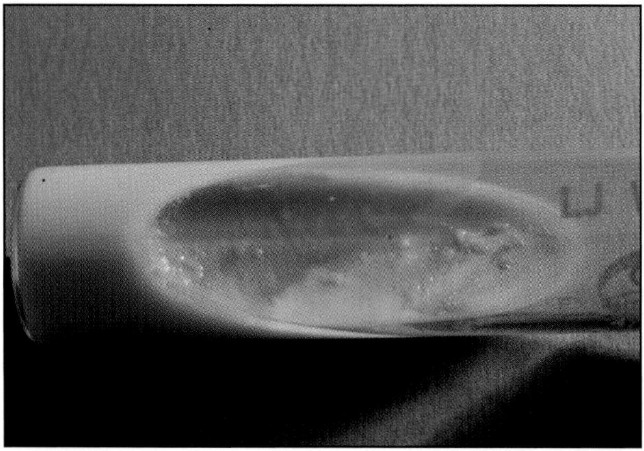

Plate 55 *Mycobacterium kansasii,* the "yellow bacillus." When grown in the light, the photochromogen produces yellow colonies that may intensify to orange to red when exposed to a constant light source.

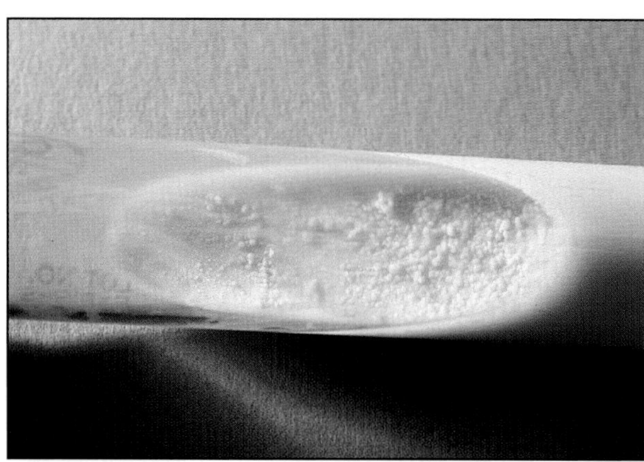

Plate 58 *Mycobacterium fortuitum,* a rapid grower, showing smooth, heaped, nonpigmented colonies.

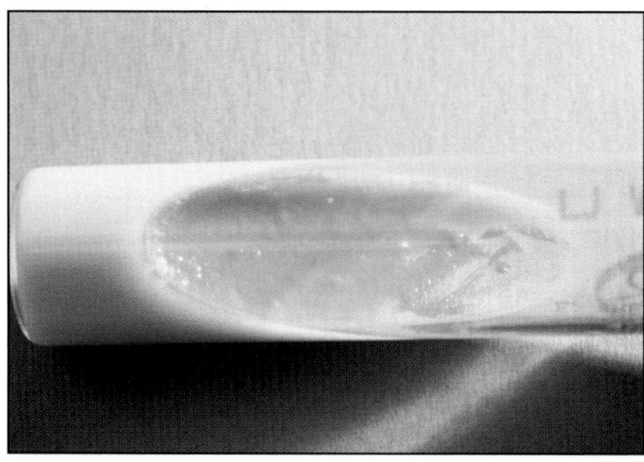

Plate 56 *Mycobacterium marinum,* a photochromogen, is nonpigmented when grown in the dark but pigmented yellow when exposed to a constant light source.

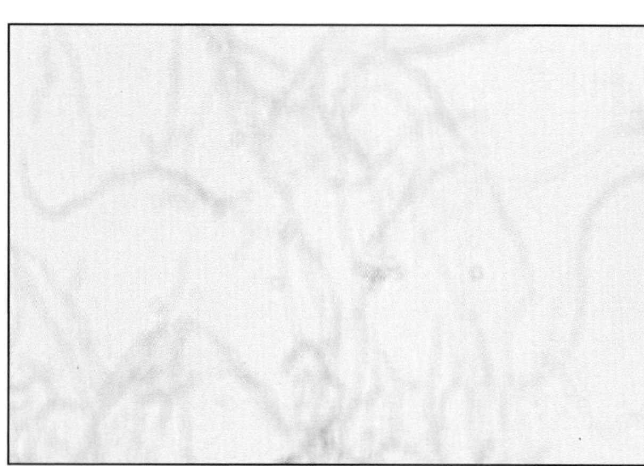

Plate 59 *Streptomyces* showing moderate acid fastness.

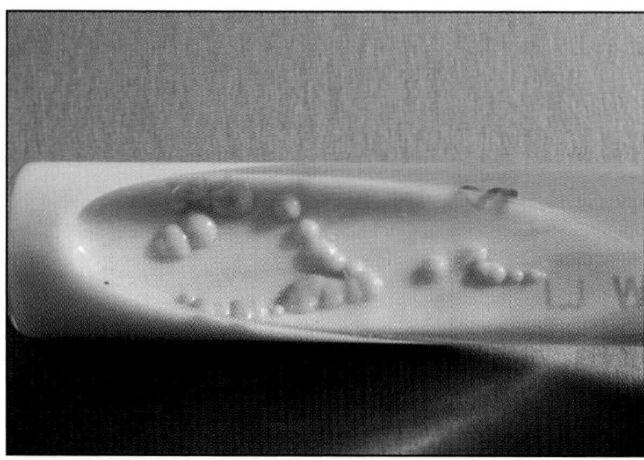

Plate 57 *Mycobacterium gordonae,* the "tap water bacillus," produces smooth, glistening yellow colonies in both the absence and the presence of light.

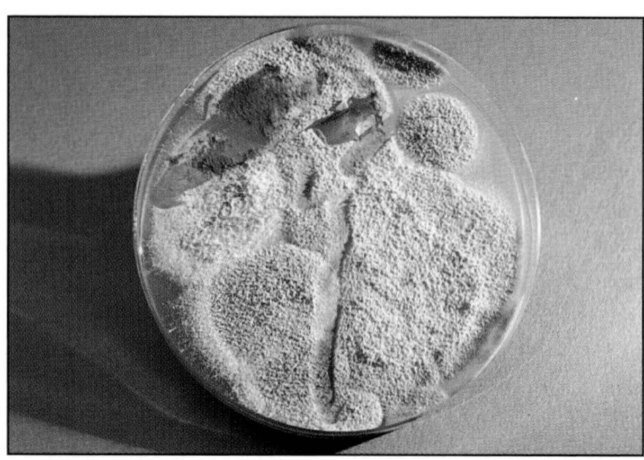

Plate 60 *Microsporum gypseum* on Sabouraud dextrose agar (SDA). Note the cinnamon-brown pigment and granular nature.

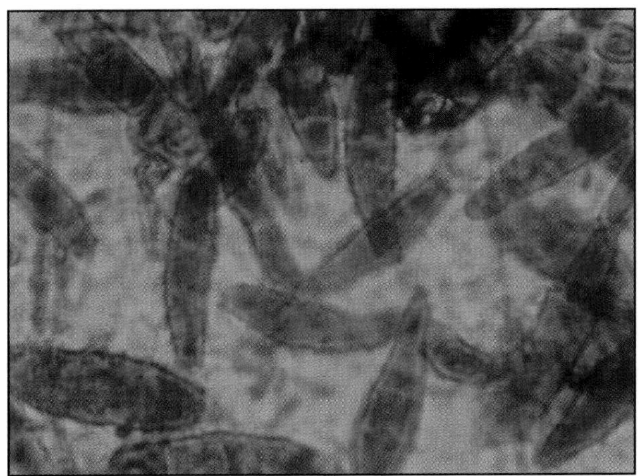

Plate 61 *Microsporum:* microscopic. Note abundance of large, multiseptate macroconidia.

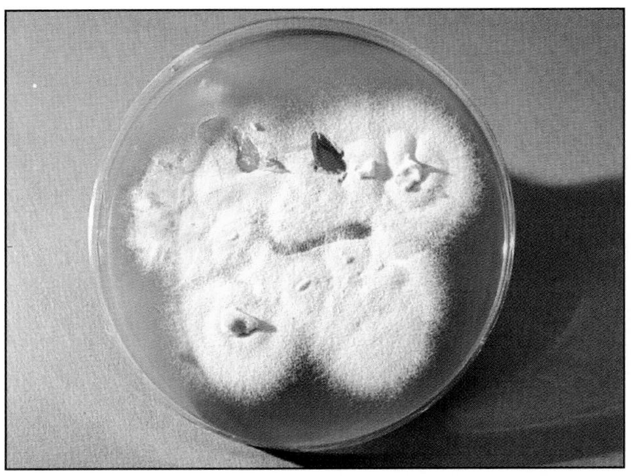

Plate 62 *Trichophyton tonsurans:* on SDA. Note creamy tan color and presence of radical rugose folds.

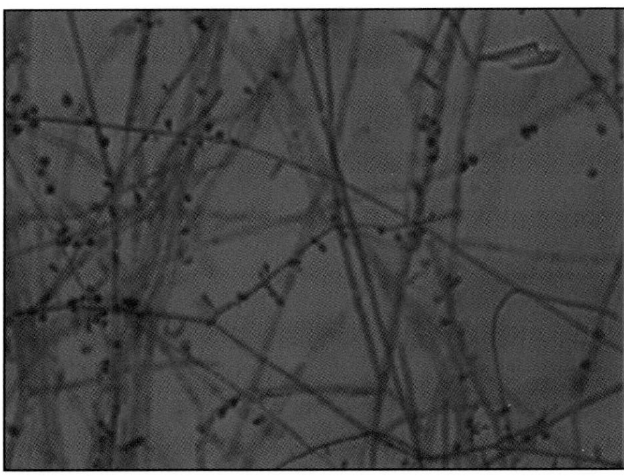

Plate 63 *Trichophyton tonsurans:* microscopic LPCB. Note abundance of piriform microconidia.

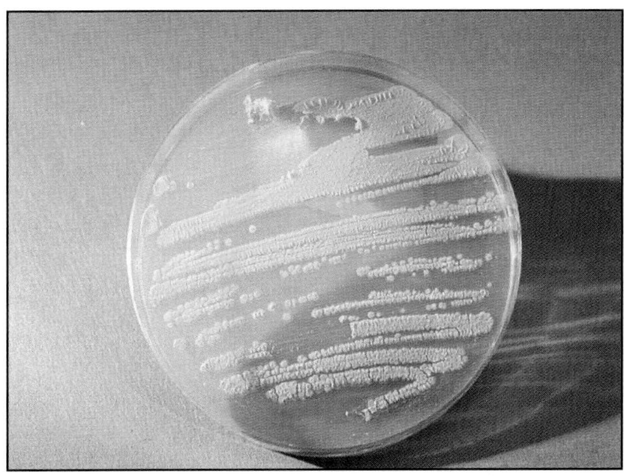

Plate 64 *Malassezia furfur* on SDA overlaid with olive oil. Colonies are creamy and yeastlike and require oil for growth.

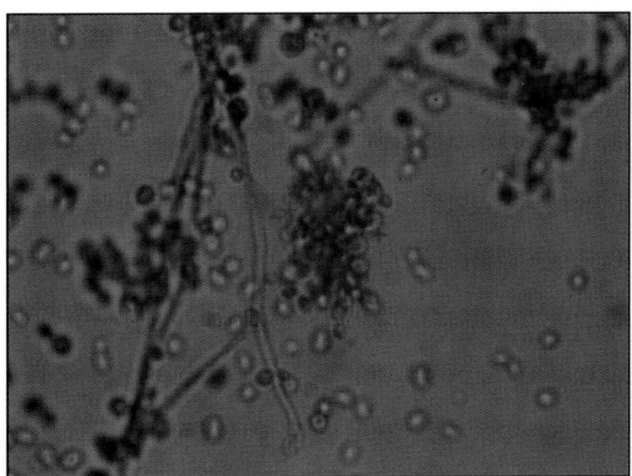

Plate 65 *Exophiala:* microscopic, prepared from a young colony showing budding yeast cells with annellations.

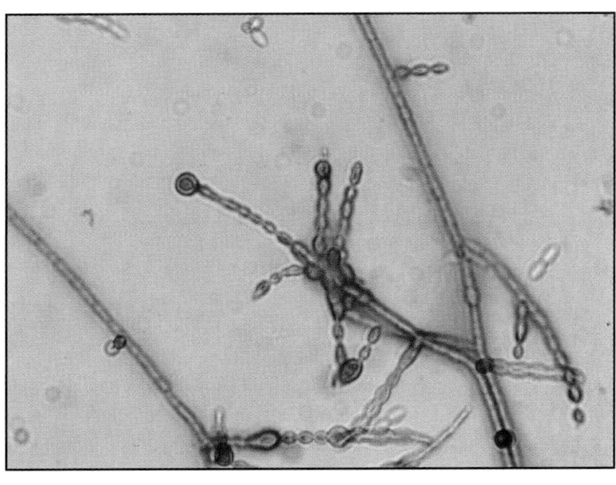

Plate 66 *Cladosporium:* microscopic, showing long chains of elliptoidal conidia.

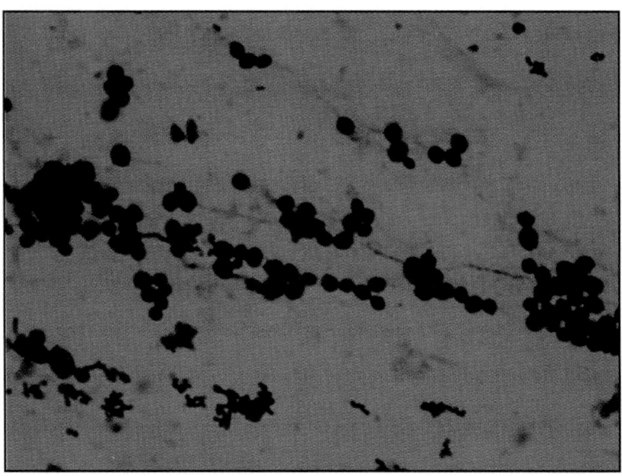

Plate 67 Gram stain of *Candida albicans,* showing blue-black oval yeast cells with some budding.

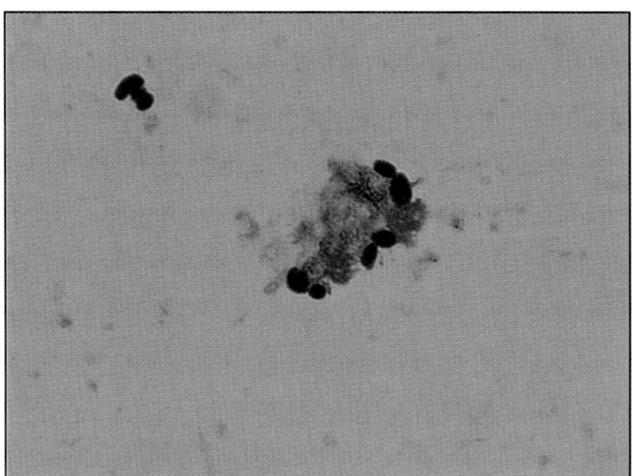

Plate 68 *Candida albicans:* showing budding yeast cells with gram-negative bacilli.

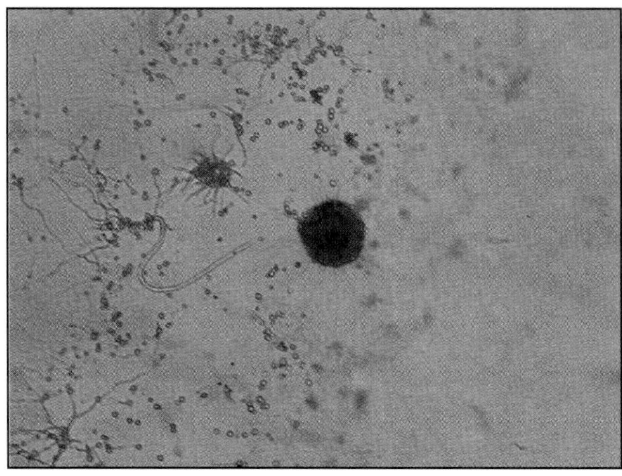

Plate 69 *Aspergillus fumigatus:* microscopic, showing chains of conidia covering the sterigmata.

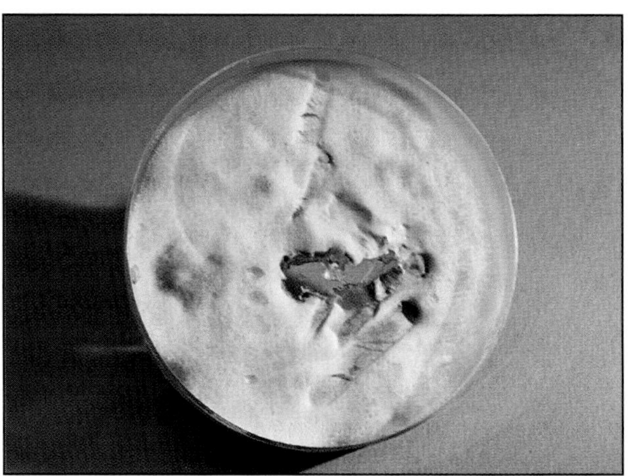

Plate 70 *Fusarium* on SDA showing fluffy mycelium with violet pigment. *Fusarium* species typically are deeply pigmented red, lavender, pink, or violet.

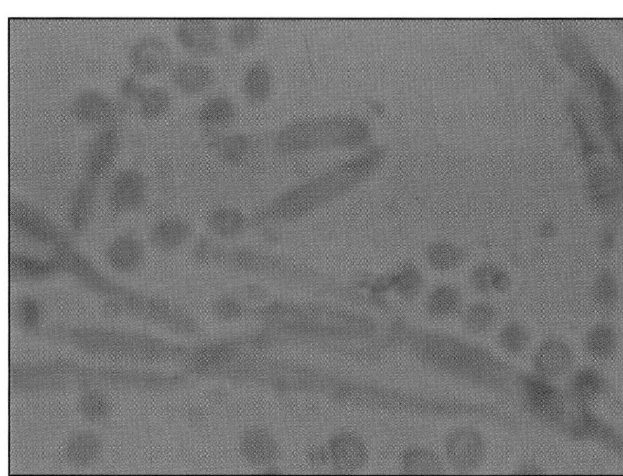

Plate 71 *Penicillium:* microscopic, showing septate hyphae, brushlike conidiophores, and chains of conidia from phialides.

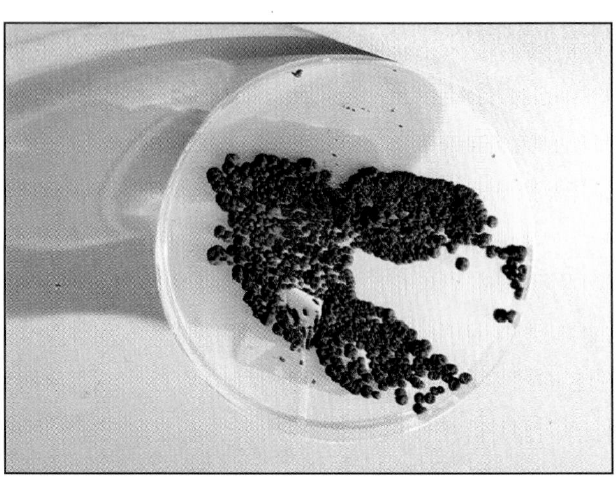

Plate 72 *Aureobasidium* on SDA showing flat, black, yeast-like colonies.

Plate 73 *Curvularia:* microscopic, showing multicellular, curved conidia with a central cell.

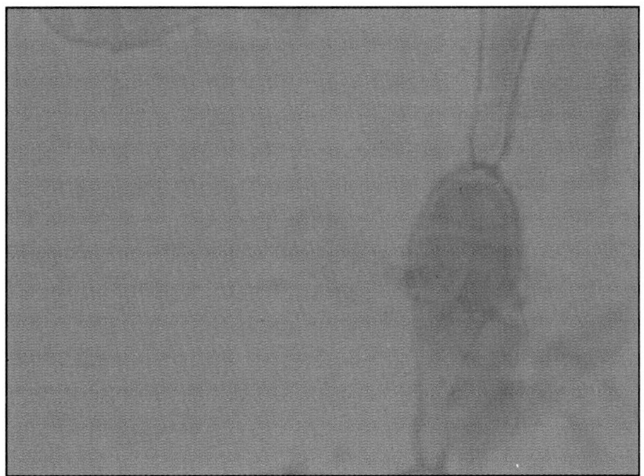

Plate 74 *Alternaria:* microscopic, showing septate hyphae, branched conidiophores, and drumstick-shaped conidia.

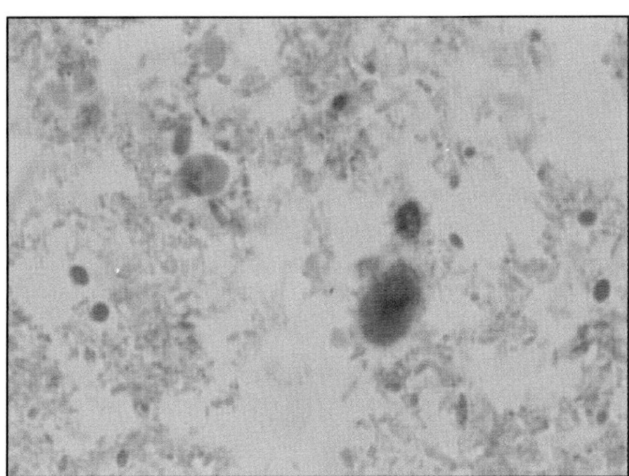

Plate 75 *Giardia lamblia* in concentrated stool, showing typical morphology of the flagellate.

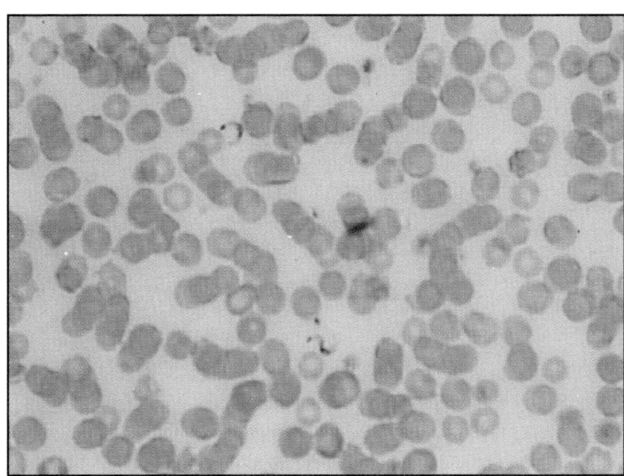

Plate 76 Peripheral blood smear showing extracellular trypanosome.

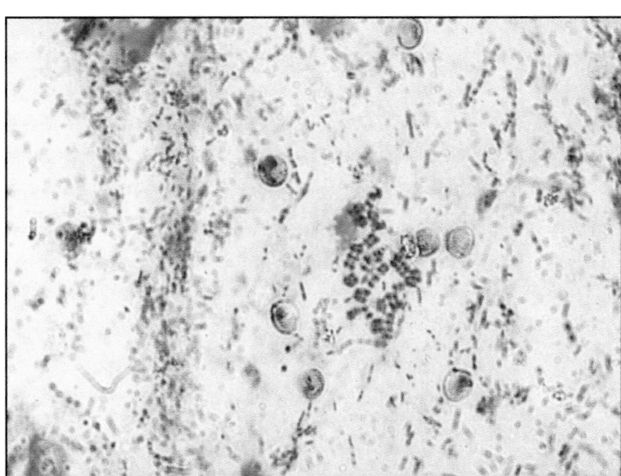

Plate 77 Modified acid-fast stain of oocysts of *Cryptosporidium parvum.* (From Baron EJ, Peterson LR, Finegold SM: *Bailey and Scott's diagnostic microbiology,* ed 9, St Louis, 1994, Mosby.)

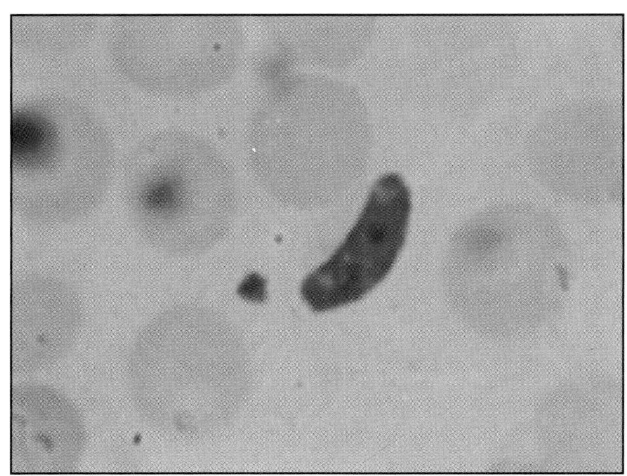

Plate 78 Crescent-shaped gametocytes of *Plasmodium falciparum.* (From Howard BJ et al: *Clinical and pathogenic microbiology,* ed 2, St Louis, 1993, Mosby.)

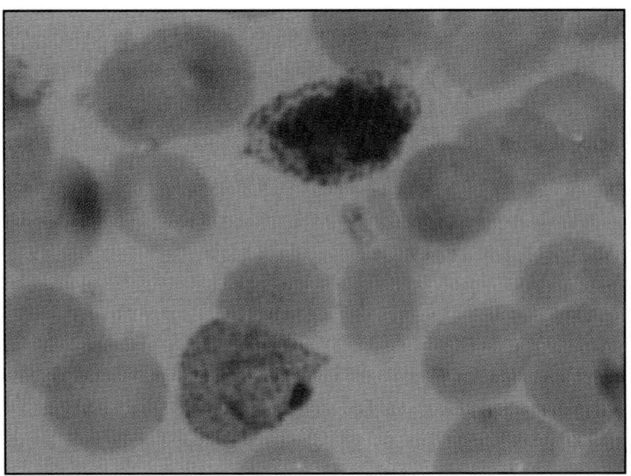

Plate 79 Schuffner's dots of *Plasmodium vivax.* (From Howard BJ et al: *Clinical and pathogenic microbiology*, ed 2, St Louis, 1993, Mosby.)

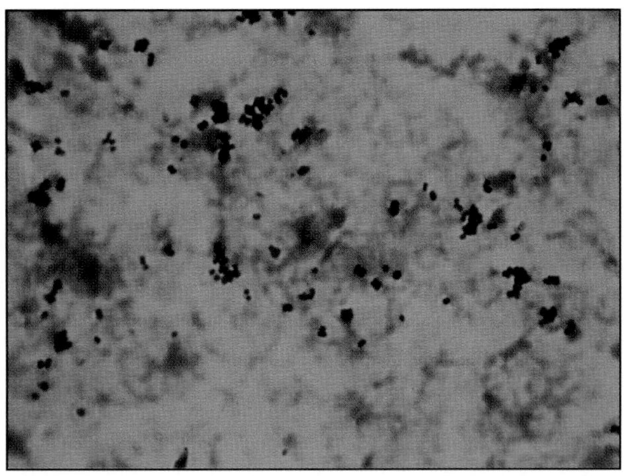

Plate 80 Gram stain from positive blood culture that grew gram-positive cocci resembling the morphology of *Staphylococcus.*

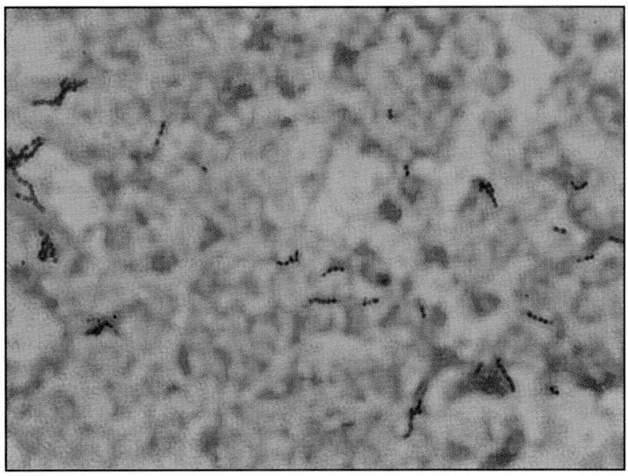

Plate 81 Gram stain from positive blood culture that grew gram-positive cocci resembling *Streptococcus.*

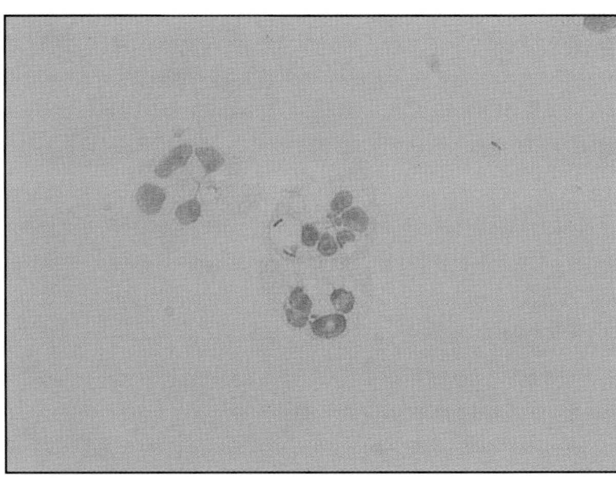

Plate 82 Gram-negative bacilli and segmented neutrophils in a Gram stain made from centrifuged CSF.

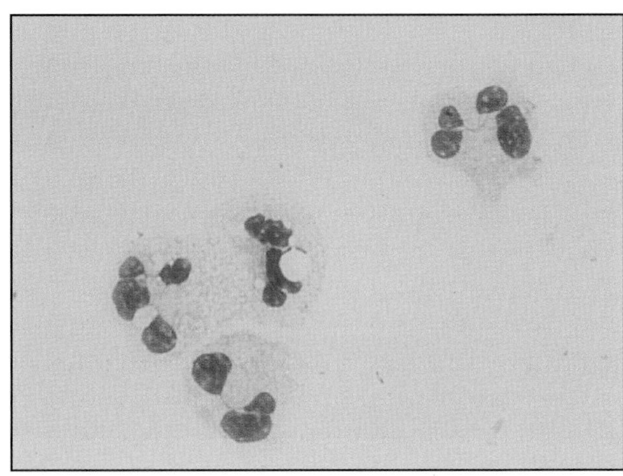

Plate 83 Specimen from Plate 82 in a Wright's stain smear showing bacilli and segmented neutrophils.

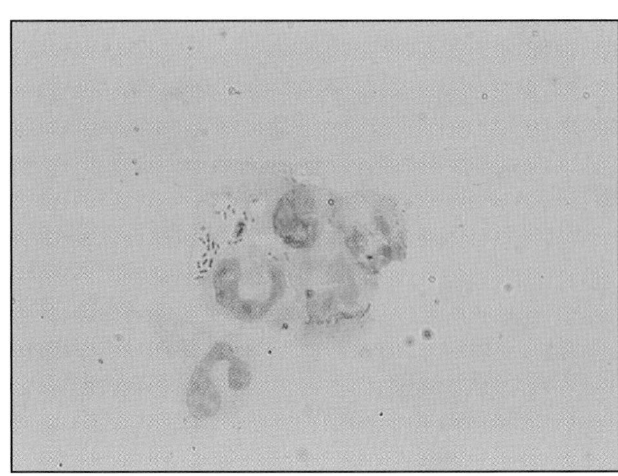

Plate 84 Gram-negative diplococci from a Gram stain of centrifuged CSF.

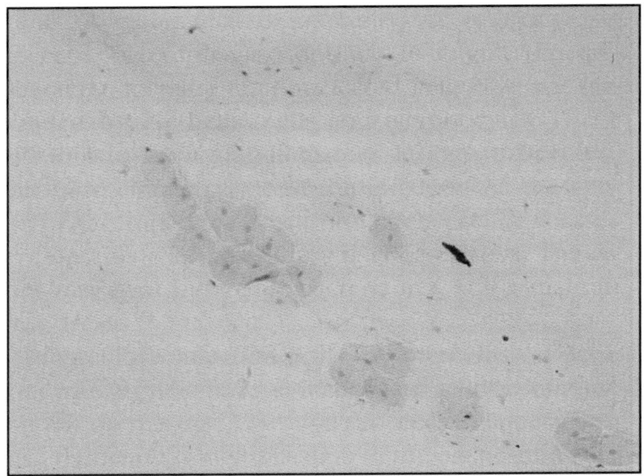

Plate 85 Gram stain of contaminated sputum showing squamous epithelial cells.

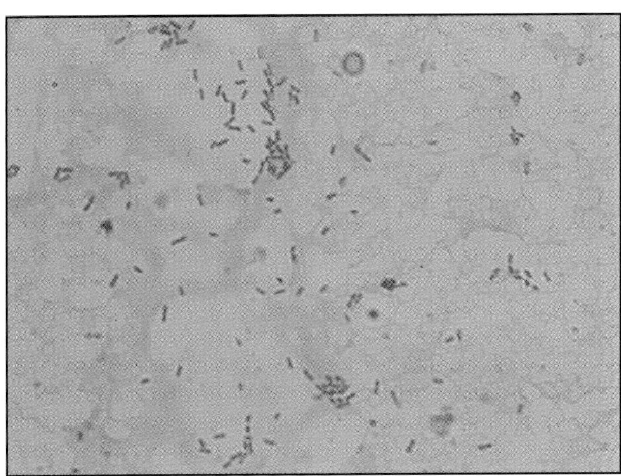

Plate 88 Gram stain of an uncentrifuged urine specimen showing gram-negative bacilli.

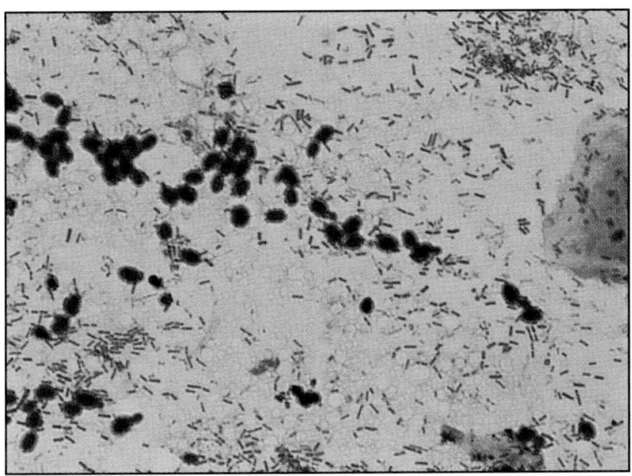

Plate 86 Gram stain of an acceptable sputum sample with gram-positive bacilli, gram-negative bacilli, and yeast. No WBCs are seen, which can be attributed to neutropenia or a diminished immune response.

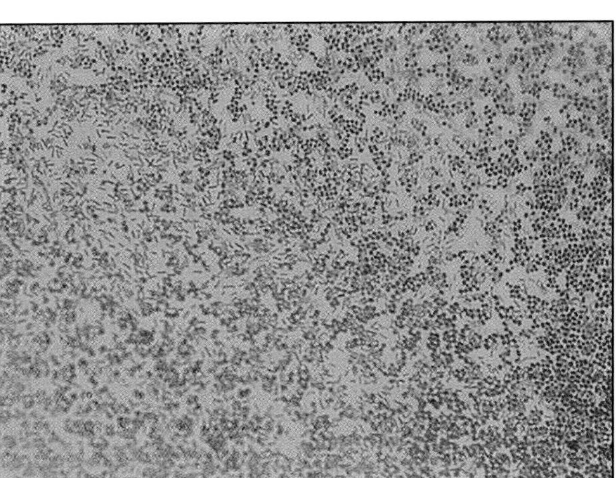

Plate 89 Gram stain of an uncentrifuged urine specimen showing mixed infection of gram-negative bacilli and gram-positive cocci.

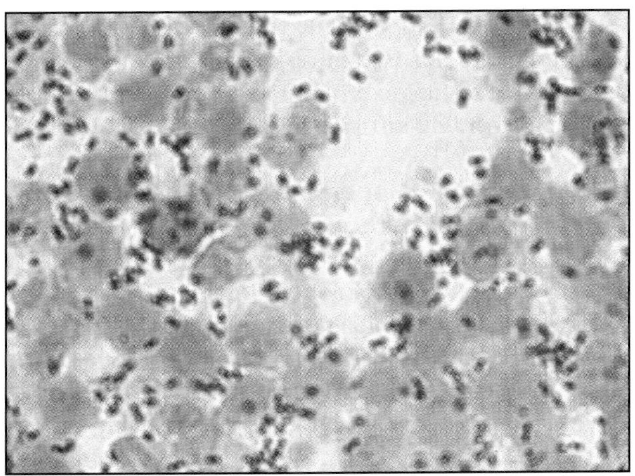

Plate 87 Gram stain of an acceptable sputum sample showing a moderate amount of gram-positive diplococci, some segmented neutrophils, and many red blood cells.

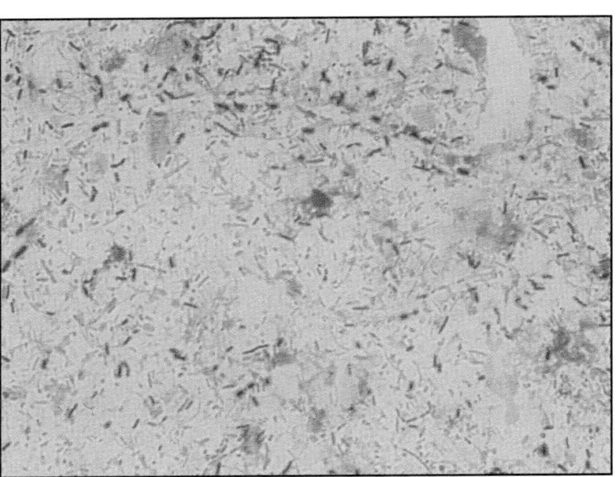

Plate 90 Gram stain of a normal stool specimen showing mixed flora of coliforms, gram-positive cocci, and anaerobic gram-negative bacilli.

TABLE 17–2

Differentiation of Clinically Important *Mycobacterium*

M. TUBERCULOSIS COMPLEX

TEST	M. TUBERCULOSIS	M. BOVIS	M. AFRICANUM
Niacin accumulation	+	–	–
Nitrate reduction	+	–	–
Heat-Stable catalase	–	–	–
Urease	+	+	+
Tween 80 hydrolysis	V	–	–
Arylsulfatase (3 days)	–	–	–
5% NaCl (growth)	–	–	–
Iron uptake	–	–	–
Growth on MacConkey agar (without crystal violet)	–	–	–
Pyrazinamidase	+	–	–

SCOTOCHROMOGENS

TEST	M. SCROFULACEUM	M. SZULGAI	M. GORDONAE	M. THERMORESISTIBLE	M. FLAVESCENS
Niacin accumulation	–	–	–	–	–
Nitrate reduction	–	+	–	–	+
Heat-stable catalase	+	+	+	+	+
Urease	+	+	–	+	+
Tween 80 hydrolysis	–	Slow +	+	+	+
Arylsulfatase (3 days)	–	–	–	–	–
5% NaCl (growth)	–	–	–	–	+
Iron uptake	–	–	–	–	–
MacConkey agar (without crystal violet)	–	–	–	–	–
Pyrazinamidase	V	–	–	NA	+

PHOTOCHROMOGENS

TEST	M. KANSASII	M. MARINUM	M. SIMIAE	M. ASIATICUM
Niacin accumulation	–	V	+	–
Nitrate reduction	+	–	–	–
Heat-stable catalase	+	–	+	+
Urease	+	+	+	–
Tween 80 hydrolysis	+	+	Slow +	+
Arylsulfatase (3 days)	–	V	–	–
5% NaCl (growth)	–	–	–	–
Iron uptake	–	–	–	–
MacConkey agar (without crystal violet)	–	–	–	–
Pyrazinamidase	–	+	+	–

*+ , Most reactions positive; – , most reactions negative; V, variable reaction; NA, test not applicable or insufficient data available.

TABLE 17-2

Differentiation of Clinically Important *Mycobacterium*

(Continued)

NONPHOTOCHROMOGENS

TEST	M. AVIUM-INTRACELLULARE	M. TERRAE-TRIVIALE	M. MALMOENSE	M. HAEMOPHILUM	M. GASTRI
Niacin accumulation	−	−	−	−	−
Nitrate reduction	−	+	−	−	−
Heat-stable catalase	+	+	+	−	−
Urease	−	−	−	−	+
Tween 80 hydrolysis	−	+	+	−	+
Arylsulfatase (3 days)	−	*	−	−	−
5% NaCl (growth)	−	*	−	−	−
Iron uptake	−	−	−	−	−
MacConkey agar (without crystal violet)	−	−	−	−	−
Pyrazinamidase	+	V	+	+	−

RAPID GROWERS

TEST	M. FORTUITUM	M. CHELONEI	M. PHLEI	M. SMEGMATIS
Niacin accumulation	−	−	−	−
Nitrate reduction	+	−	+	+
Heat-stable catalase	+	+	+	+
Urease	+	+	NA	NA
Tween 80 hydrolysis	V	−	+	+
Arylsulfatase (3 days)	+	+	−	−
5% NaCl (growth)	+	−	+	+
Iron uptake	+	−	+	+
MacConkey agar (without crystal violet)	+	+	−	−
Pyrazinamidase	+	+	−	NA

* *M. terrae* is negative, whereas *M. triviale* is positive.

cats, swine, and rabbits, *M. bovis* grows at 35° to 37°C, but not at 24°C or 42°C. Growth is evident on Middlebrook medium in approximately 3 weeks, while 6 to 8 weeks are necessary for growth to occur on LJ media. The colonies are buff and small and may be rough or smooth. The organism resembles "water droplets" on Middlebrook media.

M. bovis may be differentiated from the similar *M. tuberculosis* by its negative niacin and nitrate reactions.

MYCOBACTERIUM LEPRAE

M. leprae, the agent of Hansen's disease, or leprosy, cannot be cultured in vitro. Leprosy is an infection of the skin and mucous membranes that is spread through direct contact with infected lesions. The organism is predominantly found in southeastern Asia, China, Africa, and Latin America, although it is also found in the United States in California, Texas, and Florida. Identification is made through observation of AFB in characteristic skin lesions.

PHOTOCHROMOGENS

Mycobacterium kansasii

M. kansasii, or "yellow bacillus," produces a yellow pigment when exposed to light due to the presence of beta-carotene pigment. The color darkens to red with prolonged incubation and exposure to light (Figure 17-3 [Color Plate 55]). The organism grows best at 37°C, and growth is evident in 14 to 28 days. It grows slowly at 24°C but does not grow at 42°C. Important reactions to identify *M. kansasii* include its rapid Tween 80 hydrolysis (positive reaction in 3 days), strong reduction of nitrates to nitrites, rapid catalase activity, and negative pyrazinamidase reaction.

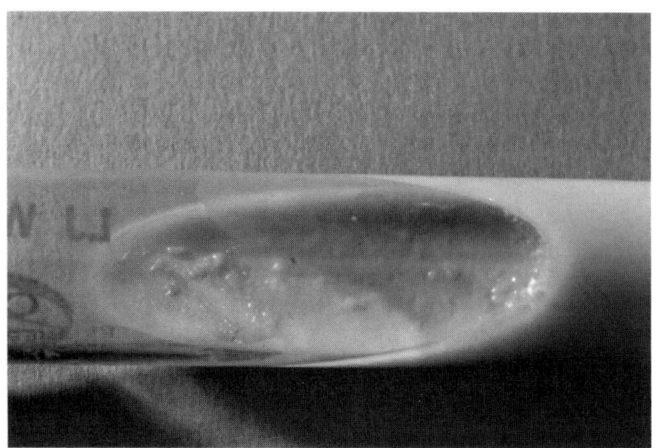

FIGURE 17-3
Mycobacterium kansasii, the "yellow bacillus." When grown in the light, this photochromogen produces yellow colonies, which may intensify to orange or red when exposed to a constant light source.

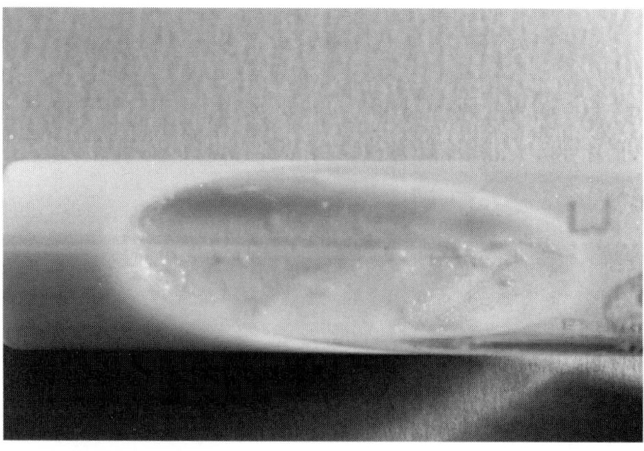

FIGURE 17-4
Mycobacterium marinum, a photochromogen, is nonpigmented when grown in the dark but pigmented yellow when exposed to a constant light source.

The organism causes a chronic pulmonary disease, similar to tuberculosis, that rarely disseminates. Infections are found in the southern and midwestern areas of the United States. AIDS-related cases, involving the bowel and lymph nodes, have recently been seen.

Mycobacterium marinum

M. marinum ("of the sea") grows optimally at 30° to 32°C. Growth at 24°C and 32°C occurs in 2 weeks, whereas the organism grows poorly or fails to grow at 35°C to 37°C. The organism appears as nonpigmented colonies that develop a deep-yellow pigment when exposed to a constant light source (Figure 17-4 [Color Plate 56]). Important reactions to identify *M. marinum* include positive niacin accumulation by some strains, positive hydrolysis of Tween 80, failure to reduce nitrates to nitrites, positive urease and pyrazinamidase activity, and failure to produce heat-stable catalase.

M. marinum is associated with skin infections occurring as red to blue lesions. Infection most often results from contact with poorly chlorinated or unchlorinated fresh or salt water. Water sources that may harbor *M. marinum* include swimming pools, fish aquariums, and water-cooling towers. **Swimming pool granuloma,** a more serious form of the infection, involves the formation of nodules on the elbows, knees, toes, or fingers. These nodules may ulcerate. Those at increased risk of infection include fishermen and lifeguards.

Mycobacterium simiae

M. simiae was first recovered from the *Macaca* rhesus monkey. Growth is observed in 2 to 3 weeks. Most strains are classified as photochromogens. Important reactions include positive accumulation of niacin, a slow hydrolysis of Tween 80 (positive reaction in 10 days), and high heat-stable catalase activity.

M. simiae is a rare cause of pulmonary infections, which may disseminate into the blood.

Mycobacterium asiaticum

M. asiaticum, rarely isolated in the United States, is similar to *M. simiae* but is negative for niacin accumulation.

SCOTOCHROMOGENS

Mycobacterium scrofulaceum

M. scrofulaceum produces smooth, buttery, yellow to orange colonies in 4 to 6 weeks. Pigment production is evident in both the absence and the presence of light. Showing no temperature preference, it grows at 25°C, 32°C, and 37°C. Important reactions include negative results for Tween 80 hydrolysis and nitrate reduction and positive heat-stable catalase activity.

The organism has been implicated as a cause of cervical lymphadenitis, particularly in children.

Mycobacterium szulgai

M. szulgai can be classified as both a photochromogen and a scotochromogen. When grown at 25°C, the organism is classified as a photochromogen, but when grown at 35° to 37°C, it is classified as a scotochromogen. The organism grows in 2 weeks at 35° to 37°C and produces an orange pigment when exposed to constant light. Important reactions include positive nitrate reduction, a slow positive reaction for Tween 80 hydrolysis, and failure to grow in 5% NaCl. The last reaction is important in its differentiation from *M. flavescens,* which is able to grow in 5% NaCl.

M. szulgai has been isolated as an agent in pulmonary and cutaneous disease.

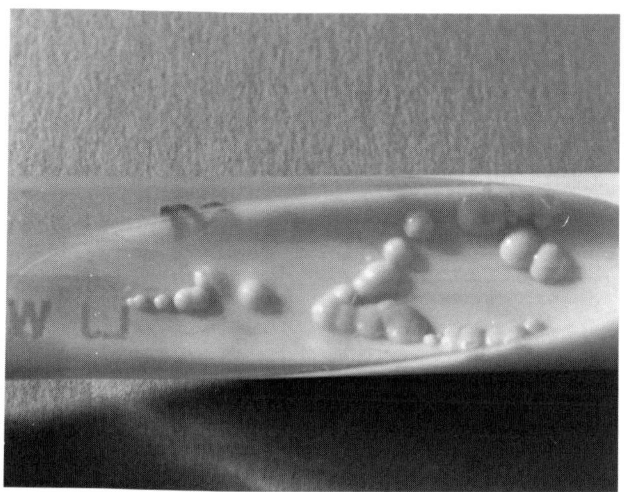

FIGURE 17-5

Mycobacterium gordonae, the "tap water bacillus," produces smooth, glistening yellow colonies in both the absence and the presence of light.

Mycobacterium gordonae

M. gordonae, the "tap water bacillus," is found in a variety of water sources. Although it is a frequent isolate, it is usually nonpathogenic except when isolated from the immunosuppressed host. The organism, previously known as *M. aquae,* grows in approximately 7 days at 37°C as yellow to orange colonies (Figure 17-5 [Color Plate 57]). Notable reactions include positive results for Tween 80 hydrolysis and heat-stable catalase.

Mycobacterium xenopi

M. xenopi, a slow-growing organism, produces small yellow colonies. Growth is optimal at 42°C. The organism also grows at 37°C, but fails to grow at 25°C. *M. xenopi* produces branching colonies with aerial hyphae on cornmeal agar, which have been described as "birds' nests." Important reactions include negative reactions for niacin accumulation and nitrate reductions and positive reactions for catalase and arylsulfatase, which become positive within 2 weeks. The organism was first isolated from the African toad and also has been isolated from birds and several hot and cold water sources. It was considered to be nonpathogenic until recent years, when *M. xenopi* has been identified as the agent of pulmonary infection in patients with preexisting lung pathologies. The organism can also disseminate into the bone marrow and lymph nodes.

Miscellaneous Scotochromogens

M. thermoresistible, a rare pulmonary isolate, is unique in its ability to grow at 52°C. The organism produces smooth yellow colonies.

N. flavescens, considered to be normal flora, produces smooth yellow colonies and grows moderately at 37°C.

NONPHOTOCHROMOGENS

Mycobacterium avium-intracellulare Complex (MAI)

M. avium-intracellulare complex is composed of slow-growing organisms that produce buff-colored colonies. The colonies are thin and transparent or smooth; asteroid margins may be present. Because of these variable morphologies, one may mistakenly conclude that it is a mixed culture. The organisms are found in the environment and have been isolated from air and water samples. MAI grows at 35° to 37°C and 42°C but not at 24°C. Identification is based on its failure to produce positive biochemical reactions. Most tests are negative, with the exception of heat-stable catalase and pyrazinamidase, which are positive.

M. avium produces disease in chickens and has been a rare cause of infection in chicken farmers. *M. intracellulare* has been considered to be nonpathogenic. The species are joined into a complex because of their similar morphological and biochemical characteristics. An increased frequency of MAI infection has been noted since 1980. The infection has been found most frequently in AIDS patients, and the disease usually involves the gastrointestinal tract. Lesions have also been found to involve the lungs, liver, and spleen of AIDS patients.

The organism is also commonly known as the "Battey bacillus," which refers to an outbreak of MAI infection in Battey State Hospital in Rome, Ga.

Mycobacterium malmoense

M. malmoense produces gray to white, smooth, raised colonies in 2 to 3 weeks when grown at 37°C. Growth is slower at 22° to 24°C and may require 7 to 12 weeks. A rare agent in pulmonary disease, important reactions include failure to accumulate niacin, nitrate reduction negative, and Tween 80 hydrolysis and heat-stable catalase positive.

Mycobacterium haemophilum

M. haemophilum grows at 28° to 32°C in 2 to 4 weeks but requires 4 to 8 weeks to grow at 25°C or 35°C. Colonies are nonpigmented. The organism cannot grow at 37°C. The organism is unique in its growth requirement for hemin, requiring chocolate agar or Mueller-Hinton agar with Fildes enrichment to grow. The organism is basically biochemically inert. *M. haemophilum* has been identified as the agent of subcutaneous lesions, ulcers, and abscesses in immunosuppressed patients.

Miscellaneous Nonphotochromogens

M. gastri is nonpathogenic and has been isolated from gastric lavage. *M. terrae-triviale* complex is a rare cause of arthritis and osteomyelitis. *M. terrae* is known

REVIEW QUESTIONS

(Continued)

b. Middlebrook 7H10
c. Petragnani
d. Mitchison's Middlebrook 7H11

20. Which statement correctly describes acid-fast staining?
a. The Ziehl-Neelsen technique does not require heat.
b. Mycobacteria stain blue with carbolfuchsin.
c. The Kinyoun method uses hot phenol.
d. Auramine O stains mycobacteria yellow-green in the fluorochrome method.

21. A sputum smear reveals an average of five acid-fast bacilli per 1000X field. According to CDC guidelines, report this result as:
a. +/−
b. 1 +
c. 2 +
d. 3 +
e. 4 +

For questions 22 to 30, place the species of mycobacteria in the proper group according to Runyon's classification (answers may be I to IV or "none"):

22. *M. fortuitum* ________________

23. *M. xenopi* ________________

24. *M. marinum* ________________

25. *M. scrofulaceum* ________________

26. *M. tuberculosis* ________________

27. *M. ulcerans* ________________

28. *M. gordonae* ________________

29. *M. kansasii* ________________

30. *M. avium-intracellulare* ________________

31. Which of the following is noted for a positive result for niacin accumulation?
a. *M. tuberculosis*
b. *M. avium-intracellulare*
c. *M. fortuitum-chelonae*
d. *M. gordonae*

32. Which of the following groups is characterized by a negative reaction for heat-stable catalase?
a. *M. tuberculosis* complex
b. Photochromagens
c. Scotochromagens
d. Rapid growers

33. In which reaction is free phenolphthalein detected using an alkaline indicator?
a. Tween 80 hydrolysis
b. Arylsulfatase
c. Pyrazinamidase
d. Urease

34. Tuberculosis is spread through:
a. Contact with contaminated inanimate objects
b. The fecal-oral route
c. Contaminated blood products
d. Contaminated respiratory droplets

35. Tuberculosis infection always results in tuberculosis disease.
a. True
b. False

36. Granulomatous lesions consisting of multinucleated cells with epithelial cells and lymphocytes are known as:
a. Caseates
b. Chancres
c. Tubercles
d. Sclerotic granules

BIBLIOGRAPHY

Barksdale L, Kim KS: Mycobacterium, Bacteriol Rev 41:217, 1977.

Curione CJ Jr et al: Gram stain evaluation of the quality of sputum specimens for mycobacterial culture, *J Clin Microbiol* 5:381, 1977.

Daley CL et al: An outbreak of tuberculosis with accelerated progression among persons infected with human immunodeficiency virus, *N Engl J Med* 326:231, 1992.

Damato JJ et al: Detection of mycobacteria by radiometric and standard plate procedures, *J Clin Microbiol* 17:1066, 1983.

Davis TE: *Mycobacterium tuberculosis:* a renewed challenge for the clinical microbiology laboratory, *Clin Microbiol Newsletter* 14:97, 1992.

Good RC, Snider DE Jr: Isolation of nontuberculosis mycobacteria in the United States, *J Infect Dis* 146:829, 1982.

Harris AD: Tuberculosis and human immunodeficiency virus infection in developing countries, *Lancet* 335:387, 1990.

Kestle DG, Kubica GP: Sputum collection for cultivation of mycobacteria: an early morning specimen or the 24-72 hour pool? *Am J Clin Pathol* 48:347, 1967.

Krasnow I, Wayne LG: Comparison of methods of tuberculosis bacteriology, *Appl Microbiol* 28:915, 1969.

Kubica GP: Differential identification of mycobacteria. VII. Key features for identification of clinically significant mycobacteria, *Am Rev Respir Dis* 107:9, 1973.

Kubica GP et al: Laboratory services for mycobacterial diseases, *Am Rev Respir Dis* 112:783, 1975.

Nardell E et al: Exogenous reinfection with tuberculosis in a shelter for the homeless, *N Engl J Med* 315:1570, 1986.

Nosocomial transmission of multi-drug resistant tuberculosis among HIV-infected persons—Florida and New York, 1988-1991, *MMWR* 40:585, 1991.

Roberts GD, Koneman EW, Kim YK: *Mycobacterium.* In Balows A, editor: *Manual of clinical microbiology,* ed 5, Washington DC, 1991, American Society for Microbiology.

Wolinsky E: Nontuberculosis mycobacteria and associated diseases, *Am Rev Respir Dis* 119:107, 1979.

Woods GL, Washington JA II: Mycobacteria other than *M. tuberculosis:* review of microbiologic and clinical aspects, *Rev Infect Dis* 9:275, 1987.

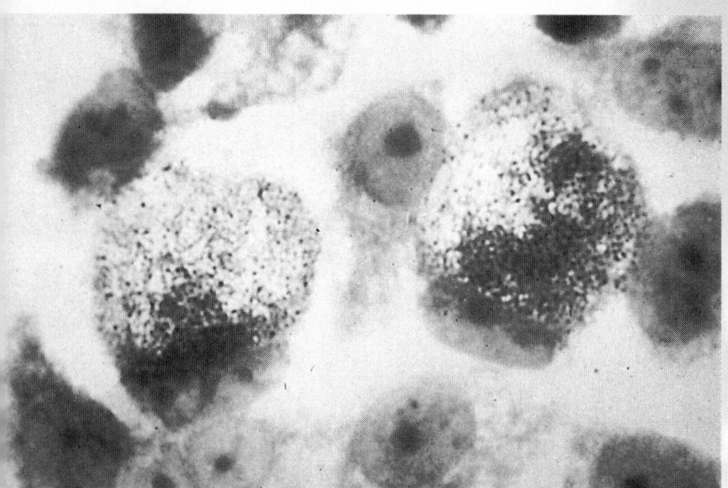

CHLAMYDIA TRACHOMATIS

CHAPTER OUTLINE

CHLAMYDIA
MYCOPLASMA
RICKETTSIAE

KEY TERMS

COLD AGGLUTININS
LYMPHOGRANULOMA VENEREUM
PRIMARY ATYPICAL PNEUMONIA
PSITTACOSIS (ORNITHOSIS)
TRACHOMA
WEIL-FELIX REACTION

Chlamydia, Mycoplasma, and Rickettsiae

LEARNING OBJECTIVES

1. State the important characteristics of the genus *Chlamydia.*
2. List the three pathogenic species of *Chlamydia* and describe the diseases associated with each.
3. State the specific serotype(s) of *Chlamydia trachomatis* that cause lymphogranuloma venereum (LGV) and nongonococcal urethritis.
4. Describe the life cycle of *Chlamydia.*
5. Explain how *Chlamydia* species are identified from clinical specimens.
6. List the important characteristics of the genus *Mycoplasma.*
7. Discuss the infectious diseases associated with *Mycoplasma pneumoniae.*
8. Explain how *M. pneumoniae* infection is diagnosed.
9. List the clinically significant genital mycoplasmas and ureaplasmas and name the associated infections.
10. For each of the following rickettsiae, name its group, species, and insect vector:
    a. Rocky Mountain spotted fever
    b. Rickettsialpox
    c. Endemic typhus
    d. Brill-Zinsser disease (recrudescent typhus)
    e. Scrub typhus
    f. Q fever
    g. Trench fever

CHLAMYDIA

Chlamydia organisms are obligate intracellular parasites originally thought to be viruses because they cannot produce adenosine triphosphate (ATP) or survive outside an animal host cell. In the past the organisms have been known as *Bedsonia,* which refers to a large virus and the trachoma inclusion conjunctivitis (TRIC) agent, one type of infection associated with this organism.

Chlamydia species possess a gram-negative-like cell wall and multiply by binary fission. The organisms contain both deoxyribonucleic acid (DNA) and ribonucleic acid (RNA) and are susceptible to a variety of antibiotics. Because of these characteristics, *Chlamydia* species are now classified as bacteria in the family Chlamydiae. The organisms have a unique life cycle (Figure 18-1) and possess intracytoplasmic inclusions.

The three species of *Chlamydia* are *C. psittaci, C. trachomatis,* and *C. pneumoniae.*

Chlamydia psittaci is the agent of psittacosis, a disease of psittacine birds, such as parrots, parakeets, and cockatoos. The infection is also known as **ornithosis,** since it is now known that *C. psittaci* can also be carried by other birds, including turkeys, pigeons, and chickens. Humans may acquire the infection by inhalation of contaminated aerosols or fomites or through person-to-person transmission. The infection incubates for 1 to 2 weeks and is characterized by chills, fever, and malaise. The severity of the infection can vary from a subclinical, mild, respiratory-type infection to a fatal pneumonia. After inhalation the organism is deposited in the alveoli and ingested by alveolar macrophages, which enter the regional lymph nodes. Dissemination to the reticuloendothelial system occurs next. The most common manifestation is a mild to moderately severe pneumonia with fever, headache, and cough. The severe form may also be associated with jaundice and endocarditis. Ornithosis is an occupational hazard for poultry workers and may pose a hazard for pet shop workers and avian pet owners.

Chlamydia pneumoniae, a relatively new species, is associated with mild respiratory tract infections. It is believed that the organism is spread from human to human without an animal reservoir. The species, also known as "TWAR" (for the first two isolates, TW-183 and AR-39) is pear shaped with a large periplasmic space and round elementary bodies.

Chlamydia trachomatis is an agent of lymphogranuloma venereum, endemic trachoma, nongonococcal urethritis, and infant pneumonitis. There are 15 serotypes; serotypes A, B, Ba, and C are associated with endemic trachoma, a leading cause of blindness. **Trachoma** is found in many areas of the world, particularly in poorly developed countries in the Middle East, North Africa, India. In the United States the disease is most frequently found in the Native-American population in the Southwest. Trachoma is spread by close contact with infected individuals. It begins as a conjunctivitis, which may persist for months to years, spreading to the cornea. Conjunctival scarring and corneal vascularization may occur, which may lead to scarring and blindness. Infants are often infected early in life through direct contact or through flies, which also transmit the organism.

C. trachomatis serotypes D, E, F, G, H, I, J, and K are associated with diseases spread primarily by the venereal routes. These infections include nongonoccal urethritis, epididymitis, proctitis, mucopurulent cervicitis, endometriosis, and salpingitis. Other types of diseases associated with serotypes D through K include neonatal pneumonitis and inclusion conjunctivitis. *C. trachomatis* is the most common cause of nongonoccal urethritis in males, surpassing gonorrhea as the most prevalent sexually transmitted disease in the United States. Chlamydial infections in females, such as pelvic inflammatory disease, may lead to severe damage to the fallopian tubes, infertility, and ectopic pregnancies. Some individuals may carry the organism asymptomatically, serving as a reservoir of infection. The infection may be transmitted from an infected mother to the infant during delivery, which may lead to conjunctivitis or pneumonia.

C. trachomatis serotypes L1, L2, L3 are associated with **Lymphogranuloma venereum (LGV),** a disease transmitted through the venereal route. The infection is endemic in Asia, Africa, and South America but is rarely seen in the United States. The initial lesion is a small, painless genital ulcer that may be unnoticed and spontaneously heal. This is followed in 2 to 6 weeks by lymphadenopathy of the inguinal lymph nodes. The lymph nodes enlarge, and buboes may occur. The infection can spread systematically, resulting in pneumonia, meningitis, conjunctivitis, or polyarthritis. It can also remain localized, causing granulomatous proctitis. The Frei test, a delayed hypersensitivity skin test that uses purified LGV antigen, can be used for disease identification. The test becomes positive as early as 10 days after infection; it also may be positive in other chlamydial diseases. Unfortunately, the test remains positive indefinitely. Since false-negative results also occur, the test is no longer considered to be very useful.

Most *Chlamydia* infections can be treated with tetracycline, erythromycin, or the fluoroquinolones. *C. trachomatis* is susceptible to the sulfonamides, but the other species are not.

Specimens to be collected to diagnose chlamydial diseases depend on the site of the infection. Scrapings are preferred over swabs whenever possible. Dacron and nylon swabs are recommended because cotton is toxic to the organism. Swabs should be placed in a suitable transport medium, which should contain sucrose and phosphate buffer and antibiotics to inhibit other

A, Elementary body (EB), the infectious particle, attaches to surface of susceptible host cell.

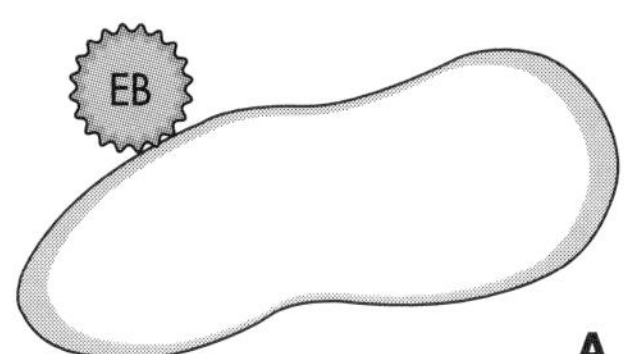

B, EB is enclosed in host cell through endocytosis. Cytoplasmic vesicle (phagosome) encloses EB.

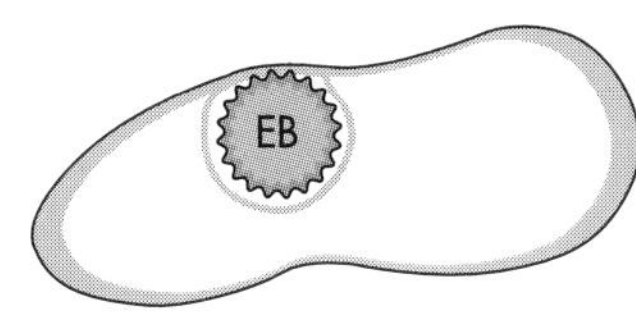

C, EB reorganizes into a more metabolically active body known as the reticulate body (RB). RBs multiply by binary fission approximately 18 to 24 hours after infection.

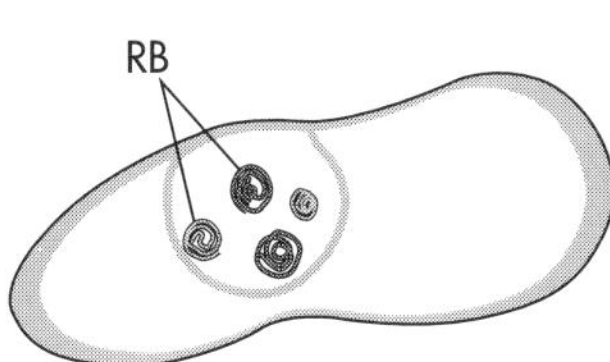

D, Another reorganization occurs, and infectious elementary bodies are formed. These bodies are still enclosed within the phagosome and appear as an intracellular inclusion, which can be stained.

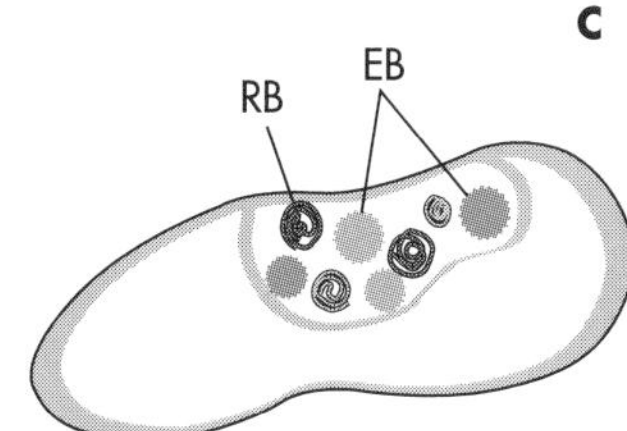

E, The cell ruptures, releasing many infectious elementary bodies.

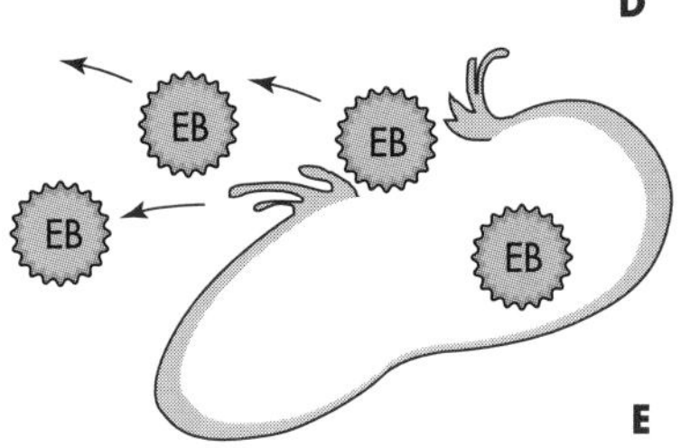

FIGURE 18–1
Life cycle of *Chlamydia.*

organisms. Two swab systems are commercially available and provide a narrow swab for conjunctival and male urethral specimens. A second, larger swab is provided for collection of the cervical specimen. Specimens include conjunctival swabs or scrapings; urethral, cervical, or rectal scrapings or swabs; and biopsy samples from the lung.

Identification of *Chlamydia* includes cytological methods that require epithelial cells scraped from the infected areas. The cells can be stained with iodine solution or Giemsa stain and examined for the presence of chlamydial inclusions. The inclusions are cytoplasmic and perinuclear and stain light to dark brown with iodine. The iodine stains the glycogen present in the inclusions, and the inclusions stain purple with Giemsa stain. The inclusions can also be detected using a fluoroscein-labeled serum with antichlamydial antibodies. Fluorescent inclusions are seen in a positive reaction. The use of monoclonal antibodies has added to the specificity of the fluorescent technique.

Chlamydia organisms require cell cultures to grow. Cell scrapings are collected and placed in a cell culture medium. The usual cell line is McCoy's heteroploid murine cells that have been pretreated with cycloheximide. Other cell lines that can be used include HeLa-229 cells, L-929 cells, and BHK-21 cells. A monolayer of the cell culture is inoculated with the culture. The cell cultures are examined in 48 to 72 hours and stained using one of the methods just described. Although extremely sensitive, cell culture is labor intensive, expensive, and difficult to perform.

Serological methods to detect antibody formation to *Chlamydia* include complement fixation, enzyme-linked immunosorbent assay (ELISA), and immunofluorescence. The usefulness of serologies may be limited, since a high prevalence of antibody to *C. trachomatis* exists in the general population. Complement fixation is more useful for diagnosis of LGV and *C. psittaci* infections. Commercially available ELISA products include *Chlamydia* Stat (Whittaker Bioproducts), which uses purified *Chlamydia* (LGV II) antigen to detect chlamydial antibody in the patient's serum. Immunofluorescent procedures can also detect patient antibody in serum or secretions through reaction with specific serotypes of chlamydial antigen. Both methods provide for serial dilutions of the patient serum so that the antibody titer can be quantitated.

Detection of chlamydial antigen can be made using a direct fluorescent antibody (DFA) technique in which antibodies to the outer membrane protein or lipopolysaccharides are bound to fluorescein-labeled isothiocyanate. The specimen is added, and in a positive reaction the fluorescein-labeled antibody binds to the elementary body in the organism. The antigen can also be detected by using a direct enzyme immunoassay, with antibodies directed against the outer membrane protein or lipopolysaccharides used to detect these components of the organism.

MYCOPLASMA

Mycoplasma species, classified as Mollicutes, are the smallest free-living organisms known and are found in several animals and plants. Mycoplasmas differ from bacteria because they lack a cell wall and are thus very pleomorphic in appearance. These organisms contain both DNA and RNA, can replicate on their own, and can grow on artificial media. Mycoplasmas cannot synthesize cell wall components and are resistant to all antibiotics that inhibit cell wall synthesis, such as the beta-lactams.

Mycoplasmas were originally known as "pleuropneumonia-like organisms (PPLOs)," since they were first discovered causing pleuropneumonia in cattle.

The family Mycoplasmataceae contains two genera: *Mycoplasma* and *Ureaplasma.* Several species of *Mycoplasma* and *Ureaplasma* exist, but only a few species are associated with human infection. These include the species *M. hominis, M. genitalium,* and *U. urealyticum,* which colonize and possibly infect the genital tract. *M. pneumoniae* is an important cause of respiratory infections, most notably primary atypical pneumonia. Several species, such as *M. orale, M. buccale, M. faucium,* and *M. salivarium,* are considered to be normal flora of the upper respiratory tract or oral cavity.

Mycoplasma organisms can be speciated on their ability to ferment glucose, utilize arginine, and hydrolyze urea. Table 18-1 lists reactions for the significant pathogens.

TABLE 18–1

Biochemical Reactions for Clinically Significant Mycoplasmas

SPECIES	GLUCOSE	ARGININE	UREASE
M. hominis	−	+	−
M. pneumoniae	+	−	−
U. urealyticum	−	−	+

Mycoplasma pneumoniae, previously known as the Eaton agent, is a frequent cause of community-acquired pneumonia and tracheobronchitis in children and young adults. It is spread through direct respiratory contact. The organism injures respiratory mucosal cells, impairing ciliary function. Infections may either be asymptomatic or manifest as a respiratory tract infection. After an incubation period of 2 to 3 weeks, the disease begins as a mild respiratory infection that may later be associated with fever, headache, malaise, and a persistent, dry, nonproductive cough. The disease is often referred to as **primary atypical pneumonia** because it is accompanied by a dry cough instead of the typical exudate associated with bacterial pneumonia. In addition, because it lacks a cell wall, *M. pneumoniae* does not respond to traditional antimicrobial therapy, such as penicillin, for bacterial pneumonias. Another common name for this infection is "walking pneumonia" since the patient may appear only moderately ill despite widespread pulmonary infiltrates. The chest x-ray film usually shows a patchy infiltration of the hilar areas of the lungs; the middle and lower portions of the lobes may be involved later. The Gram stain of sputum usually shows mononuclear inflammatory cells with normal oropharyngeal flora. Infections are most common in the autumn and winter months and are often seen in individuals who are in close contact, such as in military camps, schools, or dormitories.

M. pneumoniae is also associated with pharyngitis, rhinitis, and ear infections. Complications of *M. pneumoniae* infections include hemolytic anemia, skin rash, meningitis, and a temporary arthritis. Infections can be treated with erythromycin or tetracycline.

The "genital mycoplasmas" include *Mycoplasma hominis* and *Ureaplasma urealyticum.* The organisms can colonize adults asymptomatically and are also a cause of nongonococcal urethritis in males. *M. hominis* has also been identified as an agent in salpingitis and postpartal fever in females.

Since mycoplasmas are difficult to culture, identification most often is based on serological results. Since the organisms are surface parasites, blood, sputum, synovial fluid, vaginal discharge, urethral swabs, tissue washings, or amniotic fluid can be examined, based on the site of infection. Throat swabs may be used to isolate *M. pneumoniae,* since the organism can colonize the throat.

Because the organisms are very prone to drying and osmotic changes, specimens should be placed into a transport medium. Usually, two media are inoculated to grow mycoplasmas. A diphasic liquid medium that contains fresh yeast extract, peptone, and horse serum is used. In addition, an agar, such as E-agar or Shepard's A7-B agar, should be inoculated. The agars may be supplemented with substrates, such as glucose, arginine, or urea.

Incubation, either anaerobically or in 5% to 10% carbon dioxide (CO_2), is recommended. *M. hominis* and *U. urealyticum* grow within 1 to 5 days, whereas *M. pneumoniae* requires 1 to 2 weeks to grow. On E-agar, colonies of *M. pneumoniae* appear as a typical "fried egg" appearance, with a dense center and translucent periphery. The reactions for each substrate can be determined and used in the identification of the species.

Because of the difficulty and lengthy process of culturing mycoplasmas, serological identification methods have been the primary method for identification. **Cold agglutinins,** which are nonspecific antibodies produced in response to *M. pneumoniae* infection, develop in approximately 50% of all patients. Cold agglutinins are gamma globulins of the immunoglobulin M (IgM) type that agglutinate human group O erythrocytes at 4°C but not at 37°C. These antibodies can be detected in the patient's serum shortly after the onset of disease and peak during the convalescent period. A fourfold increase in antibody titer between the acute-phase and convalescent-phase specimens is diagnostic for current infection. Alternatively, a titer greater than 1:128 is also diagnostic for current infection.

Antibody production against *M. pneumoniae* can be detected using complement fixation, ELISA, or fluorescent antibody methods. Several of these methods are commercially available and are able to detect IgG and IgM antibodies against *M. pneumoniae.*

RICKETTSIAE

The rickettsiae include the genera *Rickettsia, Ehrlichia, Coxiella,* and *Rochalimaea.* The organisms are gram-negative, obligately intracellular bacteria that divide by binary fission and contain both RNA and DNA. Rickettsiae infect a larger variety of wild animals, including birds, small mammals, rats, cattle, sheep, rodents, and flying squirrels. The infections are spread through insect vectors, such as lice, fleas, and ticks. Table 18-2 summarizes the Rickettsiae, including group, species, disease, and insect vector.

All the rickettsiae, except *Coxiella,* cannot survive outside of the animal host or insect vector.

All rickettsial infections, except Q fever, which is caused by *Coxiella burnetii,* begin after inoculation through a bite of an infected insect vector. *C. burnetii* is transmitted through the aerosol route. The disease in-

TABLE 18–2

Clinically Significant Rickettsiae of the Genera *Rickettsia, Coxiella, Ehrlichia,* and *Rochalimaea*

GROUP	SPECIES	INFECTION	TRANSMISSION
Spotted fever	*Rickettsia rickettsii*	Rocky Mountain spotted fever	Ticks
	R. akari	Rickettsialpox	Mites
	R. australis	Australian tick typhus	Ticks
	R. conorii	Boutonneuse fever	Ticks
Typhus	*R. prowazekii*	Epidemic typhus	Lice (infected feces)
		Sporadic typhus	Flying squirrels
		Brill-Zinsser disease (recrudescent typhus)	Reactivation of latent infection
	R. typhi	Murine typhus	Fleas (infected feces)
Scrub typhus	*R. tsutsugamushi*	Scrub typhus	Chigger bites
Q fever	*Coxiella burnetii*	Q fever	Ticks, aerosols
Ehrlichiosis	*Ehrlichia canis*	Ehrlichiosis	Ticks
	E. chaffeensis	Ehrlichiosis	Ticks
	E. equi	Ehrlichiosis	Ticks
	E. sennetsu	Ehrlichiosis	Ticks
Rochalimaea	*R. quintana*	Trench fever	Lice

cubates for 3 to 14 days, and the organism multiplies in the endothelial cells of the blood vessels. The organisms are phagocytized by host cells, multiply, and are released after cell lysis. Signs of infection include fever, headache, and a characteristic maculopapular rash that first appears on the wrists and ankles. The rash spreads to the chest and abdomen and may eventually become petechial in appearance. Cell injury and eventually death can occur from vascular changes as multiplication continues in the blood vessels. Other manifestations of infection include conjunctivitis, pharyngitis, and mild respiratory distress.

Rickettsial disease is most often diagnosed through clinical signs and the patient's medical history. Because these organisms are a Biosafety Level 3 biohazard, specific safety guidelines must be followed. Aerosols can release viable organisms from blood specimens, and laboratory-acquired infections have occurred.

Rickettsial infections are most frequently identified through the **Weil-Felix reaction.** Serum from patients with suspected rickettsial infections may or may not agglutinate specific strains of *Proteus vulgaris.* The strains of *P. vulgaris* used are OX-19, OX-2, and OX-K. For example, with rickettsialpox, no agglutination is noted in any of the *Proteus* strains, whereas agglutination is observed with OX-19 and OX-2, but not with OX-K, for Rocky Mountain spotted fever. The test is lacking in specificity, and several diseases yield variable results; thus the test is only presumptive. Confirmation with a more specific method, such as microimmunofluorescence, is necessary to detect serum antibodies to rickettsiae. In this procedure, antigenic dots for rickettsial diseases are fixed on a microscopic slide, and the patient's serum is added. A fluorescein-conjugated antihuman globulin is added, which binds to the antigen-antibody complex in a positive reaction.

Alternatively, tissue samples can be cultivated in embryonated eggs or tissue culture. Tissue samples can also be directly stained with an immunofluorescent dye to detect rickettsiae in the sample.

REVIEW QUESTIONS

MATCHING

Match the correct species for each rickettsial infection listed. Then select the mode of transmission of the infection. List all responses that apply.

Species	Insect Vector			
____	____	**1. Rocky Mountain spotted fever**	a. *Rickettsia tsutsugamushi*	A. Tick bite
____	____	**2. Rickettsialpox**	b. *Rickettsia rickettsii*	B. Lice
____	____	**3. Epidemic typhus**	c. *Coxiella burnetii*	C. Chigger bites
____	____	**4. Q fever**	d. *Rickettsia akari*	D. Aerosols
____	____	**5. Scrub typhus**	e. *Rickettsia typhi*	E. Mite bite
			f. *Rickettsia prowzekii*	

MULTIPLE CHOICE

6. Which statement correctly describes the genus *Chlamydia*?
a. Classified as viruses
b. Do not contain both DNA and RNA
c. Obligate intracellular bacteria
d. Smallest free-living organisms known

7. The agent in ornithosis is:
a. *Mycoplasma pneumoniae*
b. *Chlamydia pneumoniae*
c. *Chlamydia trachomatis*
d. *Chlamydia psittaci*

8. Each of the following conditions has been associated with *C. trachomatis* except:
a. Lymphogranuloma venereum
b. Nongonococcal urethritis
c. Infant pneumonitis
d. Atypical pneumonia

9. Which of the following serotypes are associated with *Chlamydia* diseases acquired through the venereal route?
a. A, B, Ba, and D
b. D through K
c. L4, L5, and L6
d. All the above

REVIEW QUESTIONS

(Continued)

10. The iodine stain for identification of *C. trachomatis* stains:
   a. The glycogen in the inclusion brown
   b. The periplasmic space purple
   c. The cell membrane brown
   d. The DNA in the inclusion purple

11. The DFA technique for *Chlamydia trachomatis* detects:
   a. Patient's antibodies to *C. trachomatis*
   b. Elementary bodies of *C. trachomatis*
   c. Cold-agglutinating antibodies produced in response to *C. trachomatis* infection
   d. Febrile agglutinins

12. Each of the following statements correctly describes the mycoplasmas *except:*
   a. They contain both DNA and RNA.
   b. They do not have a cell wall.
   c. They cannot replicate on their own.
   d. They are the smallest free-living organisms known.

13. *Mycoplasma pneumoniae:*
   a. Responds well to penicillin therapy
   b. Is the etiologic agent of primary atypical pneumonia
   c. Is most often identified through culture and biochemical reactions
   d. All the above

14. Which of the following results for cold agglutinins would be indicative of current infection with *Mycoplasma pneumoniae?*
   a. Acute titer of 4 and convalescent titer of 32
   b. Acute titer of 4 and convalescent titer of 8
   c. Convalescent titer of 256
   d. Both a and c are correct.
   e. All are correct.

BIBLIOGRAPHY

Barnes RC: Laboratory diagnosis of human chlamydial infections, *Clin Microbiol Rev* 2:199, 1989.

Cassall GH, Cole BC: Mycoplasmas as agents of human disease, *N Engl J Med* 304:80, 1981.

Crosse BA: Psittacosis: a clinical review, *J Infect Dis* 21:251, 1990.

Gallo D: Isolation and identification of *Chlamydia trachomatis:* a comparative study, *Lab Med* 15:481, 1984.

McCormack WM, guest editor: *Chlamydia,* Chicago, 1990, Abbott diagnostics educational services. Abbott Diagnostics, a division of Abbott Laboratories.

McTighe AG: *Chlamydia trachomatis:* review of human chlamydial infections and laboratory diagnosis, *Lab Med* 13:638, 1982.

Nelson JA, Bouseman JK: Human tick-borne illnesses: United States, *Clin Microbiol Newsletter* 14:105, 1992.

Philip A: *Mycoplasma pneumoniae:* disease characteristics and laboratory diagnosis, *Lab Med* 11:241, 1980.

Phillips LE, Goodrich KH, Turner RM et al: Isolation of *Mycoplasma* species and *Ureaplasma urealyticum* from obstetrical and gynocological patients using commercially available medium formulations, *J Clin Microbiol* 24:377, 1986.

Rikihisa Y: The tribe Ehrlichiae and ehrlichial diseases, *Clin Microbiol Rev* 4:286, 1991.

Taylor-Robinson D: Mycoplasma and ureaplasma. In Murray PA, editor: *Manual of clinical microbiology*, ed 6, Washington, DC, 1995, American Society for Microbiology.

Taylor-Robinson D, McCormack WM: The genital mycoplasmas, *N Engl J Med* 302:1003, 1980.

Walker DH: Rocky Mountain spotted fever: a disease in need of microbiological concern, *Clin Microbiol Rev* 2:227, 1989.

crowded quarters; intravenous drug users; institutionalized persons, including prisoners and mentally retarded patients; those who receive frequent IV procedures; and homosexuals.

Before the screening of blood donors for HBV, the virus was the major cause of posttransfusion hepatitis. Disease control is through careful screening of blood donors, sterilization of dental and medical instruments, and passive immunization through the HBV vaccine. The HBV vaccine is a series of three intramuscular (IM) doses of synthetic HBV. It is recommended for all health care workers at risk.

After exposure, HBV may incubate for 50 to 180 days, with an average incubation time of 90 days. The infection can be mild and asymptomatic, symptomatic, fulminant, or chronic. The disease has an insidious onset, with initial signs of fever, rash, or arthritis. Jaundice may occur shortly after initial signs and may usually persist for 4 to 6 weeks. Fulminant, fatal hepatitis and chronic hepatitis are possible complications of primary infection. An individual may test positive for HBsAg for years without evidence of liver disease, whereas other chronic carriers may develop hepatitis. HBV may also result in primary hepatocellular carcinoma.

Patients with HBV infection typically have abnormal liver function, as evidenced by increased levels of the liver enzymes. Serum bilirubin level is also elevated. Diagnosis is accomplished through clinical signs and serological testing. Currently, six HBV markers can be used in the diagnosis of infection. Tests for HAV may also be necessary if a differential diagnosis is to be made. The serological tests available for the diagnosis of HBV infection currently are as follows:

- **HBsAg.** HBsAg is present at the onset of infection. It is the first serological marker to appear, and it disappears as the patient recovers. Persistence more than 6 months may indicate chronic infection. It is present in acute, active, chronic, and carrier states of HBV infection.
- **Anti-HBsAg.** Total antibody to HBsAg appears 2 to 6 weeks after HBsAg is gone and usually persists for life. Its presence generally indicates recovery or immunity after the HBV vaccination.
- **Anti-HBcAg-IgM.** Anti-HBcAg-IgM is an indicator of recent acute infection; it is usually present for 6 months. Acute infection is indicated when anti-HBcAg-IgM is present with HBsAg.
- **Anti-HBcAg.** Total antibody to HBcAg (IgG and IgM) appearing after HBsAg but before anti-HBsAg appears; thus it sometimes is referred to as the "core window." It is present in high levels at the onset of symptoms but drops to low levels, and levels may persist for 5 to 6 years. Anti-HBcAg indicates current or previous infection and is not associated with recovery or immunity.
- **HBeAg.** HBeAg is present in acute and chronic hepatitis and is a marker of infectivity; persistence usually indicates chronic liver disease.
- **Anti-HBeAb.** Anti-hepatitis B e antibody does not appear until HBeAg disappears; it is usually associated with a favorable outcome.

Hepatitis C virus (HCV). The agent of NANB hepatitis is an **RNA-containing** virus with a lipid envelope. HCV seems to be most related to the viral family Flaviviridae. Formerly known as NANB hepatitis, HCV was first isolated in 1984. HCV may be acquired parenterally through contaminated blood products, organ transplantation, hemodialysis, or IV drug use. Nonparenteral routes have also been described.

Before the development of a marker for its detection, HCV was the most frequent cause of posttransfusion hepatitis, responsible for approximately 90% of all cases. Before 1990, elevation of the liver enzyme ALT and the presence of anti HBcAg were used as markers for HCV infection. In 1990 the first ELISA test to detect antibody to HCV was available. The test has subsequently been improved to detect earlier antigens.

HCV incubates 2 to 26 weeks after exposure, with an average incubation of 8 weeks. Disease is usually milder than HBV, although persistent chronic infection may occur.

Hepatitis D virus (HDV), or **delta virus,** is a small virus with a size of 35 to 37 nm that possesses **single-stranded** RNA and is infective only in the presence of HBV infection. It is transmitted through routes similar to HBV. Serological testing to detect HDV antigen, IgM antibody to HDV, and total antibody to HDV are available.

Hepatitis E virus (HEV) possesses **single-stranded** RNA and has a size of 32 to 34 nm. It is associated with enterically transmitted NANB hepatitis, which is spread through contaminated water in underdeveloped countries. HEV has been associated with hepatitis outbreaks in several parts of the world, including Mexico, Pakistan, India, and Indonesia. The disease resembles HAV, and laboratory diagnosis is not yet routine because it involves Western blot assays, PCR, and electron microscopy.

Herpesviruses

The Herpetoviridae **(herpesviruses)** are **enveloped, DNA-containing viruses with icosahedral symmetry** of approximately 100 nm in size. This viral family produces **latent viral infections** that can be reactivated and cause disease after months or years. Known sites where the virus may remain latent include the white blood cells (WBCs) and peripheral nerves. Reactivation seems to be associated with immunosuppressed patients, those with underlying medical problems, and patients undergoing chemotherapy or corticosteroid therapy.

Infections of the herpesviruses are generally more severe in adults than in children. Asymptomatic infection is common, and patients may unknowingly shed the virus.

Subfamily Alphaherpesvirinae include HSV-1 and HSV-2, as well as VZV.

Herpes Simplex Virus (HSV)

HSV infections occur throughout the world. HSV-1 infection is common in childhood, and most adults have antibody to this virus. HSV-1 generally produces more mild infections and is less resistant to treatment compared with HSV-2. Transmission of the virus is through active ulcerations of the mucous membranes or the genitalia. The general rule that HSV-1 causes infections above the waist, whereas HSV-2 causes infections below the waist, may hold true, but cross-infections are increasingly more common.

HSV-1 is associated with gingivostomatitis, ulcerative mouth lesions, and fever blisters. The virus may spread to the lips and cheeks. Primary lesions may be accompanied by fever, malaise, and cervical lymphadenopathy. Most cases are mild or asymptomatic and resolve without treatment. Approximately 90% of all cases of primary herpes gingivostomatitis are attributed to HSV-1.

HSV-2 produces 80% to 90% of all cases of genital herpes, a common sexually transmitted disease (STD). Early signs of infection include fever, malaise, and inguinal lymphadenopathy, although some primary infections are asymptomatic. Primary lesions typically appear on the vagina, cervix, glans, or penile shaft. Recurrent lesions may occur. A link between HSV-2 and cervical carcinoma has been established.

Neonatal HSV-2 infections may result if the infant acquires infection during delivery from an actively infected mother. The virus typically attacks the infant's CNS, and developmental difficulties may be seen.

Other infections associated with HSV include herpetic keratitis; herpetic whitlow, which infects the fingers and is an occupational hazard for those who have contact with patients who excrete the virus; and CNS infections, including sporadic encephalitis. HSV infections in AIDS patients and those with other immunosuppressive states have been increasing.

Specimens that may be collected for diagnosis of HSV include lesions or conjunctival scrapings. Direct examination for the virus can be accomplished through electron microscopy, the Papanicolaou smear, DFA, indirect fluorescence, immunoperoxidase techniques, cell cultures, and SVCE detection. CPE is typically observed within 7 days as round, clumping, syncytial, giant cells. Serological testing is not very helpful, since uninfected individuals may possess antibody and because antibody against HSV-1 and HSV-2 cannot be differentiated.

Varicella-Zoster Virus (VZV).

VZV is the agent of **varicella**, or chickenpox, and herpes zoster, or shingles, which is a reactivation of latent varicella infection. Chickenpox is generally a childhood disease, with most cases occurring in children less than 10 years of age. The infection is characterized by a generalized skin rash with raised, fluid-filled lesions. Infection is transmitted through the respiratory route, and the virus may incubate for 10 to 20 days. VZV multiplies in the respiratory tract and regional lymph nodes and is then disseminated by the blood to the skin. Headache, fever, and rash may be associated symptoms. The lesions first appear on the scalp and trunk and other warm areas of the body, followed by lesions on the arms and legs. Lesions pass through several stages before healing. The lesion first appears as a vesicle with clear fluid, resembling a "dewdrop on a rose petal." The lesions then develop into pustules with purulent fluid that eventually rupture. The final stage is the scab or crusting phase. Individuals are contagious 24 to 48 hours before the eruption of the rash and remain infectious until all lesions have scabbed. The association between Reye's syndrome and aspirin use to treat viral infections, including chickenpox, is widely known. Primary varicella is much more serious in immunosuppressed children, including those with leukemia or solid tumors and transplant recipients. In these patients the rash may be more severe, and pneumonitis, hepatitis, and encephalitis may occur. Vaccination with VZV immune globulin is recommended for these children. Primary varicella is often more serious in adults than in children, with pneumonitis being a concern.

Reactivation of VZV may occur in the form of herpes zoster. It is believed that the virus remains latent in the dorsal root ganglia of peripheral or cranial nerves after the primary infection. Shingles is predominantly a disease of elderly and immunosuppressed patients. Factors involving reactivation are not entirely understood, but trauma and an altered host immune system seem to play a role. Herpes zoster is accompanied by fluid-filled skin vesicles and pain along the areas of the rash. Complications include neuralgia, keratitis, ophthalmia, hearing loss, facial paralysis, and aseptic meningitis.

Diagnosis of VZV infections is usually made from clinical signs. The vesicular lesions can be directly examined for the appearance of intranuclear inclusions and multinucleate giant cells. Cell culture and serological tests to determine prior immunity to VZV are also available.

Cytomegalovirus (CMV)

A member of the subfamily betaherpesvirinae, CMV is an opportunistic infection that can be transmitted through direct contact with saliva, via blood transfusions, and through organ transplants. It typically produces asymptomatic or mild infection in healthy individuals, and approximately one-half the population is seropositive by age 30. Formerly known as "salivary gland virus," CMV has been isolated from saliva, urine, feces, milk, and semen. Repeated contact with the virus is necessary for infection. The virus can remain latent in WBCs, endothelial cells, and other organs.

Congenital CMV may occur as a primary infection during pregnancy if the mother lacks the antibody to the virus. Reactivation of a latent viral infection in the mother may also result in congenital CMV. Although many infants are asymptomatic at birth, developmental abnormalities, mental retardation, or deafness may occur later. Symptoms of congenital CMV include jaundice, hepatosplenomegaly, growth retardation, mental retardation, microencephaly, and lung disease. Perinatal CMV may occur during delivery if the mother is infected, or the virus may be acquired through the mother's breast milk.

CMV infection has presented a great problem to transplant recipients. CMV can be acquired if a seronegative recipient receives a transplanted organ positive for CMV. The infection manifests as a pneumonia more than 1 month after the transplant and thus is known as the "40-day fever."

CMV can also be acquired through transfused blood when the donor is seropositive and the recipient is seronegative.

Specimens for the identification of CMV include primarily urine, although saliva, tears, milk, semen, and vaginal secretions can also be collected. Direct cytological examination reveals the characteristic "owl eyes"—large cells with large, basophilic, staining inclusions within the nucleus. The virus can be isolated in cell culture and shell vials. CPE is typically observed as the rounding of cells. Early viral antigens may be detected through the use of a fluorescent antibody stain.

Serological tests often are not very helpful, since they cannot differentiate among primary, reactivated, and persistent infections. Currently, latex agglutination and ELISA are available to detect CMV antibody.

Prevention of CMV infection is through the screening of blood donors and organ donors. Seropositive products should not be transfused into seronegative recipients.

Epstein-Barr Virus (EBV)

A member of the subfamily gammaherpesvirinae, EBV was first isolated from malignant Burkitt's lymphoma cells in African children. The lymphoma is found in the lower jaw, as well as in the kidneys, liver, and adrenal glands. The virus is also the cause of infectious mononucleosis.

EBV is shed in the saliva and transmitted through oral contact. The virus incubates for 1 to 2 months, during which it disseminates to the RES, including the liver, spleen, and lymph nodes. Typical signs include fever, sore throat, enlarged lymph nodes, and enlarged tonsils. Splenomegaly, hepatomegaly, and elevated liver enzymes may also be seen. Recovery usually occurs in 2 to 3 weeks; however, complications may include splenic rupture, hemolytic anemia, encephalitis, and chronic EBV infection.

The role of EBV in chronic fatigue syndrome (CFS) continues to remain controversial. CFS is accompanied by overwhelming fatigue, muscle aches, low-grade fever, and mild lymphadenopathy. Patients generally are positive for antibody to EBV.

Infectious mononucleosis is diagnosed clinically and through hematology and serological testing. The differential WBC count typically shows greater than 50% lymphocytes with the appearance of "atypical lymphocytes." The presence of heterophile antibody can be detected using one of several commercially available slide tests. Heterophile antibody occurs in one species but reacts with antigens of different species. This antibody may be present in the serum of those with infectious mononucleosis or serum sickness, as well as in some healthy individuals (Forssmann antibodies). Heterophile antibodies in all three cases will agglutinate sheep and horse red blood cells. Guinea pig cells are used to absorb human serum. The cells will remove the agglutinins of serum sickness and Forssmann antibodies, leaving the agglutinins of infectious mononucleosis to remain.

Human Herpesvirus Type 6 (HHV-6)

Another member of the subfamily gammaherpesvirinae, HHV-6 was first known as *human lymphotropic virus* since it first was detected infecting B cells in vitro. The virus was first isolated in saliva and mononuclear cells of peripheral blood in 1986. It is now known that the virus primarily infects T lymphocytes, where it is known to remain latent. The route of infection is most likely through respiratory contact.

HHV-6 is the agent of **exanthem subitum** or **roseola,** also known as **sixth disease.** Roseola is a benign childhood disease most frequently seen in children ages 6 months to 3 years. The infection is characterized by a sore throat and high fever that persist for 3 to 5 days. A nonspecific maculopapular rash of the trunk and neck develops 24 to 48 hours after the fever subsides. The virus rarely produces infections in adults.

Papovaviruses

The family Papovaviridae is characterized by having **double-stranded DNA, icosahedral symmetry, no envelope,** and a size of 45 to 55 nm. Members of this family include papillomavirus (pa), the cause of common warts, polyomavirus (po); and simian vacuolating virus (va); thus the name "papova."

More than 60 genetic types of human papillomavirus (HPV) exist, which are primarily associated with a variety of cutaneous lesions and benign growths, including plantar warts, common warts, and sexually transmitted venereal warts. Genital infections may be associated with neoplastic lesions, including cervical carcinoma.

Polyoma strains JC and BK produce mild or asymptomatic infections. The infection is most likely spread through respiratory secretions.

Parvoviruses

Parvovirus is a small (18 to 26 nm), **DNA-containing, nonenveloped virus with icosahedral symmetry.** Parvoviruses are known to infect mice, hamsters, cats, and dogs; however, only parvovirus B-19 is known to cause human infection. The virus is the agent of erythema infectiosum, or fifth disease (after measles, rubella, varicella-zoster, and roseola), a childhood illness. The virus is spread through the respiratory route and is characterized by fever and a unique "slapped-cheek rash." The virus has an affinity for RBC precursors, which may lead to a mild anemia in normal patients or a severe, chronic anemia in patients who have malignancies or hematological abnormalities.

Poxviruses

The poxviruses are large (225 × 300 nm) **DNA-containing viruses** that are **enveloped with complex coats.** The family includes variola, the smallpox virus, and vaccinia virus, as well as the agents of cowpox and monkeypox.

Smallpox is an ancient disease that killed millions during our recorded history. The virus was spread through direct respiratory contact and multiplied in the lymph nodes. This was followed by the viremic phase with dissemination to various organs; the pox lesions developed next. The rash occurred in a single crop, in contrast to chickenpox. Vaccinations were administered to those who lived or worked in potentially hazardous areas. The disease is now eradicated, and in 1979 the World Health Organization (WHO) declared that the world was free of smallpox.

Arboviruses

The arthropod-borne viruses or arboviruses, include the families **Togaviridae, Flaviviridae,** and **Bunyaviridae.** All three viral families have **single-stranded RNA** and are **enveloped.** The alpha viruses, or group A togaviruses, are the agents in various types of encephalitis. **Western equine encephalitis (WEE)** is found in the Western United States and Canada, **eastern equine encephalitis (EEE)** is found in the Eastern and Southern United States, and **Venezuelan equine encephalitis (VEE)** is found in South and Central America. All these viruses are transmitted to animals, including horses and birds, by the mosquito vector; humans serve as accidental hosts.

The **flavivirus** of the family Flaviviridae is the agent of **St. Louis encephalitis (SLE),** which is found sporadically in southern and southern-central United States. Birds constitute the major reservoir, and mosquitoes are the vector in SLE. Epidemics seem to occur every 10 years in Texas or the Gulf Coast area. Flaviviruses are also the cause of **Japanese B encephalitis,** a severe form of the disease, found in the Far East, Korea, and Japan, as well as of **yellow fever** and **dengue fever.** The vector in yellow fever is the mosquito, and the disease, characterized by headache, backache, and nausea, can produce severe liver damage. Dengue fever, found in the Caribbean and Southeast Asia, is characterized by headache, backache, fatigue, and chills. Rash and arthritis may also be symptoms.

Animal inoculation is often necessary for the identification of the arboviruses, although some of the viruses can be isolated in cell culture.

Rubivirus, also a togavirus, is unique in this viral group because no insect vector is needed. The virus is the agent of **rubella (German measles),** an acute febrile disease that once was responsible for minor epidemics every 5 to 7 years. The virus has **single-stranded RNA, icosahedral symmetry,** a diameter of 60 to 70 nm, and surface projections, including hemagglutinins. The infection is spread through respiratory secretions, incubates for 2 to 3 weeks, and then invades the nasopharyngeal mucosa, multiplying in the lymph nodes. It is then disseminated by the blood, and a mild fever, rash, and lymphadenopathy develop. The maculopapular rash has a duration of 3 to 4 days. The virus is shed for approximately 1 week before clinical signs of infection.

Since the virus can cross the placenta, rubella may infect the baby in utero. Congenital infection may be mild and asymptomatic or severe, causing cataracts, glaucoma, deafness, heart abnormalities, mental retardation, or death.

Today the rubella vaccine is given to children at 15 months of age as a part of the MMR (measles-mumps-rubella) immunization. The vaccine is live and attenuated and confers lifelong immunity in approximately 95% of those immunized.

Serodiagnosis is usually the method for identification. IgG and IgM appear a few days after the onset of the rash. A hemagglutinin inhibition test to identify and quantitate the antibody is available. The virus can also be isolated from the throat and urine in cell culture.

The family Bunyaviridae includes bunyavirus, the agent of LaCross virus or California encephalitis, and phlebovirus, the agent of Rift Valley fever. Hantavirus, the agent of Korean hemorrhagic fever, and Nairovirus, the agent of Crimean-Congo hemorrhagic fever, are also members of this family.

Picornaviruses

The Picornaviridae are a large, diverse viral family that includes the enteroviruses and rhinoviruses. The family is characterized by the presence of **single-stranded RNA, icosahedral symmetry,** and **absence of an envelope.** The viruses have a very small size of 20 to 30 nm, thus the prefix "pico." The Picornaviridae are associated with CNS disorders, which may result in paralysis or death, and with aseptic meningitis, myocarditis, and mild or asymptomatic respiratory disease. Often, poor hygiene, overcrowding, or poor sanitation are factors in the acquisition of these infections.

The enteroviruses consist of poliovirus, echovirus, and coxsackieviruses, as well as HAV, which has been discussed previously.

Poliovirus occurs naturally only in humans and is disseminated through the fecal-oral route and through respiratory secretions. Primary infection is of the respiratory tract, followed by viremia to various parts of the body, including the skin, heart, and meninges. The most common type of polio is abortive poliomyelitis, which is mild or asymptomatic with rapid recovery. Poliovirus may also cause an aseptic meningitis, which may extend into paralytic poliomyelitis, the most severe type of polio infection. It is characterized by destruction of large motor neurons in the spinal cord and is usually accompanied by paralysis.

Historically, two types of polio vaccines have been administered. The Salk vaccine is formalin-killed virus and stimulates antibody production in the serum, but not in the mucosa. The Sabin vaccine is a live, attenuated vaccine given orally. The Sabin vaccine stimulates the production of both IgA and IgG and is the preferred vaccine today. However, the virus can be excreted through the stool, which can serve as a route of infection in susceptible individuals.

Coxsackie viruses are named for Coxsackie, NY, where the viruses were first isolated. Coxsackievirus A and coxsackievirus B are associated with aseptic meningitis, paralysis, pharyngitis, myocarditis, and rash; coxsackievirus A is also the agent of hand-foot-and-mouth disease.

Echovirus has been isolated in cases of aseptic meningitis, fever, respiratory infections, and paralysis.

Enteroviruses may be isolated from throat swabs, feces, CSF, urine, blood, and conjunctival swabs, depending on the site of the infection. Direct detection and serological testing is not recommended, and identification is most often accompanied through clinical signs and virus isolation in cell culture.

Rhinoviruses, agents of the common cold, usually produce mild respiratory infections without a fever. More than 100 serotypes are known. Rhinovirus can survive at room temperature for 24 hours. The virus seems to be transmitted through the contaminated hands of those infected with the virus and not through sneezing. The virus may invade the lower respiratory tract, resulting in a more serious infection. Rhinoviruses grow best at 33°C, and identification is not attempted due to the large number of serotypes and because the infections are most often mild. Rhinovirus infection is prevented through good handwashing and the avoidance of hand-to-eye or hand-to-nose contact.

Orthomyxoviruses

The family Orthomyxoviridae includes the genus *Influenza,* which has as its members **influenza viruses A, B, and C.** The viruses contain **single stranded RNA,** possess **helical symmetry,** and are **enveloped.** Influenza viruses range in size from 80 to 120 nm. Important characteristics of this family include the presence of **hemagglutinin antigen (HA)** and **neuraminidase antigen (NA).** HA allows the virus to attach to glycoproteins on the surface of RBCs and respiratory epithelial cells. NA permits the virus entry into the host cell.

Influenza viruses are spread through aerosols and respiratory droplets. The infections are characterized by an abrupt onset, fever, chills, headache, muscle aches, and a dry cough. Typical types of infections include the common cold, tracheobronchitis, and pneumonia.

Influenza pandemics occur approximately every 10 years. The surface antigens of type A influenza virus are constantly changing. Regional or national influenza outbreaks occur in the winter and are named for the viral structure and location of the outbreak. Pandemics of note include A_2 Asian (1957), A_3 Hong Kong (1968), and the A_1 outbreak of 1978. Type A infections may be accompanied by secondary bacterial pneumonias.

Vaccination of high-risk populations is recommended, with a new vaccine prepared annually based on the type of virus isolated from outbreaks the previous year.

Specimens collected for identification of influenza viruses include throat swabs and nasopharyngeal washing. Direct immunofluorescence can be performed on nasopharyngeal washings, and the virus can be isolated in cell culture and hemadsorption assay.

Serological diagnosis through hemagglutination inhibition, a measure of the patient's antibody titer against the HA, can be used. Antibodies to NA may also be detected. Both antibodies appear 1 to 2 weeks after infection and may persist for up to 4 months. Paired sera for acute and convalescent antibody titers are recommended. Indirect immunofluorescent methods to detect IgG and IgM in influenza A and B are also available.

Paramyxoviruses

The Paramyxoviridae includes the genera Paramyxovirus, Morbillivirus, and Pneumovirus. The family possesses single-stranded RNA, helical symmetry, an envelope, and an average size of 150 to 300 nm.

Paramyxovirus includes the parainfluenza viruses, mumps virus, and New Castle virus. Parainfluenza virus causes mild upper respiratory tract infections as well as pneumonia, hepatitis, and meningitis. Parainfluenza virus type 1 produces croup, an infection seen in infants and characterized by difficulty in breathing and a hoarse, barking cough. Parainfluenza infections are spread by direct contact from infected persons or through respiratory droplet infection.

Respiratory tract specimens are collected for identification of the parainfluenza viruses. Direct immunofluorescence can be performed on nasopharyngeal washings, and the virus can be isolated in cell culture. Hemadsorption is recommended because not all the viruses produce CPE. Serological diagnosis is not recommended due to recurrent infections.

Mumps is an infection of the parotid glands characterized by swelling behind the ears and difficulty swallowing. Mumps virus possesses both HA and NA antigens and a hemolysin. The virus is transmitted through respiratory secretions in contaminated saliva. It is most contagious just before and immediately after the parotid glands swell. The virus multiplies in the upper respiratory tract and adjacent lymph nodes.

Once a common childhood disease, infections have steadily declined due to widespread vaccine use. The mumps vaccine was first introduced in 1967; today the MMR is given to infants at 15 months of age. Most cases today are seen in nonimmunized children. A complication seen in adult males affected with mumps is inflammation of the gonads, which may lead to sterility.

Mumps virus can be isolated in cell culture. Serological detection of IgM and IgG antibodies through immunofluroescence is also available.

Morbillivirus, the cause of **rubeola** (measles), possesses HA and a hemolysin but does not possess NA. Once a severe, acute, highly contagious childhood disease with epidemics seen every 2 to 3 years, the incidence has dramatically decreased due to vaccination. The virus is spread via respiratory secretions, through nasal secretions or coughing. Measles virus incubates approximately 10 days, multiplying in the respiratory tract, before the first symptoms of fever, nasal drainage, headache, cough, and sore throat. A primary viremia occurs, and the virus is spread to the RES and viscera, where it multiples a second time. This is followed by a secondary viremia and the appearance of a rash, initially on the head. The rash characteristically moves down the body.

Measles vaccination is a part of the MMR given to infants at 15 months of age. Because of vaccination, measles is seen much less frequently in children but is seen more frequently in older children, adolescents, and young adults. Outbreaks at college campuses were seen in 1989 and 1990, prompting the recommendation of a second measles immunization at either 4 to 6 years of age or before entrance to middle or high school.

Complications of measles infection are common and include pneumonia and encephalitis.

Measles is diagnosed through clinical signs and is usually not cultured because the virus is shed very early in the infection. The virus may be isolated in cell culture. Serological testing is available to determine if an individual is seropositive to the virus.

Respiratory syncytial virus (RSV), a member of the genus Pneumovirus, is a small virus with single-stranded RNA. RSV is pleomorphic and enveloped and does not contain HA. Types of infections range from mild respiratory tract infections and ear infections to pneumonia and other severe respiratory diseases. The infection is most common and most serious in infants and young children. RSV is spread through droplets of contaminated respiratory secretions, which enter through the eyes or nose.

Diagnosis is achieved by clinical signs and cultures, including nasal aspirates, throat swabs, nasopharyngeal specimens, or sputum. The RSV antigen can be detected directly using immunofluorescence on the specimens or in cell culture. Serological testing includes immunofluorescence or complement fixation; the IgM antibody is present within 1 to 2 days.

Rhabdoviruses

The **Lyssavirus** in the family Rhabdoviridae is the agent of **rabies.** The virus is bullet shaped and ranges in size from a diameter of 60 to 95 nm and a length of 130 to 350 nm. The genetic material is **single-stranded RNA,** the **symmetry is helical,** and the virus is **enveloped.** Rabies is found in both wild and domestic animals, including skunks, foxes, coyotes, raccoons, bats, dogs, and cats. Infection is transmitted through contaminated respiratory secretions, most frequently from the bite of an infected animal. Cutaneous transmission from infected secretions is another route of infection. Once introduced through the wound, the virus next travels to the CNS. Once in the CNS, an often fatal encephalitis accompanied by coma, convulsions, and death occurs.

Diagnosis is usually made through clinical signs and the medical history of a bite or direct contact with secretions of a possibly infected animal. The virus can be detected using direct immunofluorescence to detect viral antigen. Characteristic Negri bodies are found in the cytoplasm of infected brain cells.

The rabies vaccine is administered in animal bite cases when it cannot be determined if the bite or contact occurred with a rabid animal or from a domestic animal that has not had the proper immunizations.

Reoviruses

The family Reoviridae includes the genera ***Reovirus, Rotavirus,*** and ***Orbivirus.*** Characteristics of the family include **double-stranded RNA, icosahedral symmetry, no envelope,** and a diameter of 60 to 80 nm.

Rotavirus is a common cause of gastroenteritis and is associated with both sporadic and epidemic outbreaks. Infants ages 6 months to 2 years are most frequently affected. In fact, rotavirus is the most common cause of gastroenteritis in this age group. Rotavirus is named for its appearance under electron microscopy as a double-shelled capsule that resembles a wheel (Latin *rota*). The virus is spread through the fecal-oral route and also may be associated with food-borne or waterborne infections.

Identification has been accomplished in the past only through electron microscopy. However, rapid latex agglutination and ELISA are now commercially available for detection of the viral antigen.

Calciviruses

Calcivirus, commonly known as **Norwalk** or **Norwalk-like viruses,** are in the family Calciviridae. Characteristics of the Calciviridae include **single-stranded RNA, icosahedral symmetry, no envelope,** and a diameter of 25 to 35 nm. The virus is named for Norwalk, Ohio, where an outbreak of diarrhea in 1968 occurred in schoolchildren, their teachers, and their families. The virus is associated with epidemics of mild gastroenteritis, predominantly in children 6 years of age or older. The virus is spread by the fecal-oral route, with virus shedding occurring in the stool as well as through contaminated food and water. Identification, when necessary, is usually accomplished using electron microscopy or ELISA.

Retroviruses

The family Retroviridae includes the subfamilies Oncornavirinae and Lentivirinae. The Retroviridae possess **single-stranded RNA, icosahedral symmetry, an envelope,** and a diameter of 80 to 130 nm. The **retroviruses** possess the enzyme **reverse transcriptase,** or **RNA-dependent DNA polyermase,** which can transcribe RNA into DNA. This is the "reverse" of the normal transcription of DNA into RNA.

The **Oncornavirinae** includes the genus ***Oncornavirus,*** of which human T cell lymphotropic virus type 1 (HTLV-1) and human T cell lymphotropic virus type 2 (HTLV-2) are members. HTLV-1, the first human retrovirus to be identified, is an oncogenic virus and the cause of adult T cell leukemia, lymphoma, and tropical spastic paraparesis. T cell leukemia is a malignancy of specific subtypes of T lymphocytes that is characterized by dermal and bone involvement, including lesions of the bone. The second retrovirus to be isolated, HTLV-2, was isolated from a patient with hairy cell leukemia. Prevalence of both viruses is low in the United States but has a higher incidence in other areas of the world. Transmission of the HTLV viruses is believed to occur through similar routes as HIV infection.

The **Lentivirinae** (Latin *lenti,* or "slow") include human immunodeficiency viruses types 1 and 2 (HIV-1 and HIV-2), which are associated with slow viral diseases with neurological manifestations. First named *HTLV-3* and *LAV (lymphadenopathy virus)* by researchers who discovered the virus in the United States and France in 1983, respectively, the virus was eventually named HIV-1. A second HIV virus (HIV-2) was subsequently isolated.

HIV has a complex structure and possesses various proteins, including the following:

- **Group-specific antigen ("gag") proteins,** which code for core proteins. These are a part of the viral nucleocapsid and provide stability for the capsule.
- **Polymerase ("pol") proteins,** which are important in the viral life cycle. These include RNA-dependent DNA polymerase (reverse transcriptase) and endonuclease.
- **Envelope ("env") proteins,** which are glycoproteins that adhere to target cells and produce cytopathic cell fusion. The envelope includes cell wall components of the host as the virus "buds."

HIV-1 is the agent of **acquired immunodeficiency syndrome** (AIDS), which is characterized by loss of immune competency, opportunistic infections, and unusual neoplasms. Through 1990, more than 1 million cases of AIDS have occurred in the United States, with approximately 100,000 deaths resulting from the virus from 1981 through 1990. Of reported cases, more than one-half have been reported in homosexual men and approximately one-fourth in those injecting illicit drugs. Other routes of infection include heterosexual contact with an infected person and congenital transmission. Before detection methods for the virus, HIV-1 was also transmitted through contaminated blood and blood products, including factor VIII concentrates used to treat hemophilia.

AIDS is a fatal disease with no known cures or recoveries. Clinical symptoms include flu-like symptoms, which may occur 6 to 8 weeks after infection. Circulating virus is present at this time, and antibodies develop within a few months of infection. This is followed by a long, asymptomatic phase that may range from months to years. During this time the level of CD4-positive T cells declines and the characteristic symptoms indicate AIDS infection, including opportunistic infections, neoplasms, or other signs.

AIDS patients acquire several opportunistic infections, including *Pneumocystis carinii* pneumonia, CMV infections, cryptosporidosis or isosporiasis diarrhea, candidiasis, toxoplasmosis, and mycobacterial infections. Other symptoms include fever, night sweats, loss of weight, and lymphadenopathy. The development of unusual neoplasms, in particular Kaposi's sarcoma, as well as anal carcinomas and B cell lymphomas, may also occur. Neurological damage, including encephalopathies, may also be present.

Today the main routes of infection are through sexual intercourse and injection of illicit drugs. No evidence indicates that the virus is spread through the aerosol route or through casual contact. Universal precautions have been established to decrease the incidence of HIV-acquired infections in the health care setting.

Diagnosis of HIV infection is based on clinical symptoms and serological testing. Several commercially available ELISAs are available as screening tests. These tests are very useful in screening blood donors for the presence of HIV, and all positive units are discarded. Careful interviewing and screening of blood donors also decreased the incidence of possible HIV-positive units.

The confirmatory test for HIV, however, is the **Western blot,** which identifies antibodies for various HIV antigens; antibodies to HIV p24 (a "gag" protein and either gp41 or gp160 (envelope antigens) usually confirm HIV infection. The criteria to interpret a positive Western blot test for HIV are established by health organizations such as the CDC or the American Red Cross. PCR methods are also available.

Treatment of HIV infections involves the treatment of the secondary opportunistic infections. Also, antiviral agents such as AZT (3′azido-3′-deoxythymidine) have been shown to prolong the life of HIV patients.

HIV-2 infections, although rare in the United States, are found more frequently in West Africa, South America, and parts of Europe. HIV-2 produces an infection similar to HIV-1, with different opportunistic pathogens seen and a milder disease course.

REVIEW QUESTIONS

MATCHING

For the following serological markers of HBV infection, match the marker with its correct description:

_____ **1. HBsAg**
_____ **2. HBeAg**
_____ **3. Anti-HBcAg**
_____ **4. Anti-HBsAg**

a. Total antibody to hepatitis B surface antigen is associated with immunity or recovery.
b. Marker of infectivity and persistence usually indicates chronic liver disease.
c. Total antibody to hepatitis B core antigen appears between HBsAg and anti-HBsAg.
d. Recent acute infection is indicated.
e. First serologic marker to appear, persistence may indicate chronic infection.

Match the virus with its associated infection:

_____ **5. VZV**
_____ **6. EBV**
_____ **7. HHV-6**
_____ **8. HSV-1**
_____ **9. Human papillomavirus**
_____ **10. Parvovirus**
_____ **11. Togavirus**
_____ **12. Variola**
_____ **13. Flavivirus**
_____ **14. Rubivirus**
_____ **15. Enterovirus**
_____ **16. Morbillivirus**
_____ **17. Pneumovirus**
_____ **18. Lyssavirus**
_____ **19. Human T cell lymphotropic virus**
_____ **20. HIV**

a. Adult T cell leukemia
b. Gingivostomatitis
c. Chickenpox
d. Warts
e. Rabies
f. Measles (rubeola)
g. Rubella
h. AIDS
i. Infectious mononucleosis
j. Smallpox
k. Respiratory syncytial virus
l. Roseola
m. Erythema infectiousum
n. Equine encephalitis
o. Polio
p. Yellow-fever

MULTIPLE CHOICE

21. Properties of viruses include:
a. Presence of both DNA and RNA
b. Presence of an ATP-generating system
c. Multiplication of binary fission
d. Obligate intracellular parasites

22. The protein coat of the virus is known as the:
a. Virion
b. Capsid
c. Nucleocapsid
d. Envelope

23. Although dependent on the virus to be isolated, optimal specimen collection time to detect most viral infections is:
a. Early in the course of the disease
b. During the convalescent phase
c. During the latent phase
d. 1 week after the onset of symptoms

24. When specimen delay is anticipated, virology specimens are optimally maintained:
a. At room temperature
b. Incubated at 35°C
c. Frozen immediately at −20°C
d. Held at 4°C and "snap-frozen" to −70°C

REVIEW QUESTIONS

(Continued)

25. Each of the following groups of viruses may be associated with aseptic meningitis *except:*
a. Enterovirus
b. Echovirus
c. Influenza viruses
d. Varicella-Zoster virus (VZV)
e. Mumps virus

26. Viral agents of gastroenteritis include:
a. Cytomegalovirus (CMV), rotavirus, and Epstein-Barr virus (EBV)
b. Rotavirus, calcivirus, and Norwalk agent
c. Herpes simplex virus (HSV), human immunodeficiency virus (HIV), and enterovirus
d. Parvovirus, rhinovirus, and echovirus

27. "Owl's eye" cytological inclusions are characteristic of infection caused by:
a. HIV
b. CMV
c. HSV
d. VZV

28. Heteroploid cell lines:
a. Contain at least 75% of cells with same karyotype of normal original cells
b. Include such examples as HEK and RMK
c. Are directly derived from parent tissue
d. Are usually derived from malignant or transformed cells

29. Which statement best describes normal antibody response to viral infection?
a. IgG appears within 2 weeks of primary infection.
b. IgM peaks in 3 to 6 weeks.
c. IgG is usually undetectable by 6 weeks.
d. None of the above is correct.

30. Which of the following hepatitis viruses is *not* transmitted through contaminated blood or blood products?
a. HAV
b. HBV
c. HCV
d. HDV

31. Which of the following viral families are associated with reactivation of latent infections?
a. Hepatitis viruses
b. Influenza viruses
c. Parvoviruses
d. Herpesviruses

32. A positive ELISA test for HIV-1 and a Western blot test with bands at p24 and gp41 most likely indicate:
a. False-positive ELISA and inconclusive Western blot
b. False-positive ELISA and Western blot
c. Positive ELISA and Western blot, indicating HIV infection
d. Lack of HIV infection

33. Which of the following are characteristic of EBV infection?
a. Failure to agglutinate sheep RBCs after absorption with guinea pig cells
b. Presence of greater than 50% lymphocytes and atypical lymphotyces on WBC differential
c. Presence of heterophile antibody
d. b and c are correct.
e. a, b, and c are correct.

Arrange the sequence of steps of viral replication in the correct order. Number the responses 1 through 5.

34. ____ Assembly
35. ____ Adsorption
36. ____ Penetration
37. ____ Release
38. ____ Uncoating

For each of the following viruses, indicate if the nucleic acid is DNA or RNA:

39. ____ HAV
40. ____ HBV
41. ____ HSV-1
42. ____ Adenovirus
43. ____ HIV
44. ____ Influenza virus
45. ____ VZV
46. ____ CMV

BIBLIOGRAPHY

The A to F of viral hepatitis, *Lancet* 336:1158, 1990.

Abbott Laboratories: *Principles in practice: testing for viral hepatitis,* Chicago, 1992, Abbott Laboratories.

Appleton H: Foodborne viruses, *Lancet* 336:1362, 1990.

Bartlett AV III, Bednarz-Prashod AJ, DuPont HL et al: Rotavirus gastroenteritis, *Annu Rev Med* 38:399, 1987.

Blacklow NR, Greenberg HB: Viral gastritis, *N Engl J Med* 325:252, 1991.

Bradley DW: Hepatitis E: epidemiology, aetiology, and molecular biology, *Rev Med Virol* 2:19, 1992.

Brandt CD, Kim HW, Rodriguez WJ et al: Adenoviruses and pediatric gastroenteritis, *J Infect Dis* 151:437, 1985.

Breinig MK, Zitelli B, Starzi T et al: Epstein-Barr virus, cytomegalovirus, and other viral infections in children after liver transplantation, *J Infect Dis* 156:273, 1987.

Calisher CH: Medically important arboviruses of the United States and Canada, *Clin Microbiol Rev 7:89,* 1994.

Centers for Disease Control: Increase in rubella and congenital rubella syndrome—United States, 1988-1990, *MMWR* 40:93, 1991.

Centers for Disease Control: Measles prevention: recommendations of the immunization practices advisory committee, *MMWR* 38:1018, 1989.

Centers for Disease Control: Protection against viral hepatitis, *MMWR* 39:1, 1990.

Chou S, Scott KM: Latex agglutination and enzyme-linked immunosorbent assays for cytomegalovirus serologic screening of transplant donors and recipients, *J Clin Microbiol* 26:2116, 1988.

Cohen S, Tyrrell AJ, Smith AP: Psychological stress and susceptibility to the common cold, *N Engl J Med* 325:606, 1991.

Croen KD: Latency of the human herpesviruses, *Annu Rev Med* 42:61, 67, 1991.

Dennehy PH, Gauntlett DR, Tente WE: Comparison of nine commercial immunoassays for the detection of rotavirus in fecal specimens, *J Clin Microbiol* 26:1630, 1988.

Dock NL: The ABC's of viral hepatitis, *Clin Microbiol Newsletter* 13:17, 1991.

Epstein MA, Achong BG: Pathogenesis of infectious mononucleosis, *Lancet* 2:1270, 1977.

Evans AS: Infectious mononucleosis and related syndromes, *Am J Med Sci* 276:325, 1978.

Field AK, Biron KK: "The End of Innocence" revisited: resistance of herpesviruses to antiviral drugs, *Clin Microbiol Rev* 7:1, 1994.

Fung JC: Pitfalls of IgM antibody testing, *Clin Microbiol Newsletter* 7:41, 1985.

Gallo RC: Retroviruses: a decade of discovery and link with human disease, *J Infect Dis* 164:235, 1991.

Hamilton JR: Viral enteritis, *Pediatr Clin North Am* 35:89, 1988.

Heilman CA: Respiratory syncytial and parainfluenza viruses, *J Infect Dis* 161:402, 1990.

Ho M: Epidemiology of cytomegalovirus infections, *Rev Infect Dis* 12:S701, 1990.

Hojvat SA: Diagnostic tests for viral hepatitis, *Clin Microbiol Newsletter* 11:33, 1989.

Johnson FB: Transport of viral specimens, *Clin Microbiol Rev* 3:120, 1990.

Kuo G, Chou O, Alter HJ et al: An assay for circulating antibodies to a major etiologic virus of human non-A non-B hepatitis, *Science* 244:362, 1989.

Kinney JS, Onorato IM, Stewart JA et al: Cytomegaloviral infection and disease, *J Infect Dis* 151:772, 1985.

Marymont JH, Herrman KL: Rubella testing: an overview, *Lab Med* 13:83, 1982.

Minnich LL, Ray CG: Early testing of cell cultures for detection of hemadsorbing viruses, *J Clin Micribiol* 25:421, 1987.

Neumann MA: Viruses. In Tilton RC, Balows A, Hohnadel DC, Reiss RF, editors: *Clinical laboratory methods,* St Louis, 1992, Mosby.

Oren I, Sobel JD: Human herpesvirus type 6: review, *Clin Infect Dis* 14:741, 1992.

Palese P, Young JF: Variation of influenza A, B, and C viruses, *Science* 215:1468, 1982.

Peter G: Childhood immunizations, *N Engl J Med* 327:1794, 1992.

Proffitt MR: Overview: diagnostic virology, clinical virology update, May 24, 1993, The Cleveland Clinic Foundation.

Sabin AB: Paralytic poliomyelitis: old dogmas and new perspectives, *Rev Infect Dis* 3:543, 1981.

Salk J: Commentary: poliomyelitis vaccination—choosing a wise policy, *Pediatr Infect Dis J* 6:889, 1987.

Shamberger RJ: ELISA on the trail of viral diseases, *Diagn Med* October, 52, 1984.

Silverman AL, Gordon SC: Clinical epidemiology and molecular biology of hepatitis C, *Lab Med* 24:656, 1993.

Smith TJ: Introduction to virology. In Howard BJ, editor: *Clinical and pathogenic microbiology,* ed 2, St Louis, 1994, Mosby.

Tsoukas CM, Bernard NF: Markers of predicting progression of human immunodeficiency virus-related disease, *Clin Microbiol Rev* 7:14, 1994.

Vainionpaa R, Hyypia T: Biology of parainfluenza viruses, *Clin Microbiol Rev* 7:265, 1994.

Waner JL: Mixed viral infections: detection and management, *Clin Microbiol Rev* 7:143, 1994.

Wolcott MJ: Advances in nucleic acid-based detection methods, *Clin Microbiol Rev* 5:370, 1993.

Zoulim F, Mimms L, Floreani M et al: New assays for quantitative determination of virus markers in management of chronic hepatitis B virus infection, *J Clin Microbiol* 30:1111, 1992.

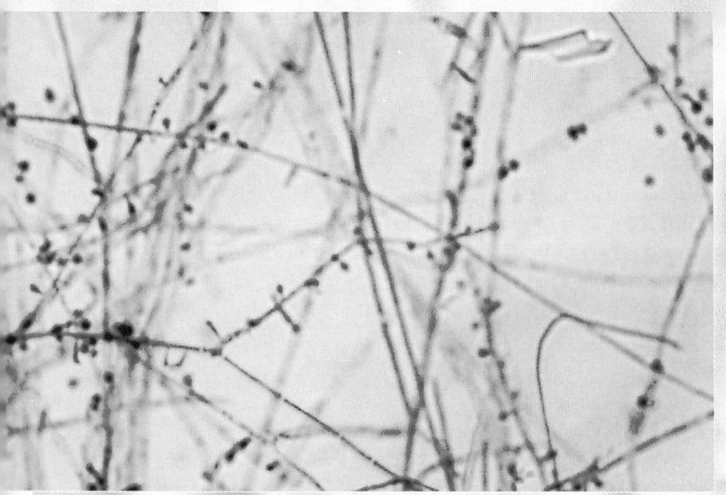

TRICHOPHYTON SPECIES

KEY TERMS

ASCOSPORE
ASSIMILATION
BASIDIOSPORE
BLASTOMYCOSIS
CHROMOBLASTOMYCOSIS
COCCIDIOIDOMYCOSIS
CONIDIA
CONIDIOGENESIS
DEMATIACEOUS FUNGI
DEUTEROMYCETES
DIMORPHIC
ECTOTHRIX
ENDOTHRIX
FUNGI IMPERFECTI
GERM TUBE
HISTOPLASMOSIS
HYPHAE
MACROCONIDIA
MICROCONIDIA
MOLD PHASE
MYCELIUM
MYCETOMA
MYCOSES
OOSPORE
OPPORTUNISTIC MYCOSES
PARACOCCIDIOIDOMYCOSIS
PENICILLIOSIS
PHAEOHYPHOMYCOSIS
PIEDRA
PITYRIASIS VERSICOLOR
SPORANGIOSPORES
SPOROTRICHOSIS
SUBCUTANEOUS MYCOSES
SUPERFICIAL (CUTANEOUS) MYCOSES
SYSTEMIC MYCOSES
THALLOPHYTES
TINEA
YEAST PHASE
ZYGOMYCOSIS
ZYGOSPORE

CHAPTER OUTLINE

SPECIMEN COLLECTION
IDENTIFICATION METHODS
- Microscopic Methods
- Culture Media
- Microscopic Examination of Growth

SUPERFICIAL OR CUTANEOUS MYCOSES
SUBCUTANEOUS MYCOSES
SYSTEMIC MYCOSES: DIMORPHIC FUNGI
YEAST AND YEASTLIKE FUNGI
OPPORTUNISTIC SAPROBIC FUNGI
SEROLOGICAL TESTING
SLIDE CULTURE
POTASSIUM HYDROXIDE (KOH) PREPARATION
TEASE MOUNT
GERM TUBE TEST
CORNMEAL AGAR WITH TWEEN 80
CARBOHYDRATE ASSIMILATION TEST FOR YEAST
RAPID UREASE TEST FOR YEAST

Introduction to Medical Mycology

LEARNING OBJECTIVES

1. Discuss the characteristics of the fungi.
2. Correctly define and describe the following:
   a. Hyphae
   b. Mycelium
   c. Septate hyphae
   d. Aseptate hyphae
3. Describe and recognize the following types of asexual reproductive structures:
   a. Blastoconidia
   b. Chlamydoconidia
   c. Arthroconidia
   d. Sporangiospores
4. Describe and recognize the following types of sexual reproductive structures:
   a. Ascospores
   b. Basidiospores
   c. Zygospores
5. Describe typical colonial textures and topographies.
6. List and describe four general considerations for proper fungal specimen collection.
7. Justify the importance of the direct examination of clinical specimens for fungi.
8. State the purpose, perform the procedure, and interpret the following microscopic techniques:
   a. Saline wet mount
   b. Lactophenol cotton blue
   c. Potassium hydroxide (KOH) preparation
9. List at least three types of primary isolation media, and state the purpose of each.
10. Describe, perform, and interpret the following laboratory techniques:
    a. Tease mount
    b. Slide culture
    c. Germ tube
    d. Carbohydrate assimilation
    e. Rapid urease
11. Identify the following dermatophytes from prepared slides, pictures, or cultures:
    a. *Microsporum audouinii*
    b. *Microsporum canis*
    c. *Microsporum gypseum*
    d. *Epidermophyton floccosum*
    e. *Trichophyton mentagrophytes*
    f. *Trichophyton rubrum*
    g. *Trichophyton tonsurans*

Continued.

12. Describe the types of tinea and the dermatophytes associated with each.
13. Discuss the clinical significance and identify the following yeasts and yeastlike fungi from prepared slides, pictures, biochemical reactions, or cultures:
    a. *Candida albicans*
    b. *Torulopsis (Candida) glabrata*
    c. *Geotrichum candidum*
    d. *Rhodotorula*
    e. *Cryptococcus neoformans*
14. Discuss the clinical significance and identify the following subcutaneous mycoses from prepared slides, pictures, or cultures:
    a. *Cladosporium carrionii*
    b. *Fonsecaea pedrosoi*
    c. *Phialophora verrucosa*
    d. *Sporothrix schenckii*
15. Discuss the clinical significance and identify the following systemic mycoses from pictures:
    a. *Blastomyces dermatitidis*
    b. *Coccidioides immitis*
    c. *Histoplasma capsulatum*
    d. *Paracoccidioides brasiliensis*
16. Describe the significance of infections attributed to the yeasts, phaeohyphomycetes, and hyalohyphomycetes.
17. Based on microscopic appearance on cornmeal–Tween 80 agar, carbohydrate assimilation patterns, germ tube results, and biochemical reactions, identify a yeast or yeastlike fungi.
18. Discuss the significance and identify the following opportunistic fungi from prepared slides, pictures, or cultures:
    a. *Rhizopus*
    b. *Absidia*
    c. *Mucor*
    d. *Aspergillus*
    e. *Penicillium*

Mycology is the study of the fungi. Although more than 50,000 species of fungi are recognized, fewer than 100 have been identified as human pathogens. The fungi are present as saprobes in the environment, relying on decaying vegetation and plants for sources of nitrogen. Humans acquire fungal infections, or **mycoses,** through inhalation of spores or through inoculation by trauma into the skin, but not through person-to-person or animal-to-person contact. Recently, increases in opportunistic mycoses have been noted in individuals with underlying medical disorders. These disorders and predisposing factors include diabetes mellitus, infection with human immunodeficiency virus (HIV), prolonged corticosteroid or antibiotic therapy, and chemotherapy. Fungi previously considered to be saprobic or contaminants may now be opportunistic pathogens.

The fungi are classified as **thallophytes;** the organisms possess true nuclei and are heterotrophic members of the plant family that lack stems and roots. The fungi do not possess chlorophyll and are larger with a more complex morphology than the bacteria. These organisms absorb nutrients through the environment.

Fungi are capable of two phases: the multicellular **mold phase,** which consists of a cottony, mycelial mass, and the unicellular **yeast phase,** which is creamy, resembling a bacterial colony. Fungi with both a yeast phase, growing at 35° to 37°C, and a mold phase, growing at 25°C, are known as **dimorphic fungi.**

The **mycelium** is an intertwining structure composed of tubular filaments known as **hyphae,** the microscopic units of the fungi. **Septate hyphae** contain cross-walls, whereas **aseptate hyphae** are continuous without cross-walls. The mycelium consists of a

vegetative portion, or **thallus,** which grows in or on a substrate and absorbs water and nutrients, and a **reproductive,** or **aerial,** part, which contains the fruiting bodies that produce the reproductive structures, known as conidia or spores. The aerial part extends above the agar surface.

Conidia and spores may remain dormant in the air or environment or may be transported through the air to other locations. The spores of pathogenic molds can be inhaled and enter the respiratory tract. This is a common route of infection, and because of this, it is imperative to practice good laboratory safety when working in mycology. All work, including the preparation of slides, plating and transferring cultures, and any biochemical work, must be performed in a biological safety cabinet. Because airborne conidia and spores are readily released from a fungal culture, one should never smell a fungal culture. Screw-cap test tubes should be used in place of test tubes with a cotton, metal, or plastic lid. In addition, Petri plates must be sealed tightly with either an oxygen-impermeable tape or Parafilm. As always, gloves should be worn and any breaks or cuts in the skin covered to prevent the transmission of the fungal infection.

Fungi may reproduce either sexually or asexually. **Sexual reproduction** requires the formation of special structures so that fertilization or nuclear fission can occur. In sexual reproduction, meiosis (reduction division of two fertile cells), followed by a merging of the cells, and nuclear fusion occur. Types of specialized spores involved in sexual reproduction include **ascospores,** which are contained in a saclike ascus; **zygospores,** which involve the fusion of two identical cells arising from the same hypha; **oospores,** which involve the fusion of cells from two separate, nonidentical hyphae; and **basidiospores,** which are contained in a club-shaped basidium. Fungi that exhibit a sexual phase are known as the **perfect fungi.**

The **imperfect fungi,** or **fungi imperfecti,** do not exhibit a sexual phase, and spores are produced asexually from the mycelium. Asexual reproduction involves only mitosis with nuclear and cytoplasmic division. **Conidiogenesis,** or conidia formation, can occur blastically or thallically. In **blastic conidiogenesis** the parent cell enlarges, a septum forms, and the enlarged portion splits off to form a daughter cell. In **thallic conidiogenesis** the septum forms first, and new growth beyond the septum becomes the daughter cell.

Conidia are asexual spores produced singly or multiply in long chains or clusters by specialized vegetative hyphae known as **conidiophores.** Conidiophores may branch into secondary segments, known as **phialides,** which then produce the conidia. Some fungi can produce conidia of two different sizes. **Macroconidia** are large, usually septate, and club, oval, or spindle shaped. Macroconidia may be thick or thin walled and have a spiny **(echinulate)** or smooth surface. Usually the entire hyphae element becomes a multicellular conidium, known as the macroconidium. **Microconidia** are small and unicellular with a round, elliptical, or **piriform** (pear) shape. Microconidia borne directly on the hyphae are known as **sessile microconidia,** and those borne on the end of a short conidiophore are known as **pedunculate microconidia.**

Other spores develop directly from the vegetative mycelium, including blastoconidia, chlamydoconidia, and arthroconidia. **Blastoconidia (blastospores)** develop as the daughter cell buds off the mother cell and is pinched off. Blastoconidia are present in yeasts, such as *Candida.* Blastoconidia may elongate to form **pseudohyphae,** which can align in an end-to-end manner. Psuedohyphae can be differentiated from true hyphae because pseudohyphae are constricted at the septae. As a result, branches form at the septation. **Chlamydoconidia (chlamydospores)** are thick-walled, resistant, resting spores produced by "rounding up" and enlargement of the terminal hyphal cells. The spores germinate into a new organism when favorable environmental conditions occur. Chlamydoconidia may occur at the hyphal tip (terminal arrangement), on the hyphal sides (sessile), or within the hyphal strand (intercalary). It is important to differentiate chlamydoconidia from **conidiospores,** which are produced by yeast, such as *Candida.* Conidiospores are thick walled but are not conidia because these structures do not germinate. **Arthroconidia (arthrospores)** involve the simple fragmentation of the mycelium at the septum into cylinder-shaped or cask-shaped spores. The spores are thick walled and may be adjacent or alternate in arrangement. In the alternate arrangement, empty spaces, or **disjunctor cells,** appear between each arthrospore. This is a useful identification characteristic of the dimorphic fungus *Coccidioides immitis* and of *Geotrichum candidium,* a yeast.

Sporangiospores are asexual spores contained in sporangia or sacs that are produced terminally or sporangiophores or aseptate hyphae. Sporulation results when the sporangial wall ruptures with the release of sporagiospores. Sporangiospores are unique to the group of fungi known as the Zygomycetes.

Figure 20-1 provides diagrams with definitions of basic structures, including hyphae, conidia, and spores.

The fungi can be classified in several ways, including the botanical taxonomy, which contains four divisions: Zygomycota, Ascomycota, Basidomycota, and Deuteromycota. *Mucor, Absidia,* and *Rhizopus* are medically important genera of the Zygomycota, whereas most other medically important fungi are classified as **Deuteromycetes,** which are characterized by septate hyphae and asexual reproduction. The fungi can also be classified by the type of mycoses; using this method, the four catagories are the **superficial and cutaneous**

TABLE 20–9

Characteristics of Some Hyalohyphomycetes and Phaeohyphomycetes

GENUS	CHARACTERISTICS
Hyalohyphomycetes (Hyaline Molds)	
Acremonium	White, spready, moist, colorless colonies that become cottony with a gray top and a yellow or rose reverse side with age Small, hyaline, septate hyphae with phialides of hyaline phialoconidia; eliptical single-celled conidia
Fusarium	Rapidly growing, white then pink to violet, fluffy, cottony growth Hyaline, two-celled or multicelled, smooth-walled fusiform macroconidia, resembling a sickle or banana; small, septate, hyaline hyphae Unicellular microconidia in balls or short chains
Penicillium	Rapid, blue-green, velvety, powdery growth Septate, hyaline or dark to blue-green hyphae that produce brushlike conidiophores that give rise to phialides, from which chains of conidia arise
Scopulariopsis	Moderately rapid growth with white, granular, glabrous colonies that later become gray and powdery. Septate, hyaline hyphae with annelides that are produced singly or in groups on a conidiophore Thick-walled, spiny, hyaline annelconidia arranged in a chain
Phaeohyphomycetes (Darkly Pigmented Molds)	
Alternaria	Rapidly growing, cottony, gray to black colonies Septate, dematiaceous conidiophores that may branch with chains of brown conidia, which are muriform and tapered
Bipolaris	Rapid grower with gray-green to dark-brown powdery, woolly, or cottony colonies Septate, dematiaceous hyphae that are simple or branching; single or grouped conidiophores with multicelled, oblong to cylindrical conidia
Curvularia	Rapidly growing, woolly, fluffy, black colonies Dematiaceous, septate hyphae with conidiophores twisted at point of attachment to conidia, which are two-celled or multicelled, and curved, with central, darkly staining, swollen cell

SEROLOGICAL TESTING

Fungal serological testing may be performed to supplement microscopic or culture methods for identification. Antigen detection may be hampered by cross-reacting components, thus requiring the testing of multiple antigens for a definite interpretation.

A very useful test is the cryptococcal antigen test for *Cryptococcus neoformans,* which detects the presence of cryptococcal polysaccharide in body fluids, such as CSF. This method uses latex particles coated with hyperimmune anticryptococcal globulin to detect cryptococcal antigen. The method is simple and reliable and has virtually replaced the India ink method for detection.

Fungal serology to detect antibody relies on correct timing of blood specimens. Antibody detection methods for blastomycosis, coccidioidomycosis, histoplasmosis, and sporotrichosis can detect active infections, but cross-reacting antigens and false-negative results are problems.

Tests are also available for the diagnosis of aspergillosis and candidiasis. Methodologies for serological testing include immunodiffusion, complement fixation, and latex agglutination.

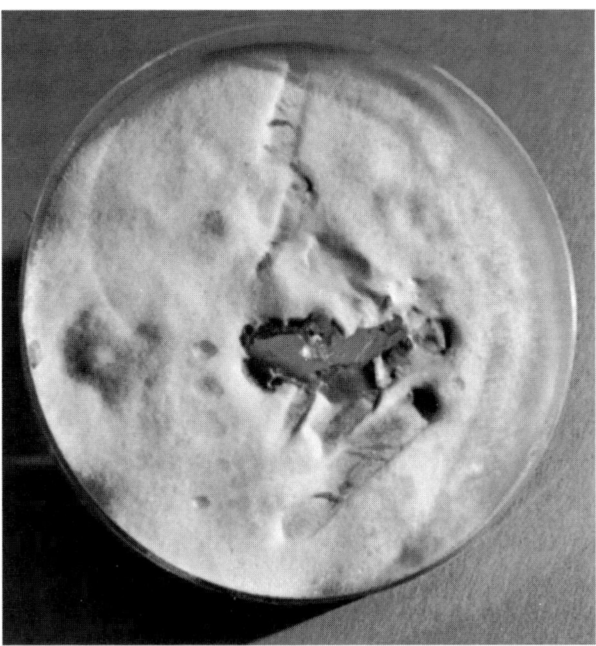

FIGURE 20–13

Fusarium on SDA showing fluffy mycelium with violet pigment. *Fusarium* species typically are deeply pigmented red, lavender, pink, or violet.

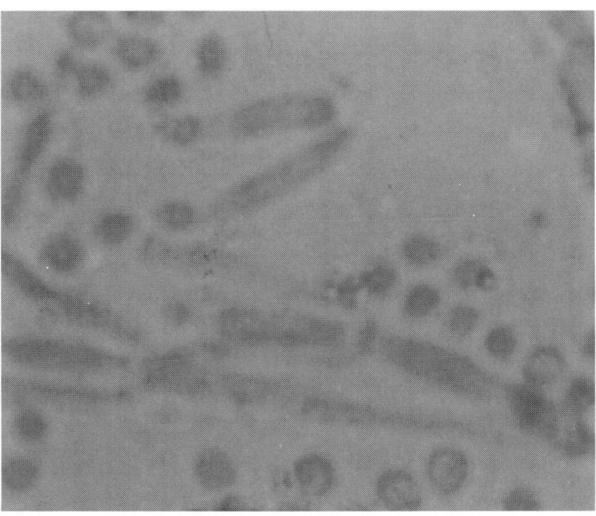

FIGURE 20–14

Penicillium: microscopic appearance showing septate hyphae, brushlike conidiophores, and chains of conidia from phialides.

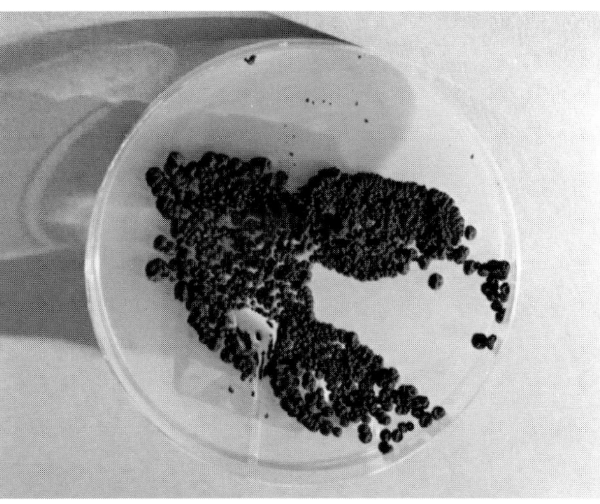

FIGURE 20–15

Aureobasidium on SDA showing flat, black, yeastlike colonies.

FIGURE 20–16

Curvularia: microscopic view showing muticellular, curved conidia with a central cell.

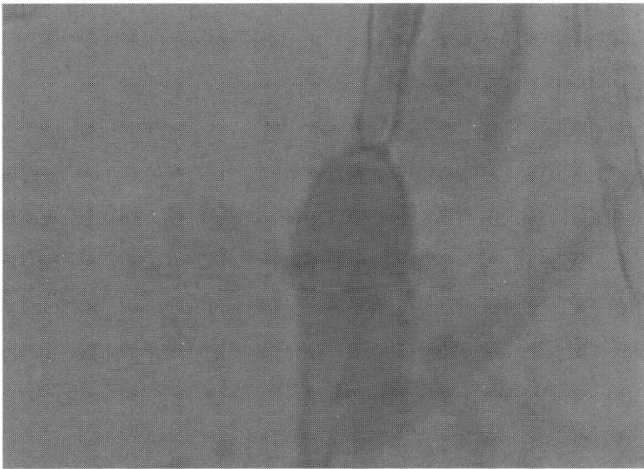

FIGURE 20–17

Alternaria: microscopic appearance showing septate hyphae, branched conidiophores, and drumstick-shaped conidia.

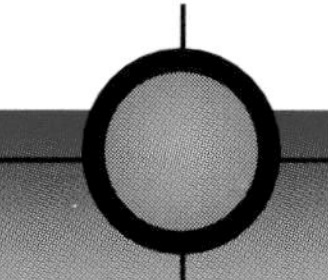

PROCEDURE
SLIDE CULTURE

PURPOSE

The slide culture is the most accurate method to preserve and observe fungal microstructure.

MATERIALS

Sterile Petri plate containing 2% agar
or
Sterile Petri plate containing filter paper and two applicator sticks (a bent glass rod, two pieces of plastic tubing, or the bent end of a flexible drinking straw can be substituted for the applicator sticks.)
Clean microscope slide and coverslip
Lactophenol cotton blue (LPCB) stain
Sabouraud dextrose agar (SDA) or other suitable agar
Sterile scalpel or sterile test tube without a lip

PROCEDURE

A wet (tease) mount should be performed before the slide culture. Work should be done under a biological safety cabinet. This procedure should not be performed on organisms suspected of being *Coccidioides, Histoplasma,* or *Blastomyces.*

1. Cover the bottom of a Petri plate with filter paper if this method is being used. Place a bent glass rod (or two sterile applicator sticks, flexible straw, or plastic tubing) in the Petri plate.
2. Place a clean microscope slide onto the bent glass rod or, alternatively, onto the surface of the agar in the Petri plate.
3. Using a sterile scapel, cut a 2 mm deep section of agar that measures approximately 1×1 mm. Alternatively, cut the block using a sterile test tube that has no lip.
4. Transfer the block of agar to the microscope slide.
5. Using either a sterile applicator stick or a heavy wire, inoculate the fungus into the center of the four sides of the agar square. If using a circular block, inoculate the four quadrants of the block.
6. Gently place a sterile coverslip over the block.
7. If using the filter paper method, add approximately 1.5 to 2.0 ml sterile water to the bottom of the Petri plate.
8. Incubate at room temperature (25° to 30°C).
9. Examine periodically for growth. Growth is usually seen on the slide's surface and underneath the coverslip. If the filter paper dries out, add additional sterile water.
10. When structures are visible, gently remove the coverslip, using sterile forceps if needed. Place the coverslip on a microscope slide containing one drop of LPCB.
11. The agar plug can be further incubated after the addition of a second coverslip, if desired.
12. Slides can be sealed with clear nail polish or Permount for later analysis, if desired.

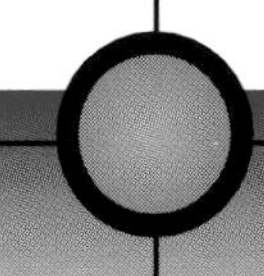

PROCEDURE

POTASSIUM HYDROXIDE (KOH) PREPARATION

PURPOSE

KOH preparations are used in the initial examination of keratinized tissue suspected of fungal infection.

PRINCIPLE

Fungal elements may be obscured by skin, hair, or nail tissue. KOH dissolves keratin in these specimens, facilitating observation of the organism's morphology.

MATERIALS

KOH solution is prepared by slowly adding 10 g KOH to 80 ml distilled water and then adding 20 ml glycerol. Mix until completely dissolved, and store in the refrigerator.

Glycerol prevents crystallization of KOH, so preparations can be examined for up to 2 days without drying.

PROCEDURE

1. Into one drop of KOH reagent on slide, place a small portion of the material (skin scrapings, hair, nail) to be examined.
2. Press coverslip down on sample.
3. Warm slide gently to dissolve keratinized cells. Do not boil.
4. Allow specimen to clear, approximately 20 minutes.
5. Examine under low (100×) and high-dry (430×) magnification.

INTERPRETATION

Observe for the presence of characteristic fungal elements, including hyphae, budding yeast, and spherules.

For hair specimens, determine if infection is ectothrix or endothrix.

NOTES

1. Do not use cotton swabs to collect specimens, since cotton fibers may resemble hyphae.
2. For nail and hard skin scrapings, it may be necessary to add dimethyl sulfoxide (DMSO) to the KOH reagent. To prepare KOH-DMSO reagent, add 40 ml DMSO with caution to 60 ml distilled water. Then carefully add 10 g KOH and mix until completely dissolved. Follow the procedure previously outlined.

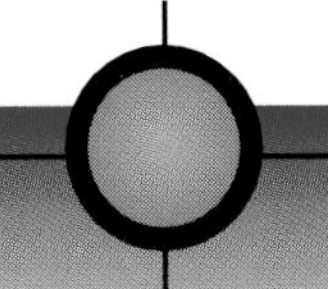

PROCEDURE
TEASE MOUNT

PURPOSE

The tease mount allows for the rapid examination of conidia, spores, and other microscopic fungal structures.

MATERIALS

Bent dissecting needle or wire bent at 90-degree angle
Lactophenol cotton blue (LPCB) stain
Clean microscope slide and coverslip
Two dissecting needles

PROCEDURE

1. With the bent dissecting needle or wire, remove a small portion of the colony from the agar surface. Select a portion midway between the center and the periphery.
2. Place a drop of LPCB on the microscope slide, and place the culture into the stain.
3. Place a coverslip over the culture, and using a pencil eraser, press down gently to disperse the mycelium. Alternatively, using two dissecting needles, gently tease apart the mycelium and then add the coverslip.
4. Observe microscopically under low (100×) and high-dry (430×) magnification for fungal characteristics.

NOTE

Although this is a rapid method, preservation of the original arrangement of spores may be disrupted due to teasing or pressure in applying the coverslip.

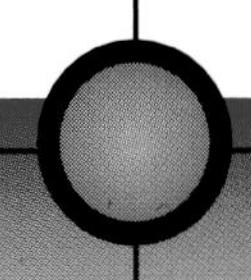

PROCEDURE
GERM TUBE TEST

PURPOSE
Candida albicans can be presumptively identified based on the production of a germ tube.

PRINCIPLE
When incubated with serum at 37°C for 1 to 3 hours, *C. albicans* will form a germ tube.

MATERIALS
Sheep, rabbit, or fetal calf serum
Test tube

PROCEDURE
1. Pipet 0.5 ml of serum into a test tube.
2. Inoculate the tube with a small amount of the organism to be tested. A large inoculum may produce false-negative results.
3. Incubate at 37°C for 1 to 3 hours.
4. Place a drop of the suspension on a slide, apply a coverslip, and examine for the presence of germ tubes.

INTERPRETATION
A germ tube is approximately half as wide and three to four times as long as the yeast cell. No point of constriction should exist where the germ tube arises from the mother cell.

QUALITY CONTROL
C. albicans: positive control; produces germ tube within 2 hours
C. tropicalis: negative control; fails to produce germ tube within 3 hours

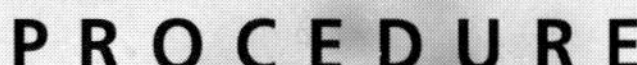

PROCEDURE
CORNMEAL AGAR WITH TWEEN 80

PURPOSE
Cornmeal agar with Tween 80 is used to distinguish the various species of *Candida* and other yeasts through examination of hyphae, blastoconidia, chlamydoconidia, and arthroconidia.

PRINCIPLE
Cornmeal agar stimulates conidiation; Tween 80 (polysorbate) reduces surface tension and enhances the formation of hyphae, blastoconidia, chlamydoconidia, and arthroconidia.

MATERIALS
Cornmeal agar with Tween 80
Inoculating wire
Coverslip

PROCEDURE
1. Using approximately one third of the plate, streak the center of the area with the organism to be identified.
2. While holding the inoculating wire at about a 45-degree angle, make three or four parallel cuts about 5 mm apart into the agar.
3. Place a coverslip on the surface of the agar, covering a portion of the parallel cuts.
4. Incubate at room temperature for 24 to 72 hours.
5. Examine by placing the plate, with its lid, on the microscope stage using the low-power (10×) and high-power (43×) objectives. The most characteristic morphology is found near the end of the coverslip.

INTERPRETATION
Note the presence and morphology of hyphae, blastoconidia, chlamydoconidia, and arthrospores.

Presence of pseudohyphae (absence of true hyphae) and blastoconidia indicates the genus *Candida:*

C. albicans: numerous chlamydospores with several tight clusters of blastoconidia evenly spaced along hyphae

C. tropicalis: fewer numbers of blastoconidia, which are arranged singly or irregularly in small clusters along the hyphae; no chlamydospores present

C. parapsilosis: colonies that appear as "spiders" or "sagebrushes" along streak lines on agar; delicate mycelium with occasional blastoconidium observed singly or in short chains

C. pseudotropicalis: elongated blastoconidia that break away from the pseudohyphae and arrange in a parallel fashion, described as "log in a stream" arrangement

Presence of true hyphae and arthroconidia may indicate *Trichosporon* or *Geotrichum.* The arthroconidia of *Geotrichum* may have a hyphal extension from one corner and are said to resemble "hockey sticks." The urease test is used to further differentiate these organisms: *Trichosporon* is urease positive, and *Geotrichum* is urease negative.

PROCEDURE

CARBOHYDRATE ASSIMILATION TEST FOR YEAST

PURPOSE

Carbohydrate assimilation of various carbohydrates can provide a definite identification for yeast and yeastlike organisms.

PRINCIPLE

The yeast's ability to utilize a particular carbohydrate is determined by using a carbohydrate-free (nitrogen-based) agar and filter paper disks that are impregnanted with various carbohydrates. Growth around the disk indicates the yeast can utilize that carbohydrate.

MATERIALS

Sterile saline tubes

Yeast nitrogen-based agar available commercially, or prepare as follows:
- Dissolve 6.5 g yeast nitrogen-based agar in 100 ml distilled water.
- Adjust pH to 6.2 to 6.4 by adding 1 *N* NaOH.
- Sterilize by filtration, and add 88 ml agar to 100 ml filtered bromcresol purple indicator to 1 L of 2% agar solution.
- Pour approximately 20 ml into sterile, plastic Petri plate.
- Prepare 2% agar by adding 20 g agar to 1 L distilled water.

Carbohydrate-impregnated filter paper disks commercially available, or prepare as follows:
- Soak 10 mm filter paper disks in 1% carbohydrate solutions.
- Allow to dry.

Carbohydrates tested may include glucose, maltose, sucrose, lactose, galactose, melibiose, cellobiose, inositol, xylose, raffinose, trehalose, and dulcitol.

PROCEDURE

1. Prepare a McFarland standard no. 4 with the yeast to be tested in a sterile tube of saline.
2. Using a sterile pipet, flood the surface of the yeast nitrogen-based agar plate with the entire suspension and allow it to soak into the medium. Remove and discard any excess suspension from the plate. Allow surface of plate to dry (approximately 5 minutes).
3. Place carbohydrate disks onto agar surface, pressing down gently with flamed forceps. For optimal results, place the disks on the four corners of the plate and in the center to form a cross.
4. Incubate plate at 30°C for 24 hours. Plates should be reincubated for another 24 hours and read again if growth is insufficient.

INTERPRETATION

Growth surrounding a disk indicates the carbohydrate has been assimilated by the yeast, indicating a positive test.

QUALITY CONTROL

Each new batch of agar and new set of carbohydrate disks should be tested with positive-reacting and negative-reacting yeasts for each carbohydrate tested.

All procedures sh
Use the followin
Sabouraud dextr
floccosum, Rhizo

Examine the colo
top and reverse s

M. gypseum —
T. rubrum —
E. floccosum —
Rhizopus —
A. fumigatus —
Fusarium —

Prepare a tease
and make a ske

M. g

Entamoeba coli

Cyst

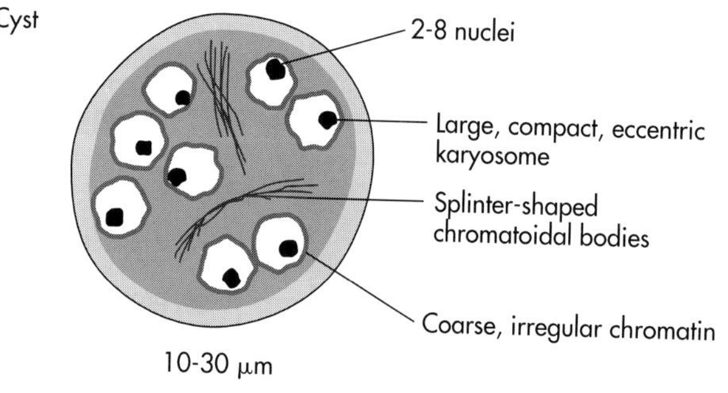

Trophozoite

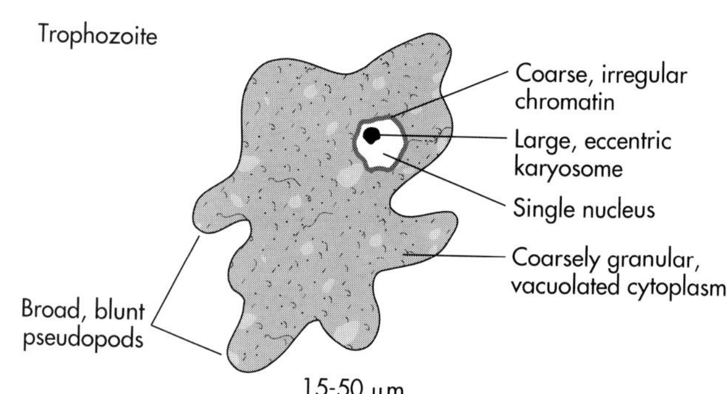

Entamoeba hartmanni

Cyst

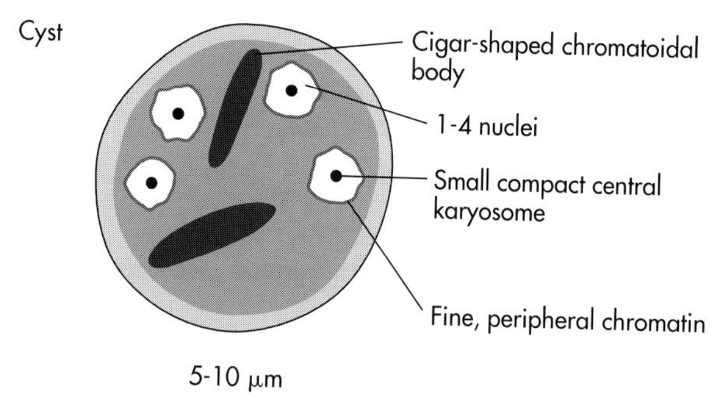

Trophozoite

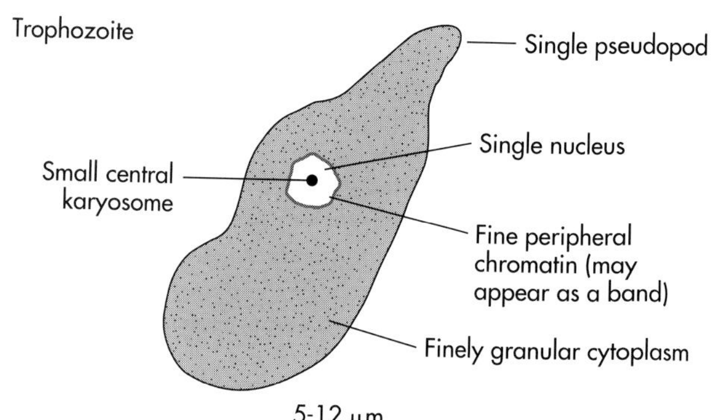

FIGURE 21–1, continued
Cyst and trophozoite forms of common intestinal amebae.

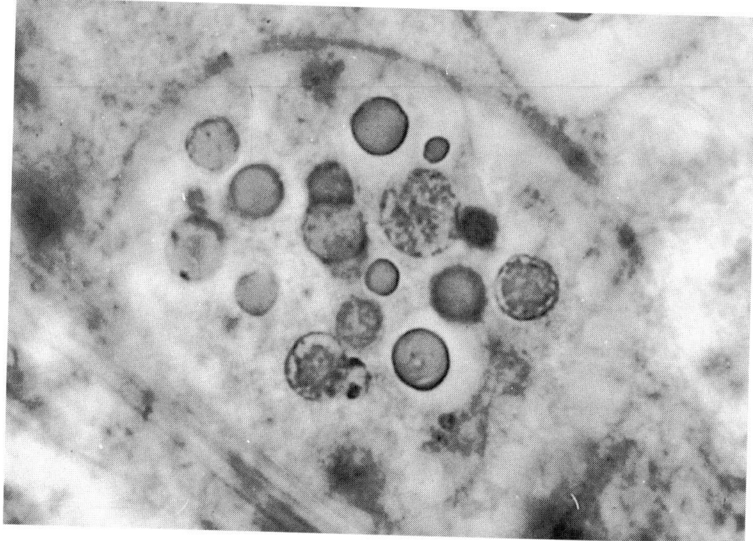

FIGURE 21–2
Trophozoite of *Entamoeba histolytica*. *(From Baron EJ, Peterson LR, Finegold SM, editors: Bailey and Scott's diagnostic microbiology, ed 9, St Louis, 1994, Mosby.)*

Free-Living Amebae

Naegleria, Hartmannella, and *Acanthamoeba* are free-living amebae found in water and soil. The parasites are found in rivers, lakes, air-conditioner systems, humidifiers, cooling towers, dust, air, compost, and vegetation. Infections may be acquired through direct contact with contaminated water, such as by swimming in nonchlorinated lakes. Infections are found worldwide, including the southern and southeastern United States.

Naegleria and *Hartmannella* species are agents of a form of meningoencephalitis that may mimic bacterial meningitis because of the predominance of neutrophils in the cerebrospinal fluid (CSF). *Naegleria fowleri* enters the upper respiratory tract through inhalation, often as a result of swimming in contaminated water. The parasite infects the nasal mucosa and spreads along the nerves to the brain and central nervous system (CNS). *Naegleria* possess broad, lobed pseudopods and exhibit active, progressive motility. The organism has a hexagonal, thin-walled cyst that lacks pores and may encyst in tissue. Of note is the organism's ability to transform temporarily into a pear-shaped flagellate when placed into water.

Acanthamoeba is associated with ulcerative, vision-threatening keratitis associated with corneal contact with contaminated water. The condition is seen most often in those who wear extended-wear contact lenses resulting from improper disinfection of the lenses or from wearing the lenses while swimming. *Acanthamoeba* organisms are larger in size and more sluggish than *Naegleria,* with spiny pseudopods known as acanthapodia. The organisms also exhibit well-defined ectoplasm and endoplasm. There is no flagellar phase, and the nuclei and cyst forms resemble those of *Naegleria. Acanthamoeba* may encyst in tissue.

Hartmannella organisms possess filamentous pseudopods and exhibit sluggish motility. They have characteristic double-walled cysts that may contain pores, are nonflagellates in water, and do not encyst in tissues.

Intestinal Flagellates

The flagellates, or Mastigophora, are motile through long extensions of cytoplasm known as flagella. When compared with the amebae, which have variable shapes, the flagellates are more rigid and maintain their shape. Infections occur in the intestinal tract, blood, and other tissues. The medically significant flagellates include *Giardia lamblia, Trichomonas vaginalis* and *T. hominis, Chilomastix mesnili,* and *Dientamoeba fragilis,* which was formerly classified as an ameba.

Giardia lamblia, the agent of giardiasis, is the most common parasite associated with gastroenteritis in the United States. The organism is found in unfiltered water and untreated lake or pond water and most often infects campers, infants and children in day care, and homosexual males. Infections are contracted after exposure to contaminated food or water. The trophozoite form, found in soft or liquid stools, contains two nuclei with large central karyosomes that may resemble "eyes." There is a large ventral sucking disk in the upper one half of the body. *G. lamblia* is bilaterally symmetrical with a pointed anterior end and a rounded posterior end, a parallel pair of axonemes, and parabasal body that is said to resemble a mouth. *G. lamblia* has four pairs of flagella and is motile with a smooth, rapid motion that has been described as a "falling leaf" or "leaf tumbling in a stream." When observed microscopically, the trophozoite form may give the appearance of a "monkey face" (Figure 21-3).

G. lamblia causes an inflammation of the intestinal mucosa that results in acute diarrhea, abdominal pain,

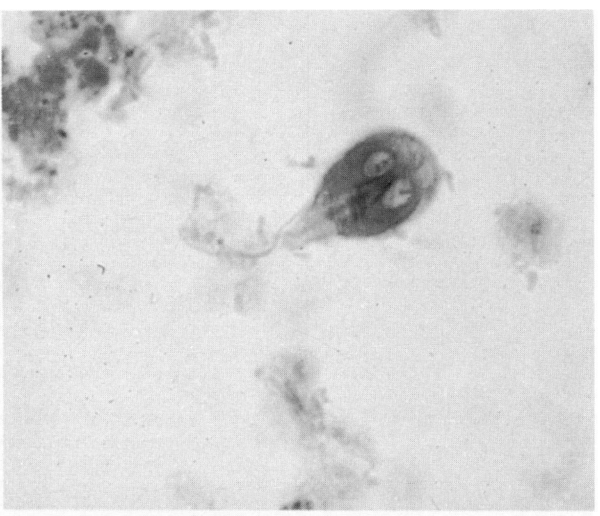

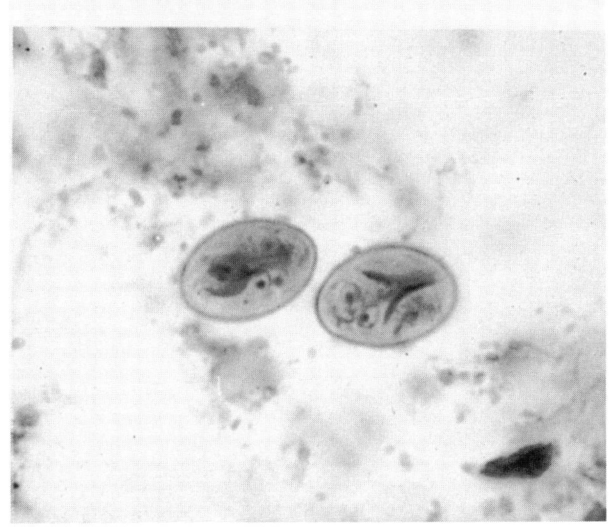

FIGURE 21-3
Trophozoite and cysts of *Giardia lamblia.* (From Baron EJ, Peterson LR, Finegold SM, editors: Bailey and Scott's diagnostic microbiology, ed 9, St Louis, 1994, Mosby.)

Giardia lamblia

Cyst

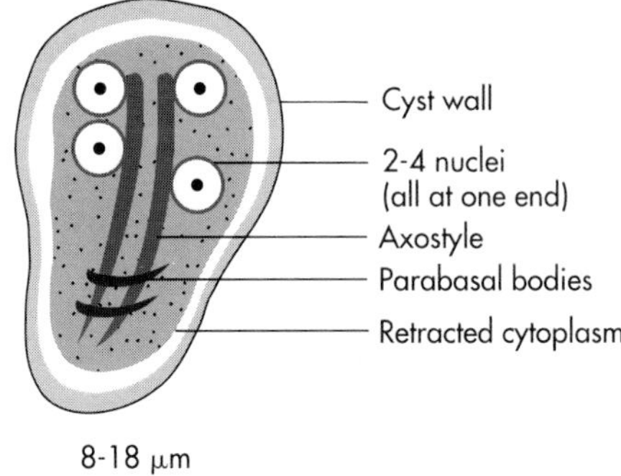

Trophozoite

Trichomonas vaginalis

No cyst form

Trophozoite

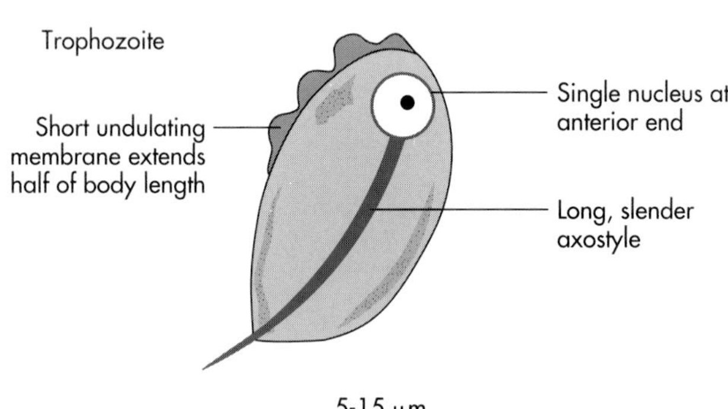

Trichomonas hominis

No cyst form

Trophozoite

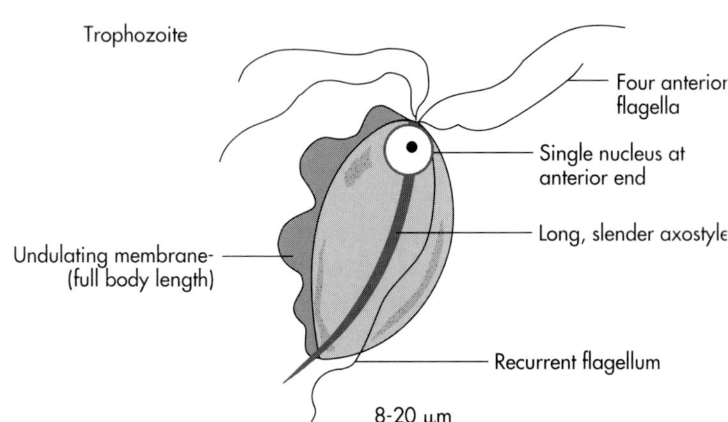

FIGURE 21–4
Clinically important intestinal flagellates.

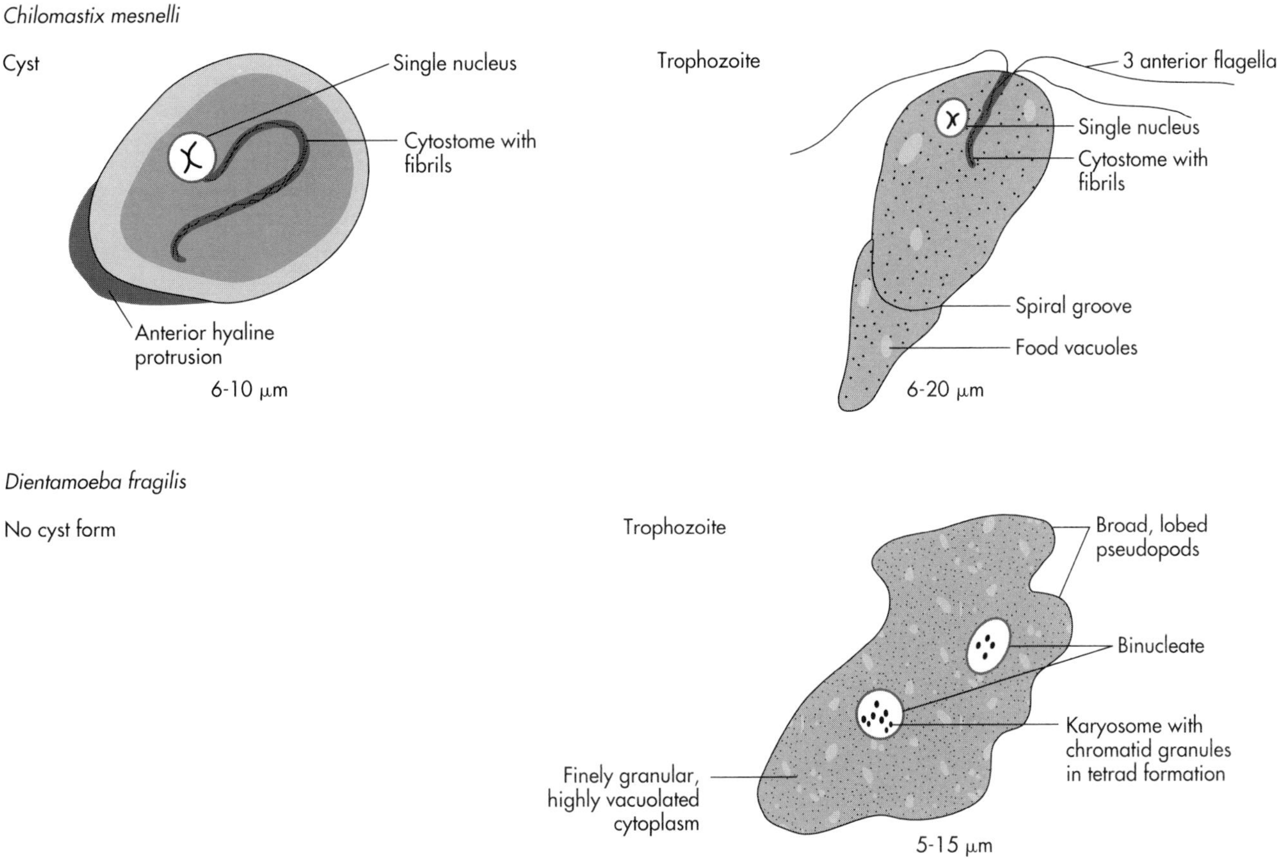

FIGURE 21–4, continued
Clinically important intestinal flagellates.

and malabsorption. More serious infections may be associated with weight loss and malnutrition.

Trichomonas vaginalis is a pear-shaped, motile parasite approximately 5 to 15 μm in length. It is the cause of vaginitis, urethritis, and prostatitis and is generally transmitted through sexual contact. *Trichomonas hominis* resembles *T. vaginalis* and also is pear shaped; it is considered to be nonpathogenic.

Chilomastix mesnili has a pear-shaped, elongated trophozoite form. A prominent, curved, cytostomal fibril borders the cytostome, resembling a shepherd's crook. It is 6 to 10 μm in diameter. The arrangement of fibrils may give the appearance of an "open safety pin." The cyst form is ingested, but the organism is considered to be nonpathogenic.

Dientamoeba fragilis is the only binucleate flagellate that infects humans. Although classified as a flagellate, the flagella are rarely, if ever, visible. The trophozoite form is 5 to 15 μm in diameter with broad-lobed pseudopods and usually two nuclei ("di"). The parasite produces a diarrheal syndrome characterized by abdominal pain.

Figure 21-4 provides descriptions and figures of the clinically important intestinal flagella.

Intestinal Ciliate

The only member of the Ciliophora, or ciliates, that infects humans is *Balantidium coli.* The largest protozoan, the trophozoite measures 50 to 100 μm long and 40 to 70 μm wide. It is oval shaped, is covered completely with cilia of uniform length, and is motile with a boring or rotary motion. The organism has a kidney-shaped macronucleus and a spherical micronucleus that appears as a crescent dot within the macronucleus. Balantidiasis results from ingestion of the cyst form in contaminated food or water. The trophozoite form multiplies in the lumen of the colon or bowel wall, resulting in the formation of lesions. The infection is seen in the tropics and is rarely observed in other parts of the world. The organism is found in pigs and rarely in other animals. Infections in humans may be asymptomatic but in heavy infestations may be characterized by bloody dysentery. Figure 21-5 provides a description of *B. coli.*

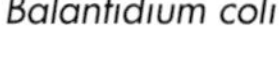

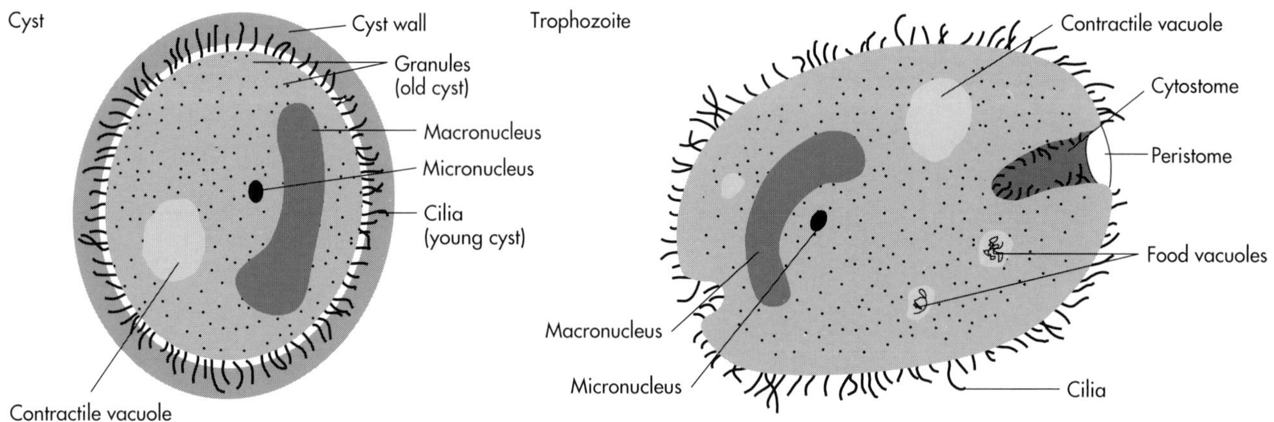

FIGURE 21–5
Balantidium coli.

Intestinal Coccidia

The coccidia are obligate intracellular parasites that have both sexual and asexual phases in their life cycles. Clinically important intestinal coccidia include *Cryptosporidium* species, *Isospora belli, Sarcocystis* species, microsporidians, and Cyanobacteria-like or Coccidia-like bodies (CLBs) such as *Cyclospora.*

Isospora belli is the agent of isosporiasis, an infection that is either asymptomatic or associated with diarrhea and malabsorption. The infection is most serious in immunosuppressed individuals, in particular AIDS patients. It is acquired through the ingestion of infective oocysts in fecally contaminated food or water. Each oocyst contains two round sporoblasts that contain four oval-shaped **sporozoites** that are released in the small intestine. The sporozoites develop into trophozoites, which then multiply asexually to form **schizonts**—groups of immature trophozoites. These organisms then either enter another asexual stage of reproduction or a sexual stage known as **sporogony** by forming **microgametocytes** (male gametes) and **macrogametocytes** (female gametes). Fertilization between the microgametes and macrogametes occurs in the intestinal lumen. After fertilization the macrogametes develop into **oocysts** that are passed in the feces. Since both the sexual and the asexual forms occur in the human GI tract, no secondary host is needed.

Diagnosis of infection with *I. belli* is made through the observation of either the immature or the mature oocyst in the stool. Immature cysts contain a single granular mass, the sporoblast which will develop into two sporozoites in the mature cyst. The mature oocyst is ellipsoidal and measures 20 to 30 μm by 10 to 20 μm in size. The oocysts may be observed in iodine preparations, although detection is enhanced by the modified acid-fast stain, in which the oocysts stain pink with bright-red sporozoites.

Cryptosporidium species are agents of enterocolitis; *Cryptosporidium parvum* is the species that most frequently infects humans. Routes of infection include direct contact with another infected individual or animal, or ingestion of fecally contaminated water or food. The infection, usually mild in an immunocompetent host, is characterized by a cholera-like, watery diarrhea with mucus production, nausea, vomiting, malabsorption, and a low-grade fever. The infection is particularly serious in the immunocompromised host, especially AIDS patients, who may develop a severe, often chronic and fatal diarrheal disease. Children may spread the infection through person-to-person contact in the daycare setting.

After ingestion of the infective oocysts, the infection may incubate for 1 to 2 weeks. Encystation, the release of the infective sporozoites, is followed by their penetration into host cells. Asexual reproduction, or **merogony,** which occurs in the host cells, results in the formation of **merozoites,** which develop through gametogony to microgametes and macrogametes, which mate to form zygotes, which in turn form thick-walled oocysts. The oocysts undergo sporogony, forming sporozoites in the oocysts, which subsequently rupture, releasing the sporozoites to complete the life cycle.

Cryptosporidiosis is diagnosed through observation of the small (4 to 5 μm), oval or spherical oocysts in the

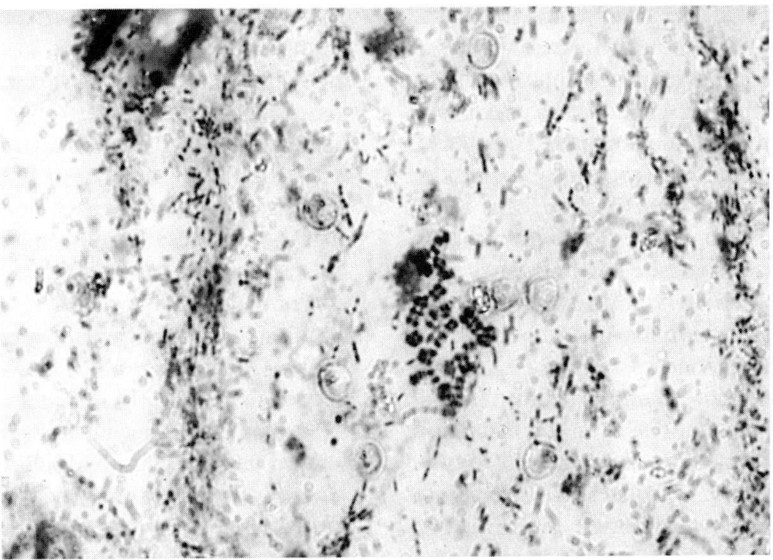

FIGURE 21–6

Modified acid-fast stain of oocysts of *Cryptosporidium parvum. (From Baron EJ, Peterson LR, Finegold SM, editors:* Bailey and Scott's diagnostic microbiology, *ed 9, St Louis, 1994, Mosby.)*

stool. The oocysts have smooth outer walls, and four sporozoites may be seen in the oocyst. Observation of the oocysts is enhanced through concentrating the stool, either through the formalin-ethyl acetate sedimentation method or through Sheather's sugar flocculation method. Sheather's sugar flocculation method uses a heavy suspension of the feces in saline, which is then strained through gauze into a centrifuge tube. An equal amount of Sheather's sugar solution (sucrose, melted phenol, distilled water) is added to the strained stool to float the oocysts to the top of the solution. A direct mount is prepared from the coverslip, which is examined using the phase-contrast microscope.

The modified acid-fast method stains the oocysts bright pink to red (Figure 21-6 [Color Plate 77]). An indirect fluorescent procedure using monoclonal antibodies is also commercially available.

The oocysts of Cryptosporodium are resistant to the effects of chlorine and other disinfectants.

Microsporidians encompass a number of genera, including *Encephalitozoon, Nosema, Pleistophora, Enterocytozoan, Septata,* and *Microsporidium.* These organisms can infect various animals, including humans, through the GI tract. Infections have been increasing in immunosuppressed hosts. Chronic, watery, nonbloody diarrhea with weight loss and malabsorption is characteristic of infection by Microsporida in AIDS patients. Microsporidians can infect several organs.

Microsporidians range from 2 to 8 μm in size and are considered to be true eukaryotes with a nucleus, nuclear membrane, and cytoplasmic membrane. A unique characteristic of Microsporida organisms is their ability to produce spores with polar tubules and inject themselves into the host cell by extruding its protoplasm. Once in the host cell, microsporidians multiply and divide repeatedly either by binary fission (merogony) or by multiple fission **(schizogony)** with spore production (sporogony). The spore, which has a thick wall, is the infective stage and is released in the stool.

Identification is made through the observation of the spores in biopsy or other specimens. The spores stain quite poorly with hematoxylin stains and acid-fast stains, and electron microscopy remains the most valuable method for identification.

Blastomyces hominis was previously classified as a yeast but is now believed to be a protozoan because it lacks a cell wall, does not grow on media used for mycology, and reproduces by binary fission and not by budding. Infection, which is usually diarrheal, is acquired through the fecal-oral route through contaminated food or water. Infection is frequently associated with immunosuppressed hosts, in particular AIDS patients, and travel abroad. It is best identified through wet mounts or trichrome stains. *B. hominis* is round and 6 to 40 μm in diameter, with a large central body and vacuole.

Miscellaneous Protozoa from Other Body Sites

Toxoplasma gondii is a protozoan parasite that has an affinity to infect the tissue of the human central nervous system. A coccidian parasite, the organism has both sexual and asexual life cycles. The sexual cycle,

TABLE 21–3

Characteristics of *Plasmodium* Species

CHARACTERISTIC	*P. FALCIPARUM*	*P. VIVAX*	*P. MALARIAE*	*P. OVALE*
Periodicity	Tertian	Tertian	Quartan	Tertian
Red blood cell (RBC) size	Normal	1.5-2 times normal	Normal	1.5 times normal; oval with irregular edges
Dots/clefts	Maurer's clefts (comma-shaped red) seen rarely	Schüffner's clots present in all stages, except early ring forms	No dots or clefts	Schüffner's dots present in all stages, including early rings; stains darker than *P. vivax*
Early ring stage	Small rings, multiple rings per cell; double-nuclei, accolé (appliqué), and signet-ring forms seen	Usually single parasite per cell; rings with two nuclei possible	Usually single parasite per cell	Usually single parasite per cell
Mature ring stage	Small and round; rarely seen in blood	Large, ameboid, with cytoplasm filling cell	Ribbon, band, or basket forms; not ameboid	Similar to *P. malariae*, but larger in size; many large, dark-staining granules
Schizonts	8-16 merozoites per schizont; rarely seen in peripheral blood	12-24 merozoites per schizont; finely granular, golden-brown malarial pigment	6-12 merozoites per schizont, which may form rosette; coarsely granular malarial pigment	8 merozoites, usually arranged around one large pigment aggregated
Gametocytes	Crescent or banana shaped	Large, round, almost filling cell; coarse malarial pigment	Round, RBCs not enlarged; coarse, unevenly distributed pigment	Similar to *P. malariae*
Comments	Stages other than early ring and gametocyte rarely seen; multiple infected RBCs common	Generally infects young RBCs; all stages found in peripheral blood	Low levels of parasitemia when compared with other species; all stages found, but generally few rings and gametocytes	Difficult to identify because *P. ovale* resembles *P. vivax* and *P. malariae;* all forms found

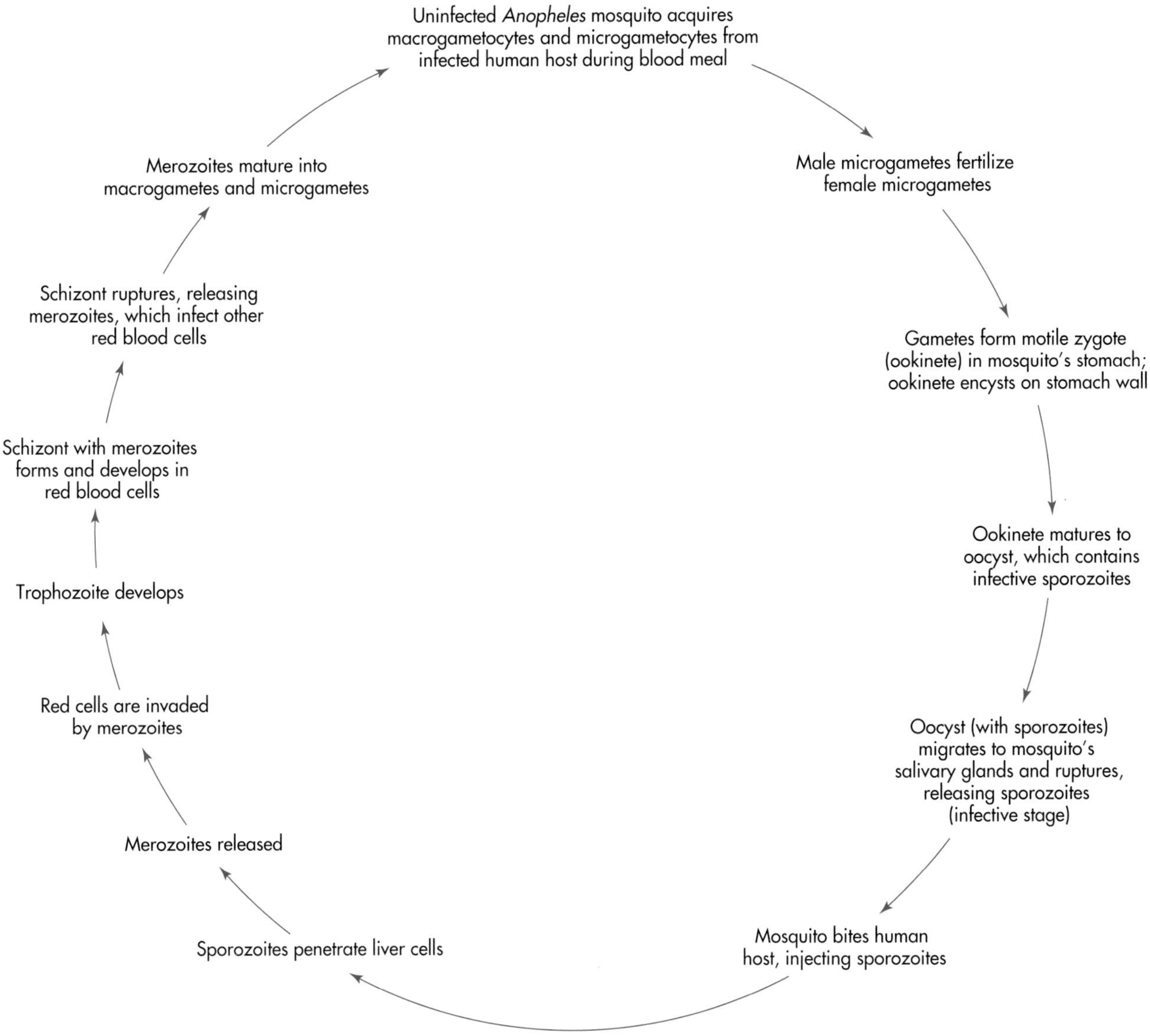

Uninfected *Anopheles* mosquito acquires macrogametocytes and microgametocytes from infected human host during blood meal

Male microgametes fertilize female microgametes

Gametes form motile zygote (ookinete) in mosquito's stomach; ookinete encysts on stomach wall

Ookinete matures to oocyst, which contains infective sporozoites

Oocyst (with sporozoites) migrates to mosquito's salivary glands and ruptures, releasing sporozoites (infective stage)

Mosquito bites human host, injecting sporozoites

Sporozoites penetrate liver cells

Merozoites released

Red cells are invaded by merozoites

Trophozoite develops

Schizont with merozoites forms and develops in red blood cells

Schizont ruptures, releasing merozoites, which infect other red blood cells

Merozoites mature into macrogametes and microgametes

FIGURE 21–7

Life cycle of *Plasmodium.*

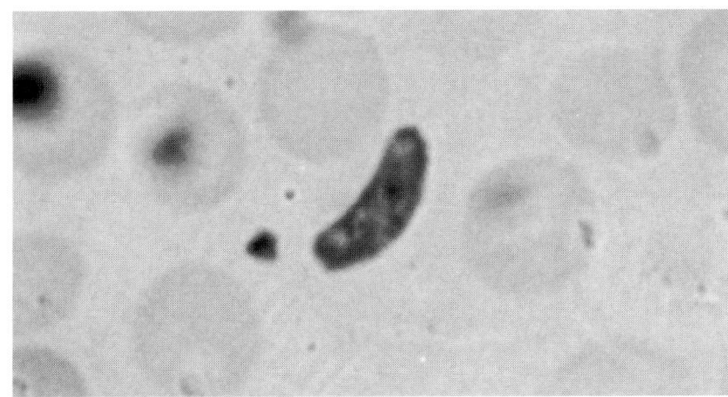

FIGURE 21–8

Crescent-shaped gametocytes of *P. falciparum. (From Howard BJ et al:* Clinical and pathogenic microbiology, *ed 2, St Louis, 1993, Mosby.)*

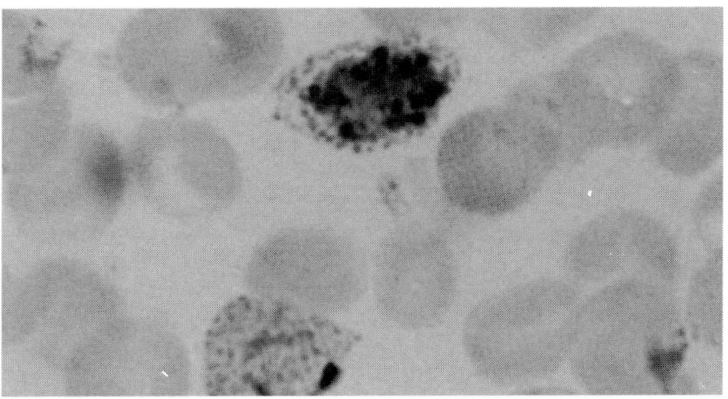

FIGURE 21–9

Schuffner's dots of *Plasmodium vivax. (From Howard BJ et al:* Clinical and pathogenic microbiology, *ed 2, St Louis, 1993, Mosby.)*

Plasmodium falciparum

Small ring forms
Accolé form
Maurer's dots
Red blood cell

Young trophozoite
(multiple rings per cell)

Red blood cell
Crescent-shaped gametocyte

Gametocyte

Plasmodium vivax

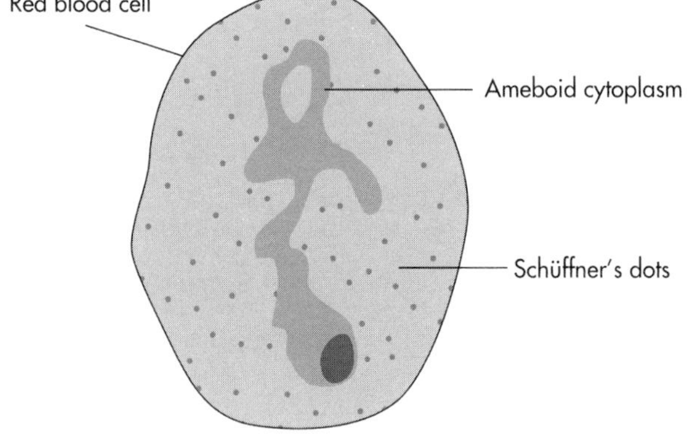

Late trophozoite

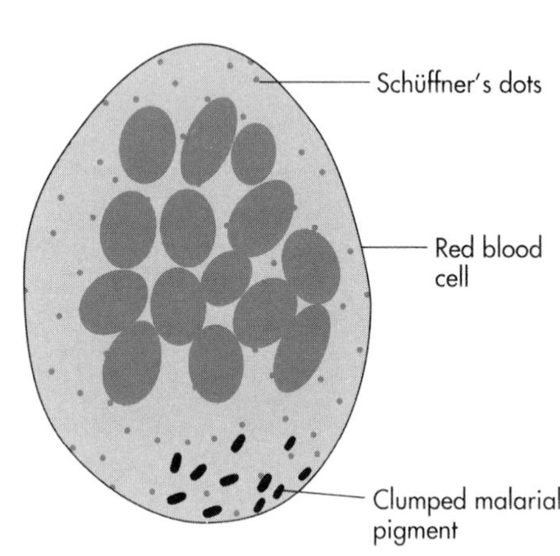

Schizont with 12 to 24 merozoites

Plasmodium malariae

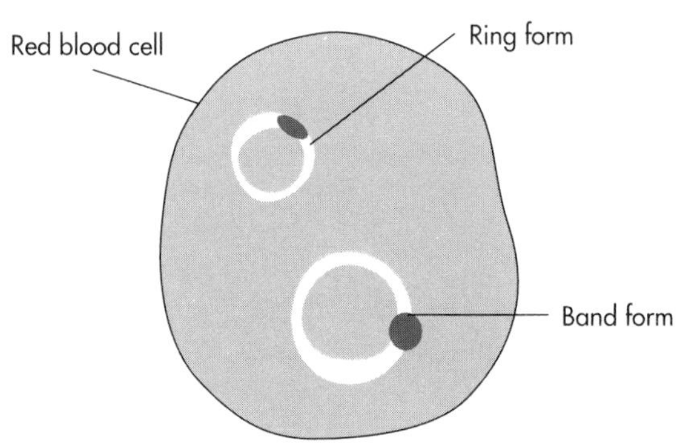

Young trophozoite
(single ring or band per cell)

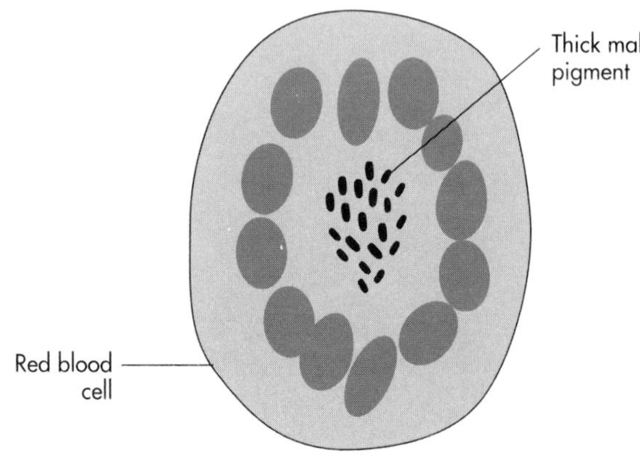

Schizont with 6 to 12 merozoites
in rosette arrangement

FIGURE 21–10
Morphology of malarial parasites (diagnostic forms).

Plasmodium ovale

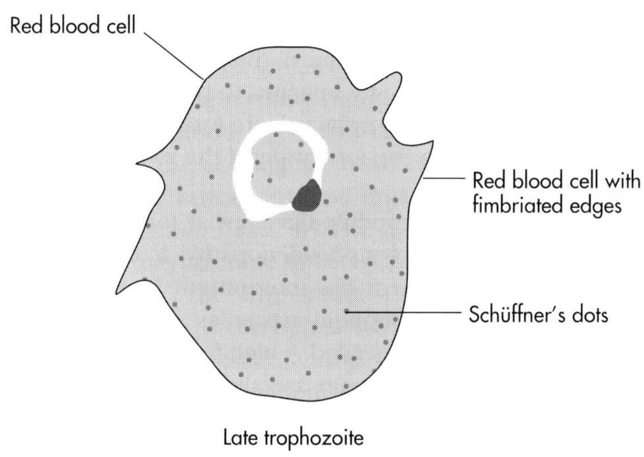

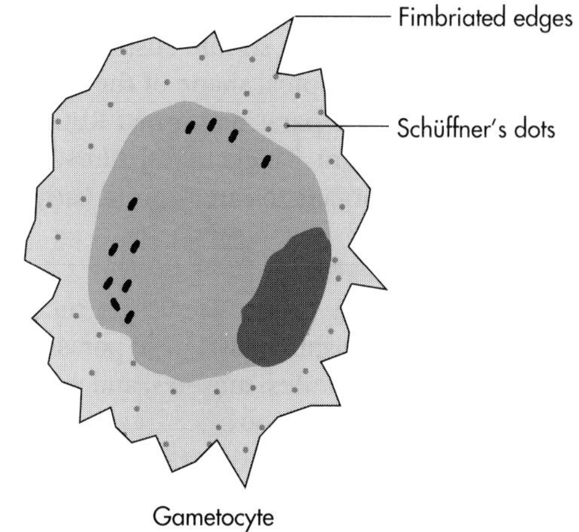

FIGURE 21–10, continued
Morphology of malarial parasites (diagnostic forms).

approximately 500 cases are reported per year, with most acquired during foreign travel or found in students and other individuals from foreign countries or in refugees. Malaria is most often found in the tropics and subtropics.

Diagnosis of malaria is accomplished through clinical symptoms and the demonstration of the organism in thick and thin Wright-stained or Giemsa-stained smears. It is best to collect the blood specimen before the fever, since the parasites are most concentrated in the RBCs at this time.

In examination of the blood smears, the clinician must first recognize the malarial parasites. The organisms are intracellular, with a red nucleus and blue cytoplasm. Second, each species has trademark characteristics that are essential in identification. Table 21-3 summarizes important characteristics of each *Plasmodium* species. Figures 21-8, (Color Plate 78), 21-9, (Color Plate 79), and 21-10 illustrate the morphology of the malarial parasites.

The first step in speciation is to identify *P. falciparum,* since it causes the most fatal and progressive form of malaria and since it is becoming increasingly resistant to chloroquine. If *P. falciparum* has been ruled out, the possibility of *P. vivax* is next investigated. *P. malariae* is often diagnosed through exclusion.

Babesia

Babesia are tick-borne sporozoan parasites that generally infect animals other than humans. Species include *Babesia microti,* which infects rodents; *Babesia equi,* which infects horses, *Babesia canis,* which infects dogs; and *Babesia bovis and Babesia divergens,* which infect cattle. Humans serve as an accidental host, with individuals who have had splenectomies at an increased risk of babesiosis. *B. microti* is endemic in southern New England, Texas, and other parts of North America. It is also the cause of Texas cattle fever. Most human infections in North America from *B. microti* occur in the coastal areas of southern New England and the eastern coastal areas, including Nantucket Island. *B. equi* is found in Europe, Russia, Africa, Asia, India, and North and South America.

Ticks are the arthropod intermediate host for *Babesia* species that occur in domestic and wild animals. Ticks may become infected by either taking a blood meal from an infected mammal or having the parasite transmitted from an infected female to her progeny. In the animal host the parasite is inoculated during the blood meal into the host, and invasion of the RBCs occurs. The trophozoite form develops, and schizogony—in this case a form of asexual reproduction resembling budding—results in the formation of a tetrad arrangement of four merozoites. On rupture of the infected erythrocytes, the merozoites are released, infecting other RBCs and continuing the life cycle.

Clinically, babesiosis resembles malaria, with an irregular fever, chills, sweats, nausea, vomiting, and fatigue. Patients also have hemolytic anemia, jaundice, and an enlarged liver and spleen. The disease is most severe and often fatal in splenectomized individuals.

Diagnosis is achieved through demonstration of the parasites in stained blood films. Within the erythrocyte the organism most often appears as a pleomorphic ringlike structure, which may resemble the ring stages of *Plasmodium.* Piriform, round, oval, elongate, and ameboid forms are possible. The piroplast form is pear shaped, with packets of two or three organisms seen, and may be described as resembling "rabbit ears." The piriform parasites may form a cross after division into

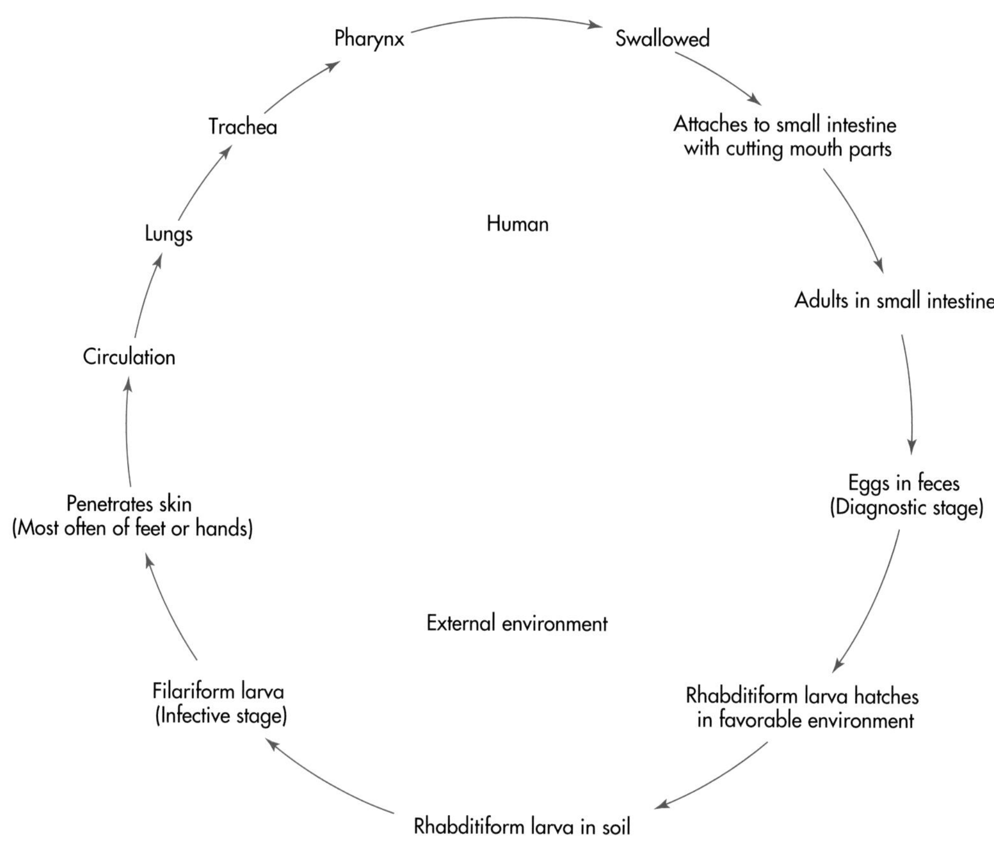

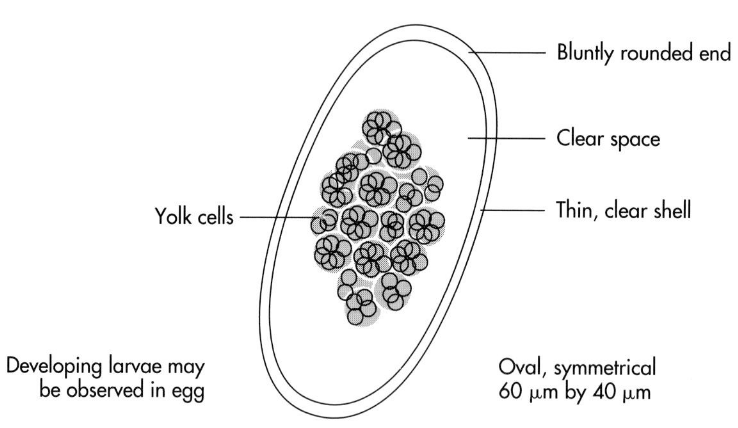

FIGURE 21–14
Life cycle and egg of hookworm.

with poor sewage disposal, which allows the eggs to remain and hatch in the soil.

Symptoms are associated with the area of infection and include a cutaneous phase known as "ground itch," a local dermatitis with redness and swelling at the site of infection. The pulmonary phase may be characterized by a pharyngitis, cough, and the production of a bloody sputum. The intestinal stage involves diarrhea, nausea, and vomiting. Since the filariform larvae have sharp-cutting mouth parts for attachment, hemorrhage may occur, with iron deficiency anemia and fatigue, weakness, edema, and congestive heart failure.

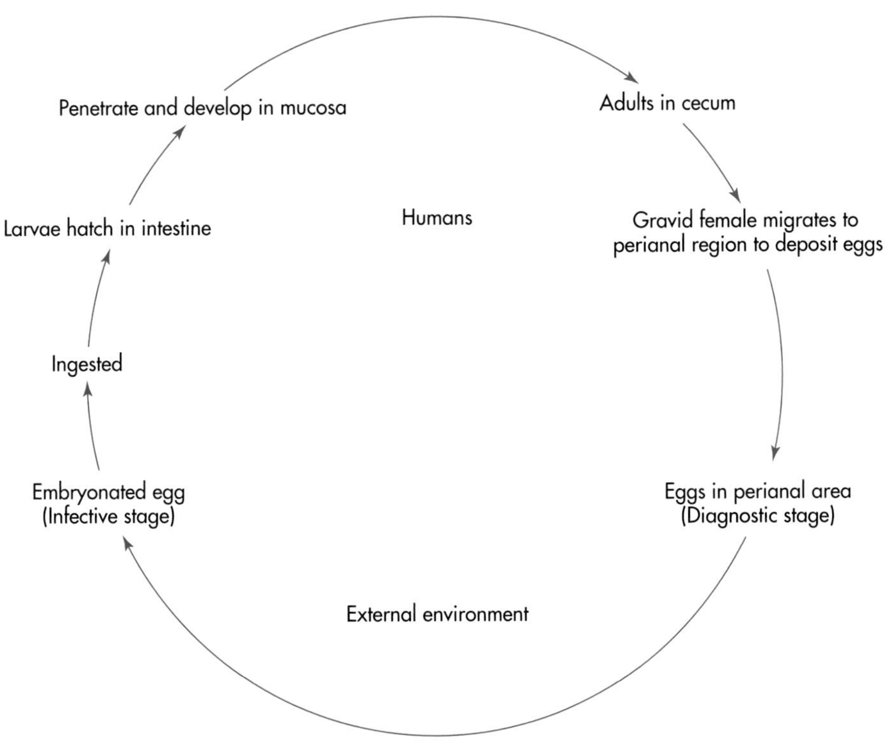

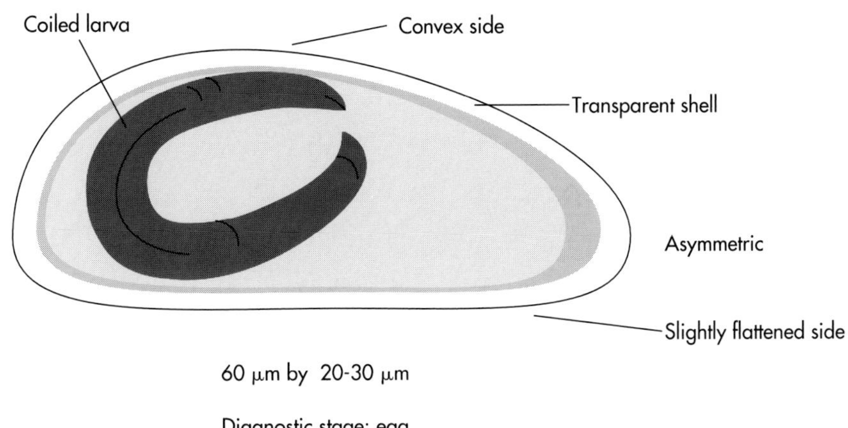

FIGURE 21–15
Life cycle and egg of *Enterobius vermicularis.*

Enterobius vermicularis

Enterobius vermicularis, pinworm, is the agent of enterobiasis, which is present worldwide, usually in temperate or colder climates. The infective form is the embryonated egg, which contains third-stage larvae that are ingested by mouth. The life cycle continues as noted in Figure 21-15. The adult worms do not have to pass through the circulatory system, as is the case for threadworm and hookworm. The mature adults are not very long, measuring approximately 5 to 10 mm in length. There is a winglike bulge at the anterior end and a long pointed tail, and thus the worm is said to resemble a "pin."

The eggs are present on the perianal folds but may not be observed in the feces. The female generally deposits the eggs at night, and thus the best specimen is obtained in the morning. The cellophane ("Scotch Tape") test may be used to collect the perianal specimen and uses a strip of cellophane tape placed on the anus, with its sticky side out to collect any eggs. The tape is then pressed onto a microscope slide with a glass coverslip and examined for the presence of eggs. The use of sticky paddles and commercially available swatches also may be used to collect the eggs. It is important to collect the specimen before bathing or a bowel movement to enhance recovery of the eggs.

The egg is the diagnostic stage (Figure 21-14). The adult worms are generally not recovered.

Pinworm infection is found worldwide and is transmitted through ingestion of infected food or contaminated hands. Children may scratch the perianal region at night, gathering eggs or larvae under their fingernails, and then transmit the parasite to other children. Infection may also be acquired after handling contaminated clothing, bedding, or other articles of the infected person. Pinworm infection is generally a mild, self-limiting infection with minimal symptoms of perianal, nocturnal itching. In heavy infestations the scratching may result in bleeding of the perianal region, nausea, abdominal pain, and irritability and nervousness. Children 5 to 10 years old are most often infected.

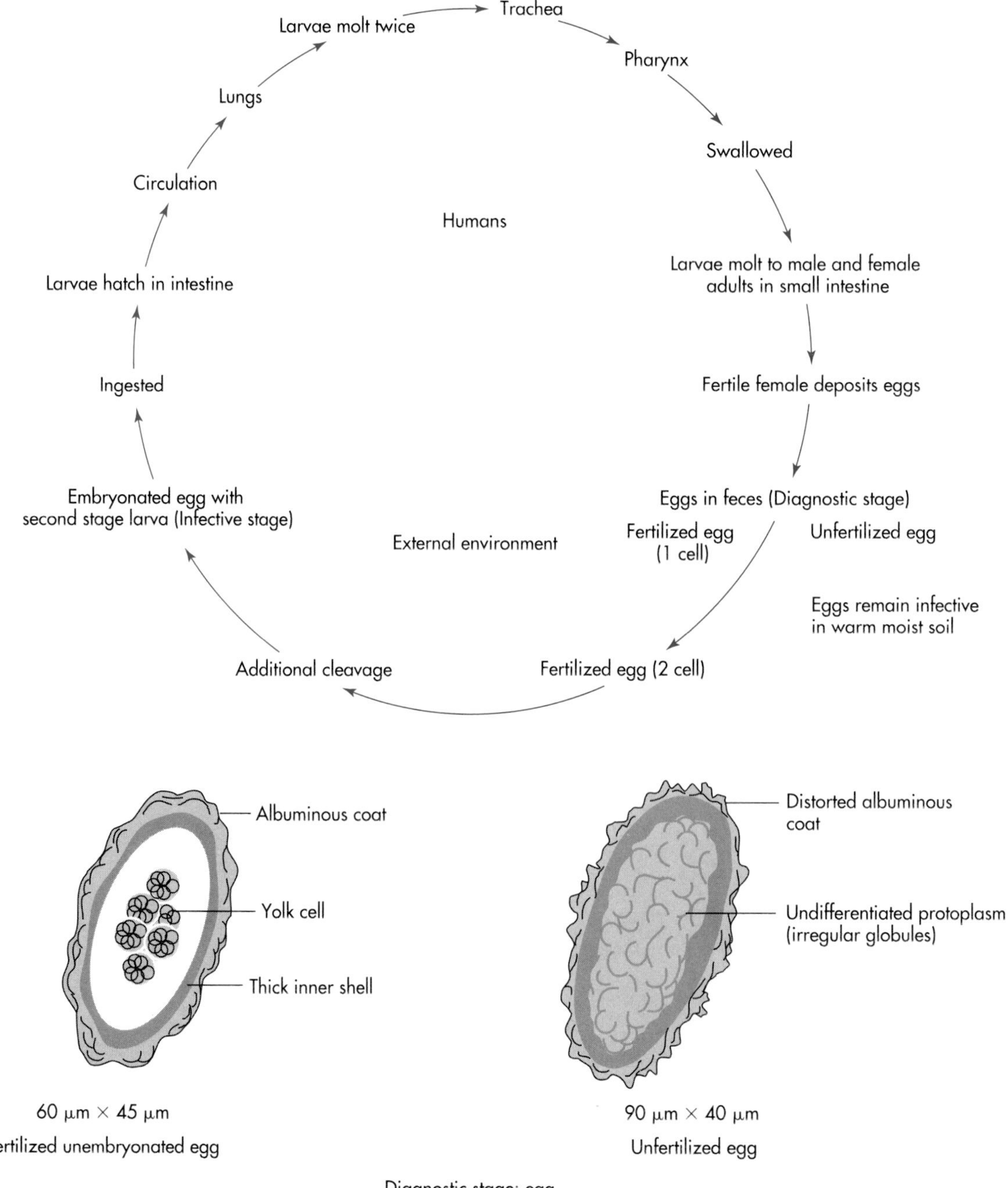

FIGURE 21–16

Life cycle and egg of *Ascaris lumbricoides*.

Ascaris lumbricoides

Ascaris lumbricoides, large intestinal roundworm, is acquired through ingestion of the embryonated eggs, which contains the second-stage larva. Figure 21-16 illustrates its life cycle and egg.

The diagnostic form is the egg, which is oval and may be observed in four different forms. A cortical layer or albuminous coat may or may not surround the egg, and the egg may be fertilized or unfertilized. The form generally observed is fertilized and unembryonated, with a thick, bile-stained coat and small, rounded projections measuring 60 × 45 μm. The unfertilized form is longer, with an undifferentiated protoplasm, brown color, and distorted coat. Figure 21-16 illustrates typical *Ascaris* eggs. Because *Ascaris* eggs are too heavy to float in zinc sulfate solution, sedimentation concentration methods are recommended for recovery.

Adult *Ascaris* worms measure 200 to 300 mm in length with a diameter of 3 to 5 mm. Male forms are shorter with a curved tail.

Ascariasis, the most common helminth infection, has a worldwide prevalence and is most frequently seen in the tropics. Infections are most often seen in young children and may be attributed to ingesting dirt or placing contaminated fingers in the mouth. Infection may result from the ingestion of raw foods that may be contaminated with soil containing contaminated human feces. Infections are generally mild and self-limiting, and

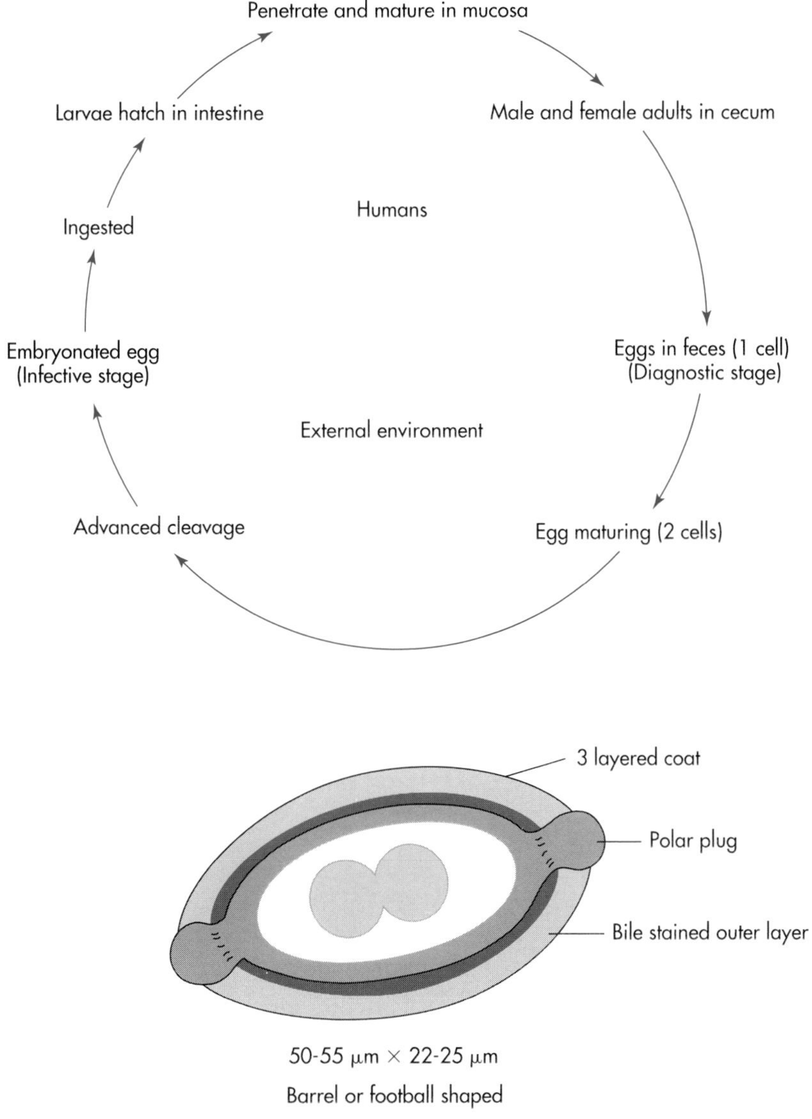

FIGURE 21–17
Life cycle and encysted larva of *Trichuris trichiura.*

the mortality rate is low. In more severe infections the lungs may be affected. Intestinal signs include abdominal pain and diarrhea. In large infestations the host may experience weight loss and malnutrition as the adult worms feed in the intestine.

Trichuris trichiura

Trichuris trichiura, or whipworm, infections are acquired through the ingestion of food or water contaminated with eggs that contain the first-stage larval form. The life cycle continues as shown in Figure 21-17. The adult worms are said to resemble a whip, with a long, thin esophagus and thick end resembling a handle, where the intestinal and reproductive organs are located.

The diagnostic form is the egg, which is characteristically elongated or lemon shaped, resembling a football or barrel (Figure 21-17). A problem in diagnosis is that there are frequently few eggs in the stool, which leads to difficulty in their detection.

Trichuriasis is most often seen in warm, humid climates with poor sanitation. It may be seen in the southeastern portion of the United States. The infection most frequently occurs in children and is related to poor handwashing practices and poor sanitary measures. The infection is usually asymptomatic or mild but may also be accompanied by abdominal pain, diarrhea, dysentery, and nausea. Malabsorption may be seen in heavy infestations.

Trichinella spiralis

Trichinella spiralis is the agent of trichinosis. Humans are considered as accidental hosts, who acquire the infection through the ingestion of contaminated raw or undercooked meat. Trichinosis is an infection of pigs and other carnivores, such as bears, and the life cycle is completed in these animals as depicted in Figure 21-18. The larvae can lodge in the myocardium, nervous tissue, or other tissue, but further development only occurs in striated muscle tissue. In striated muscle the larvae grow and molt, developing into the characteristic spiral form, for which the species is named. A host reaction occurs after the larvae are in the muscle cells for approximately 1 month to form a cyst around the larvae. The encysted larvae remain in the muscle until ingested by a new host, or they are calcified. Thus the parasitic life cycle is ultimately completed in the human host. The life cycle follows the same pathway in other animals, with its continuance through the ingestion of contaminated meat by another animal.

The prevalence of trichinosis depends on the dietary habits of the population, as well as prevention and control measures. The infection has a worldwide existence, and cases are especially found in North America and Europe, with cycles existing in bears, walruses, pigs, dogs, cats, and rats.

Measures for prevention include the use of irradiation and better agricultural control measures. These include government regulations preventing the use of garbage as feed for pigs and control of the rat population.

The infection has a low mortality rate, and symptoms may mimic other diseases. Symptoms may be absent or very severe, depending on the number of encysted larvae. The intestinal phase may be characterized by abdominal cramps and diarrhea as toxic metabolites are released by the worms. As the parasites enter the tissue, an eosinophilia develops, with the eosinophil count ranging from 10% to 90% in the first month of infection and then tapering off. The larvae then penetrate various muscle tissues, initially in the eye, which leads to periorbital swelling and edema. Headache, muscle pain, and swelling occur as the larvae penetrate the muscles of the neck, tongue, arms, legs, chest, and back. The convalescent phase may be associated with cardiac, pulmonary, or neurological symptoms.

Clinical diagnosis is made through muscle biopsy, with observation of the encysted larvae in the muscle tissue. Serodiagnosis using bentonite particles (which act as latex particles) or ELISA is typically used. A skin test can also facilitate the diagnosis.

Blood and Tissue Nematodes: Filarial Worms

The filarial worms are long, thin nematodes that parasitize the circulatory and lymphatic systems, serous cavities, and subcutaneous and deep connective tissues, including the muscles.

The life cycle begins as the infected arthropod takes a blood meal on the human host. The parasite matures in the circulatory system, connective tissue, or serous body cavity. The adult worms produce microfilariae, which may be found in the blood or skin. Ingestion by a blood-sucking insect perpetuates the life cycle.

The clinically important filarial worms include *Wuchereria bancrofti, Brugia malayi, Loa loa,* and *Onchocerca volvulus.* Diagnosis is achieved through blood films, where the motile microfilariae may be observed in fresh and thin and thick films. Skin snips may be used to diagnose infection by those worms that infect the skin and subcutaneous tissue. Identification is aided by determining if the microfilaria is sheathed or unsheathed, the shape of its tail, and the distribution of nuclei in its tail region. The sheath is an envelope over the worm that is a remnant of the ovum membrane.

Wuchereria bancrofti is found in the tropics, subtropics, Caribbean, Central Africa, and the southwestern Pacific Islands, Turkey, Hungary, Brazil, and the West Indies. The life cycle begins as infected mosquitoes take a blood meal, injecting the third-stage larval form into the host's skin. Maturation to adult forms occur in several

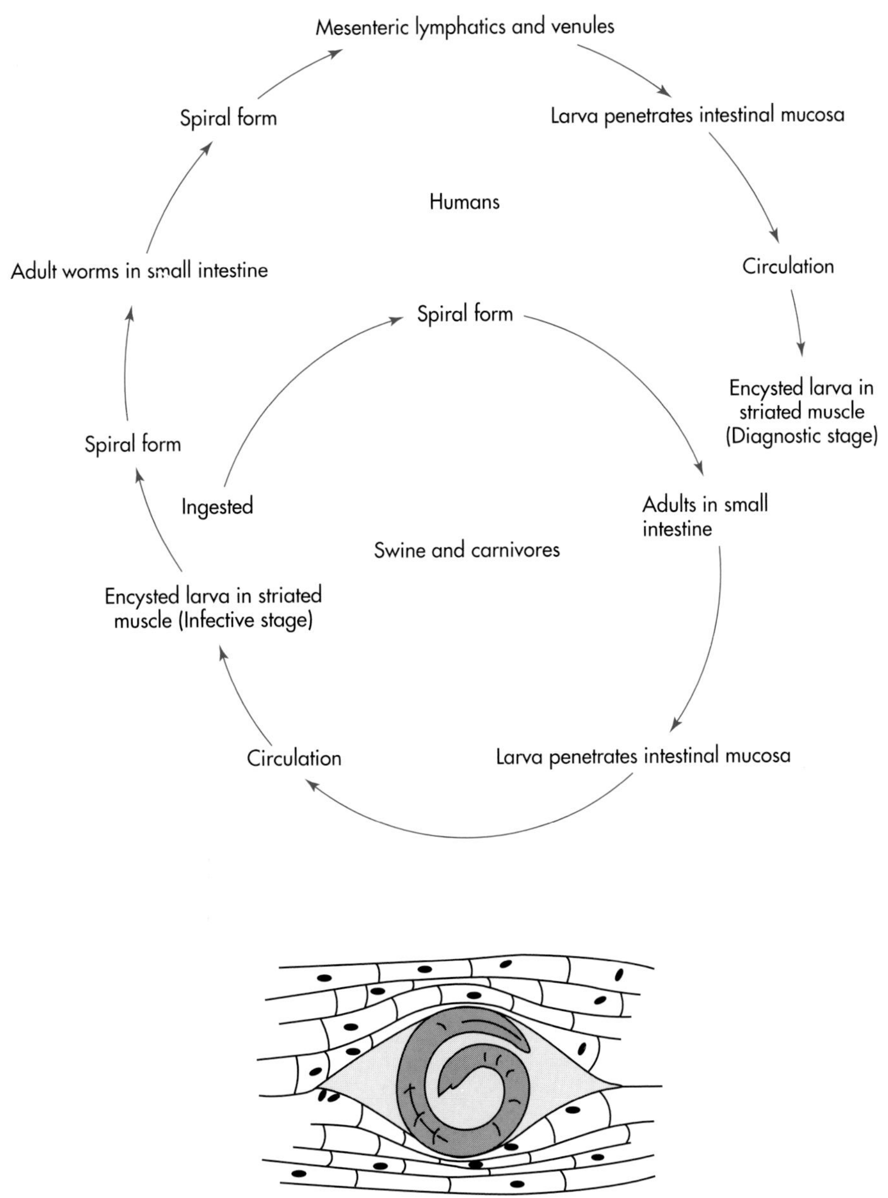

FIGURE 21–18
Life cycle and egg of *Trichinella spiralis.*

months to a year, and adult worms can survive for 10 to 15 years in coiled masses in the lymphatics. The adult male fertilizes the female, who releases hundreds of microfilariae into the peripheral blood. The microfilariae have a nocturnal periodicity, with the greatest yield in the peripheral blood from 10 PM to 2 AM. The life cycle continues if a female mosquito takes a blood meal, ingesting the microfilariae, which penetrate the gut wall of the mosquito and enter the thoracic muscles, where maturation to the third-stage larva occurs in 10 days. Migration to the proboscis follows, and during the blood meal the larvae escape into the host's skin.

The infection is known as Bancroft's filariasis or elephantiasis, and the adult worms live in the host lymphatic channels, primarily in the arms, legs, and pelvis. An acute tissue reaction occurs, with the accumulation of lymphatic fluid, swelling, and later fibrosis.

The microfilariae are sheathed with parallel rows of nuclei that do not extend into the tip of the tail. A clear, cephalic space develops at the tip of the tail. Microfilaria may be absent from the blood and found in pulmonary vessels and other organs during the day.

Brugia malayi, the cause of Malayan filariasis and elephantiasis, is found in southeast Asia, Korea, India,

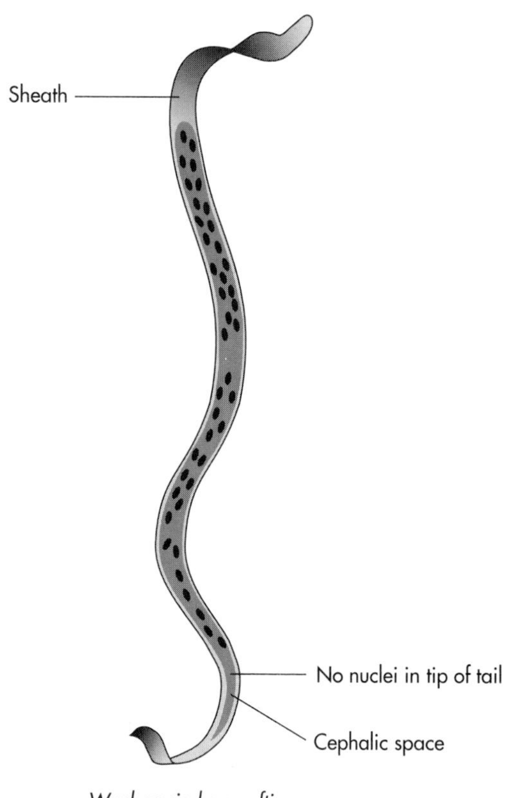

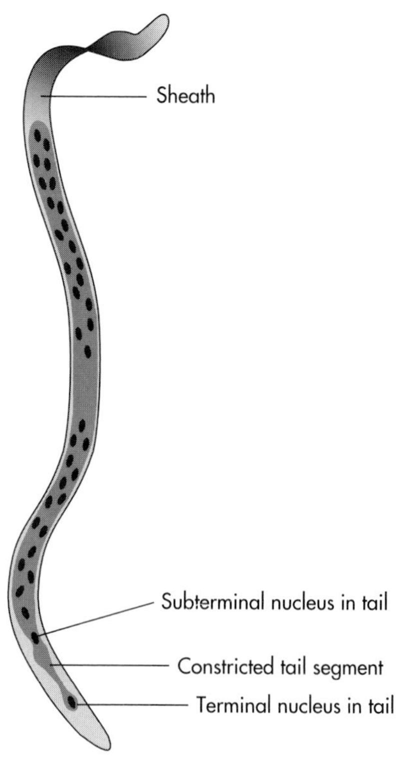

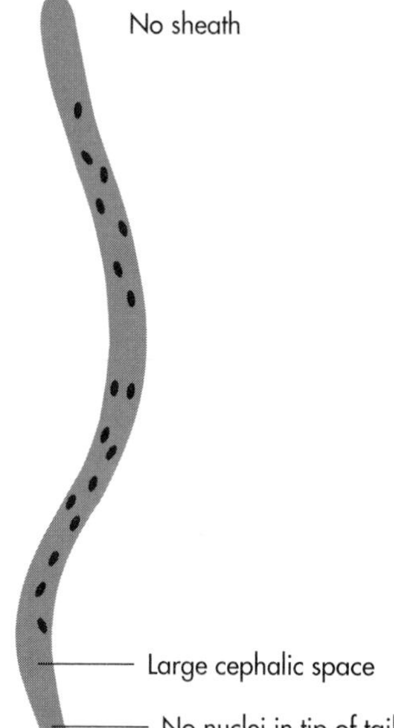
No sheath
Large cephalic space
No nuclei in tip of tail
Sharply pointed tail
Onchocerca volvulus
300-345 μm × 5-9 μm

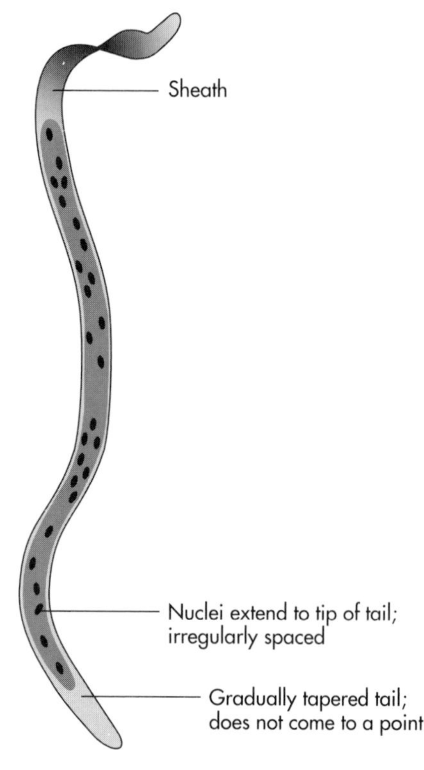

FIGURE 21–19

Diagrams and descriptions of clinically important microfilariae.

Indonesia, and China. The life cycle is similar to that of *W. bancrofti,* with the adult worms living primarily in the lymphatics but sometimes in the blood vessels. Sheathed microfilariae are produced by the adult female and are found in the blood during evening hours. Two distinct nuclei are isolated in the tail, one subterminally and the other terminally in the tail's tip. The tail is tapered, with a constriction separating the terminal nucleus from the remaining nuclei.

Loa loa, eye worm, initiates infection when the blood-sucking tabanid fly takes a blood meal, injecting the third-stage larvae into the host skin. The adults mature in the subcutaneous tissue within 6 months but can survive for up to 17 years. The fertilized female releases sheathed microfilariae into the blood. The life cycle continues if a deer fly takes a blood meal from an infected host.

Loiasis occurs as the adult worms migrate through subcutaneous tissue, releasing their toxic metabolites and resulting in inflammation. The worms typically migrate to the conjunctiva, across the bridge of the nose, and into the cornea of the eye.

Diagnosis is achieved through clinical signs and the demonstration of sheathed microfilariae in peripheral blood. The highest yield is found in specimens obtained between 11 AM and 1 PM. The microfilariae have a gradually tapered tail that does not draw to a point. The nuclei extend all the wall into the tip of the tail, with the last several nuclei irregularly spaced.

Onchocerca volvulus is the agent of onchocerciasis, or river blindness. The disease is found in South and Central America and Africa where areas for the breeding of the black fly vector are abundant. Black flies inject larvae into the wound during their blood meal. The larvae migrate to the subcutaneous tissue and mature to adults in 3 to 15 months but can survive for up to 15 years. The mature female releases unsheathed microfilariae, which are found primarily in the lymphatics of connective and cutaneous tissues.

Adult worms survive in coiled masses in the host subcutaneous tissue. The host inflammatory response results in the formation of an encapsulated nodule, or onchocercoma, which can be felt in the large bones of the arm, leg, and scalp, as well as in deeper tissue.

Diagnosis is achieved through clinical signs and demonstration of the microfilariae in skin snips; the microfilariae are usually not found in blood. The microfilariae are large and unsheathed, with a sharply pointed tail. There are no nuclei in the tip of the tail, and a cephalic space is present.

Figure 21-19 provides diagrams and descriptions of the microfilariae.

CESTODES

The members of the class Cestoda are commonly known as tapeworms because of their long, ribbonlike bodies, which appear flat in a cross section. The anterior end of the worm, or **scolex**, is used for attachment to the host through suckers and, in some parasites, hooks. The **rostellum**, crown of the scolex, may be armed and fitted with hooklets or unarmed and smooth without hooklets. The body of the worm is composed of segments known as **proglottids**. Segments form by budding at the posterior end of the worm. The chain of developing proglottids is known as the **strobila.** Each mature proglottid is **hermaphroditic**, which means that it contains both male and female reproductive organs. The organs gradually mature, and eventually the proglottids at the posterior end of the worm, known as **gravid proglottids**, have fully developed reproductive organs with a uterus filled with fertilized eggs. The embryo, which may be visible in the tapeworm eggs, is known as the **oncosphere** or **hexacanth embryo.** This first-stage larva is motile and usually contains six hooklets, which enable it to enter the intestinal tract of the intermediate host. Tapeworms lack mouths, digestive tracts, and vascular systems and absorb all nutrients and release all waste products through their outer body surface.

Table 21-5 summarizes the medically significant tapeworms.

TABLE 21–5

Cestoda: Tapeworms

SCIENTIFIC NAME	COMMON NAME
Dipylidium caninum	Cat and dog tapeworm
Diphyllobothrium latum	Broad or πfish tape-worm
Echinococcus granulosus	Dog tapeworm (hydatid cyst)
Taenia saginata	Beef tapeworm
Taenia solium	Pork tapeworm
Hymenolepsis nana	Dwarf tapeworm
Hymenolepsis diminuta	Rat tapeworm

Diphyllobothrium latum

Diphyllobothrium latum, broad or fish tapeworm, is the largest tapeworm known to infect humans, with mature adults measuring up to 10 m in length. Crustaceans serve as the first intermediate hosts, and humans are the definitive hosts and are infected by ingesting the **plerocercoid**, or second, larval form in the second intermediate host, which is raw or uncooked, contaminated fresh water fish. The scolex of the larva attaches to the intestine. The scolex is shaped like a rounded spatula ("phyllo," meaning leaf) with a pair ("di") of longitudinal shallow grooves or plates ("bothria") for sucking on its ventral surface. The individual proglottids are broader than long, and thus the organism is known as "broad tapeworm." The uterus of the gravid proglottid resembles a rosette, or flower petals, with the eggs clustered around the central opening or pore of the uterus. The unembryonated eggs, the diagnostic stage, are passed in the feces of infected humans. Figure 21-20 illustrates the life cycle and egg.

Once the eggs are passed, they must reach fresh water for the life cycle to continue. In fresh water the embryo develop in the egg and are released from the egg by "pushing" open the operculum. This free-living larval stage, or **coracidium,** further develops in water and is ingested by the first intermediate hosts, crustaceans or copepods of the genus *Diaptomus.* The first larval stage, or **procercoid,** develops in the body cavity of the first intermediate host, which is eventually ingested by freshwater fish, usually salmon, trout, pickerel, or pike. Minnows may also ingest the infected crustaceans, which may in turn be ingested by the larger freshwater fish. The life cycle continues as seen in Figure 21-20.

Infections from *D. latum* are endemic in colder climates where there are freshwater lakes. These areas include Russia, Europe, northern China, and Scandinavia,

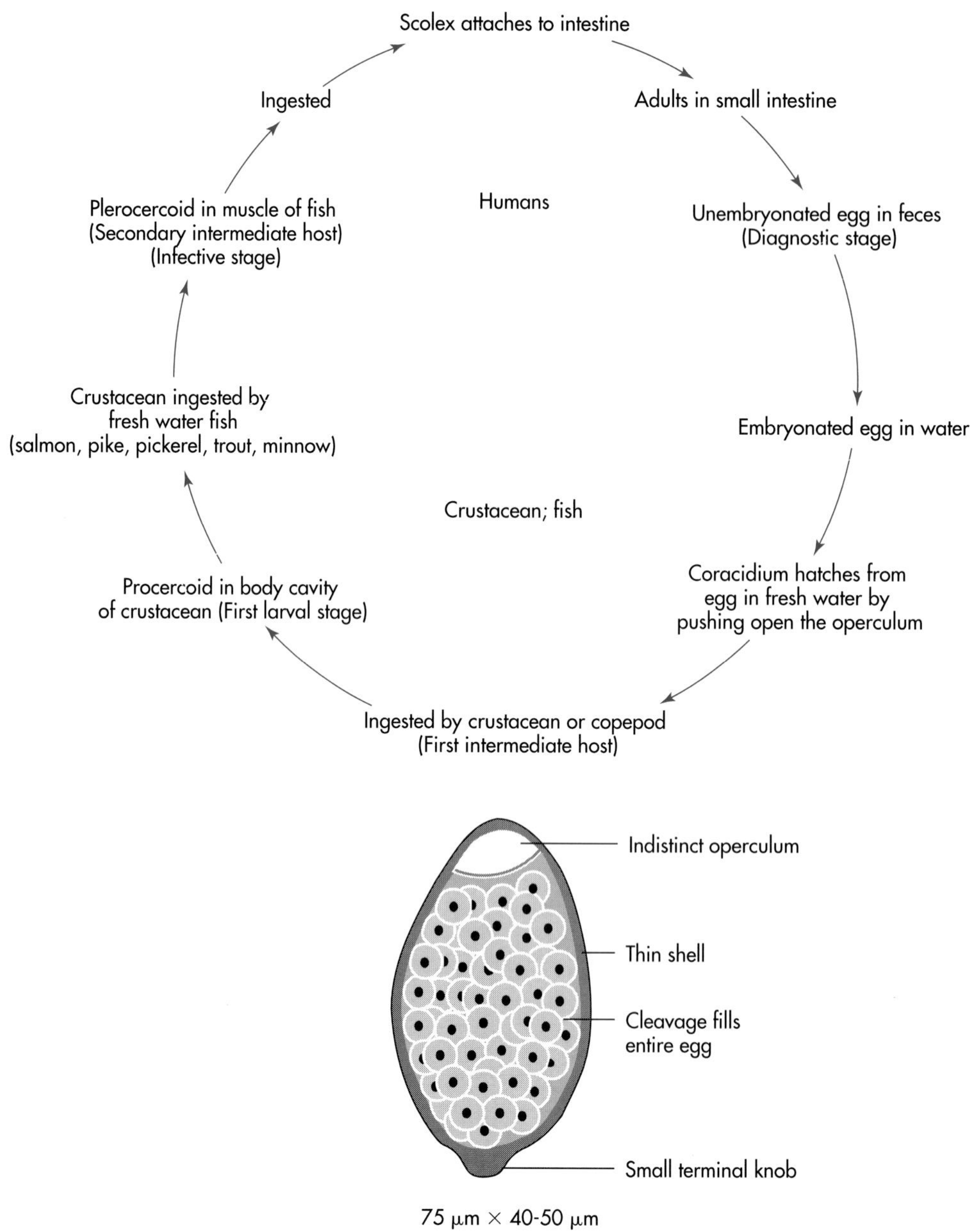

FIGURE 21–20

Life cycle and egg of *Diphyllobothrium latum.*

as well as Chile and Argentina. In North America, infections are found in Canada, Alaska, Michigan, and Minnesota. An increased incidence is associated with the consumption of raw fish, especially smoked, pickled, and kipperred freshwater fish. Other mammals, including seals and bears, are also known to harbor the parasite. Symptoms are generally minimal or absent, except in more severe infections, in which pernicious anemia caused by vitamin B_{12} deficiency from absorption by the adult worms may occur.

The diagnostic form is the egg (Figure 21-20), and since each worm may have thousands of proglottids, up to 1 million eggs may be released daily. Thus the eggs may be observed even in unconcentrated stools in wet mount preparations. The eggs resemble those of *Paragonimus westermani.* However, *D. latum* eggs are shorter, widest in the middle, with an indistinct knob and rounded operculum. *P. westermani* eggs are the widest near the operculum with no knob and measure 80 to 120 μm. The characteristic morphology of the gravid proglottid and scolex can also be used in identification when isolated.

Hymenolepsis nana

Hymenolepsis nana, dwarf tapeworm, possesses a scolex with four rounded suckers. The infective form

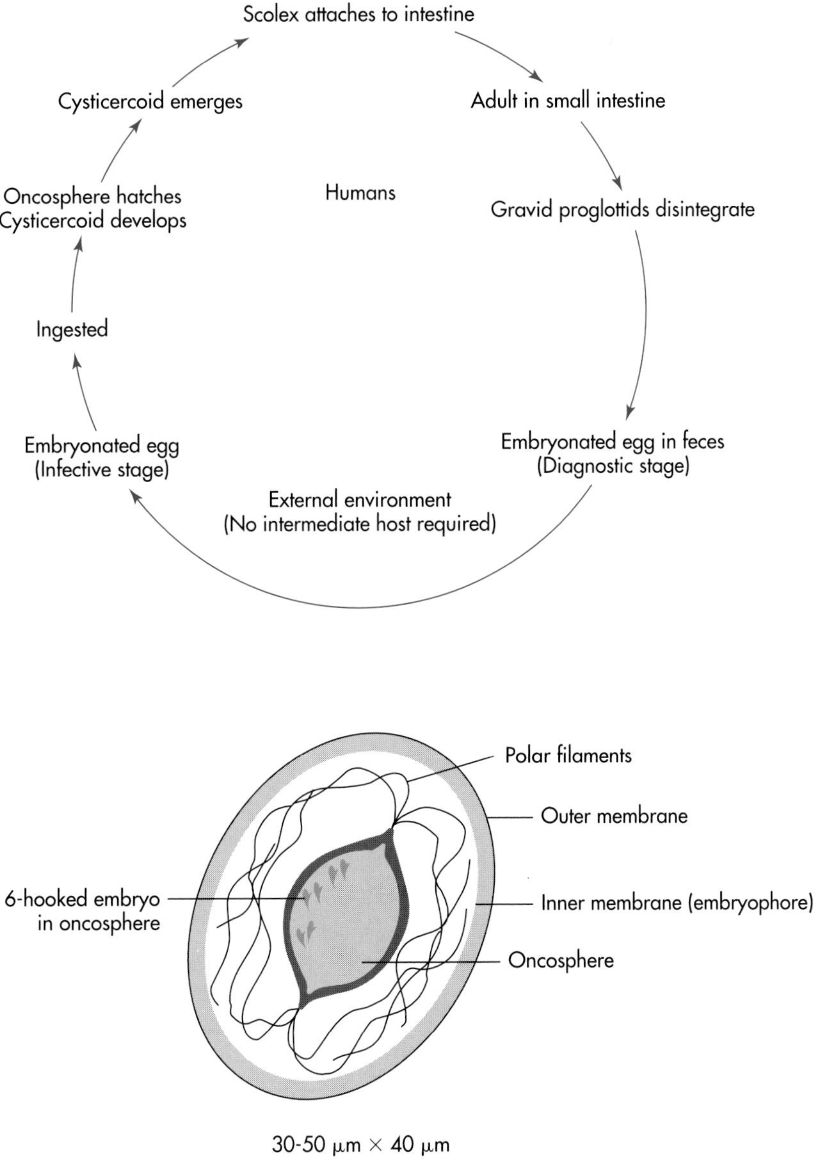

FIGURE 21-21
Life cycle and egg of *Hymenolepsis nana.*

is the egg, which is ingested by humans in food or water contaminated with the embryonated egg. The egg contains the oncosphere, or embryo, in a double-walled structure. The life cycle continues as shown in Figure 21-21. The adult worm is very small, measuring 2 to 4 cm in length, thus the name "dwarf" tapeworm.

The scolex is an armed rostellum with a ring of 20 to 30 spines and hooks, which resemble a beaklike structure. The scolex has a single row of hooklets, or sucking organs, and is very small, measuring less than 0.4 mm. The gravid proglottids may be passed in the feces. They have a narrow neck region and broaden at the distal end. The gravid uterus is a small, saclike cluster near the center of each segment. The uterine pore is central but usually not visible.

H. nana does not need a separate intermediate host, and humans serve as both the intermediate and the definitive host. The infection is acquired through the ingestion of food or water contaminated with the feces of rats or mice. The infection is seen worldwide but most often in the warmer climates, including Central America and the southeastern parts of the United States. Children can also acquire the infection from the hand-to-mouth route.

The diagnostic form is the egg, which is hexacanth or lancet shaped with six hooklets (Figure 21-21). It is round to oval, measuring 30 to 50 μm, with a thin smooth membrane ("hymen") and outer shell ("lepsis") surrounding the membrane. The oncosphere is enclosed within the thin membrane, leaving a clear space between it and the shell. Four to eight filaments emerge from the inner membrane of the egg.

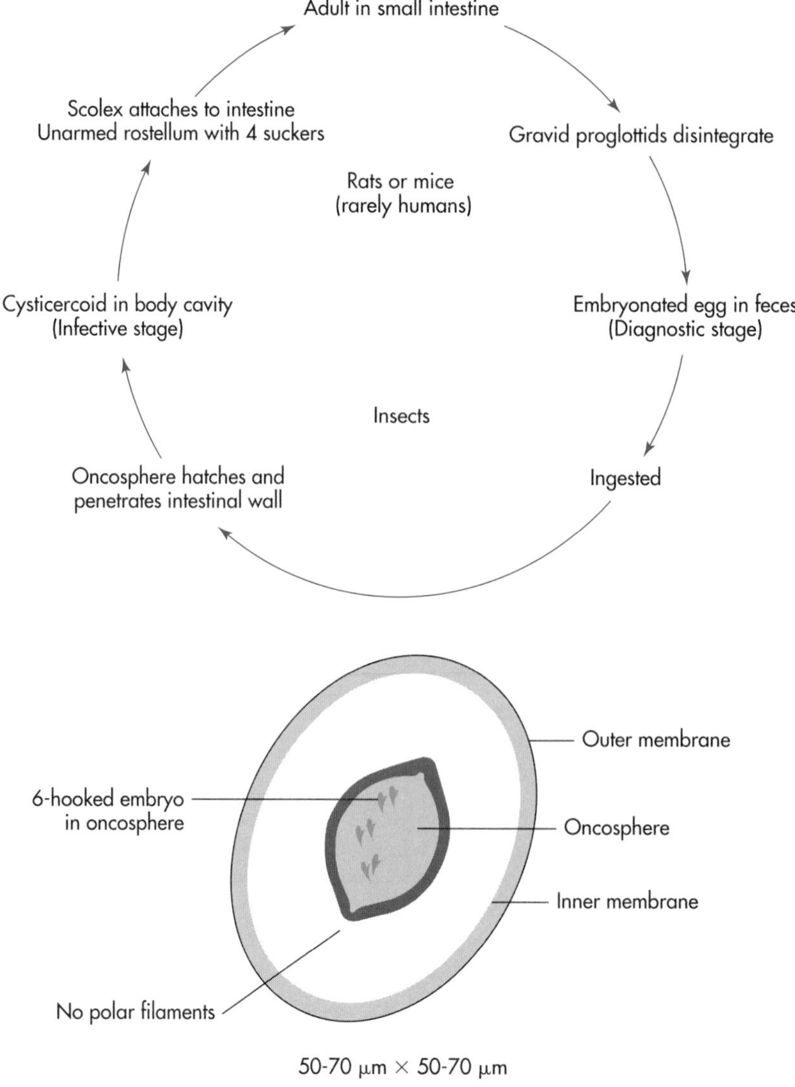

FIGURE 21-22
Life cycle and egg of *Hymenolepsis diminuta.*

Hymenolepsis diminuta

Hymenolepsis diminuta, the cause of rat tapeworm infection, is very rarely found in humans. The organism requires an intermediate host of arthropods, such as fleas or grain beetles, for the life cycle to be completed. The definitive hosts may be humans, rats, or mice. Humans may acquire the infection through ingestion of arthropods that are infected with the parasite. Grain beetles or fleas may ingest the eggs; thus they serve as an intermediate host. The oncosphere hatches within the arthropod. If the arthropod is ingested by humans, the adult worm may develop in the intestinal tract. Cereal grains containing infected arthropods may also serve as a source of infection.

To differentiate *H. nana* from *H. diminuta,* the eggs and rostellum are examined. The eggs of *H. diminuta* are slightly larger (50-70 μm) and more oval, with no filaments (Fig. 21-22). In contrast to the armed rostellum of *H. nana., H. diminuta* has an unarmed rostellum.

Dipylidium canium

Dipylidium canium, a common tapeworm of dogs and cats, may cause infections in children and household pets. Humans may acquire the infection by ingesting food or water contaminated with dog, cat, or human feces. The stroblia measure 15-75 cm long, with 50 to 150 proglottids. The scolex is conical rhomboidal, with an armed rostellum. The proglottids may detach and then migrate from the anus of the animal, appearing as small grains of rice in the external environment. Cysterceroid larva develop in the feces after ingestion of embryonated eggs. The infection is diagnosed by observation of egg packets or gravid proglottids in the feces or on the genital hair. Each egg packet is large and irregular, containing 15 to 25 globular eggs, each with a diameter of 35-60 μm, with an oncosphere with six hooklets.

Taenia saginata and Taenia solium

Taenia saginata, beef tapeworm, infection occurs as the cyst form is ingested in contaminated rare or uncooked beef. The infective form is the **cysticercus** in the muscle tissue of cattle and other herbivores. The cysts hatch in the intestinal tract and attach by four rounded suckers to the mucosa in the small intestine. The worm has hooklets and an unarmed rostellum. The life cycle continues as seen in Figure 21-23. The adult worm measures 4 to 10 m in length. The intermediate hosts, usually cattle, ingest the proglottids on contaminated grass.

Both the eggs and the gravid proglottids are the diagnostic stages (Figure 21-23). A dark-brown shell surrounds the oncosphere, and six small hooklets can be observed. The egg cannot be differentiated from that of *T. solium,* and thus the gravid proglottid should be examined for a definitive identification. The strobila of *T. saginata* measures 4 to 10 m, with up to 2000 proglottids. The gravid proglottid has 15 to 20 uterine branches, and its scolex is very small with four suckers and lacks hooks. The strobila of *T. solium* measures 2 to 4 m, with up to 1000 proglottids. Its gravid proglottid has 5 to 12 major uterine branches, with two rows of hooks located on the anterior scolex, which is armed.

T. solium, pork tapeworm, has a similar life cycle as *T. saginata.* Humans are infected through the ingestion of cysts in uncooked pork. The scolex of *T. solium* has four round suckers and two rows of hooks located at the anterior end. The adult worm measures from 2 to 6 m. Figure 21-24 depicts the life cycle and egg of *T. solium.*

One major distinction from the life cycle of *T. saginata* is *T. solium's* ability to autoinfect the human host. The eggs are infective for both pigs and humans. Once the eggs are produced by the gravid proglottids, the oncospheres may hatch in the small intestine, penetrate the intestinal wall, and enter the circulation. This can lead to cysticercus, the development of the extraintestinal encysted larval form in various organs, including the brain, lungs, eye, or connective tissue. This does not happen with *T. saginata,* since the eggs are not believed to be infectious.

Because the eggs of *T. solium* resemble those of *T. saginata,* the scolex is used to differentiate between the two species.

Infections from *T. saginata* and *T. solium* are present throughout the world, especially where human feces is disposed of improperly and where raw pork or beef is consumed. The infection is seen in Central and South America, Russia, and Africa.

Those who are infected usually harbor one adult worm and have few clinical manifestations. *T. solium* infections are usually more serious, since the entire encystment may occur in the brain or muscle, which may result in paralysis and mental disorientation.

Echinococcus granulosus

Echinococcus granulosus, the agent of echinococcosis, or hydatid cyst disease. Infection results from ingestion of embryonated eggs in the feces of dogs and other carnivores, which serve as the definitive hosts. After ingestion in humans, the oncosphere hatches, penetrates the intestinal wall, enters the circulation, and forms hydatid cysts in the liver, lungs, or other tissues, where the life cycle ends. The cysts may have a longevity up to 30 years in humans and require surgical removal.

If the embryonated eggs are ingested by sheep, pigs, or cattle, the cycle results in the formation of hydatid cysts in the viscera, which may be ingested by carnivores, such as dogs or wolves. The scolex from the cyst attaches to the intestine, and adults develop in the small intestine. The gravid proglottids then produce eggs that are released in the animal's feces. If ingested by the intermediate hosts (humans, sheep, pigs, cattle), the life cycle continues.

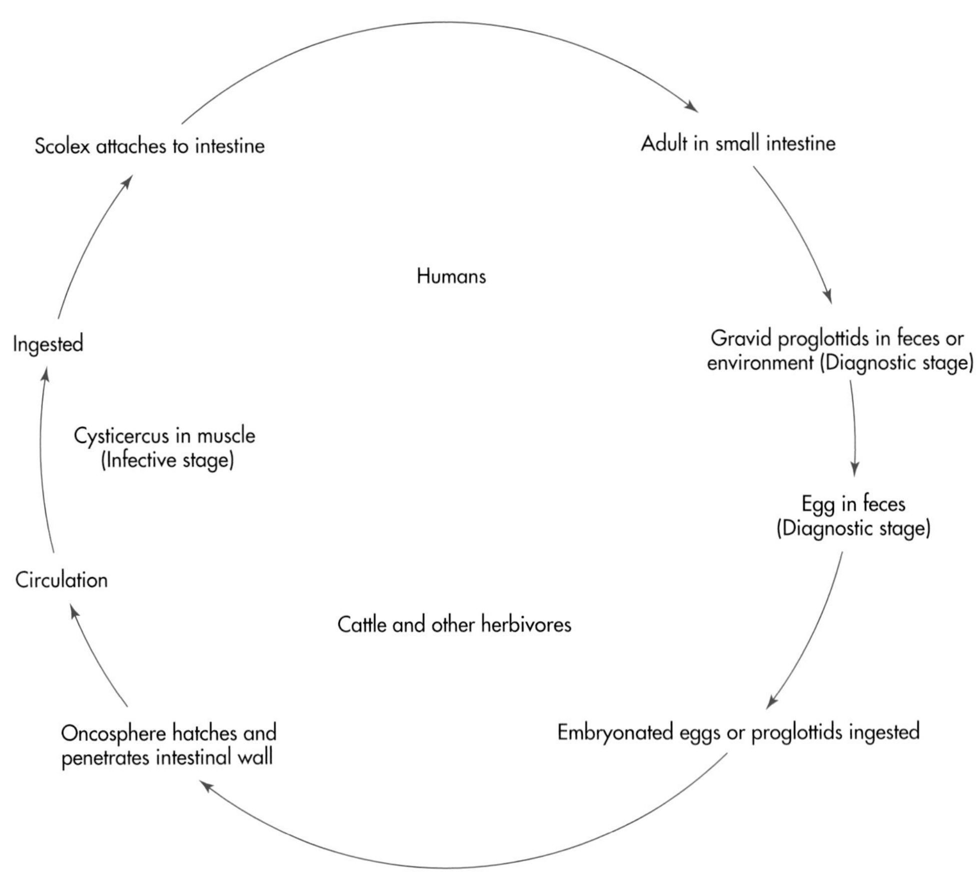

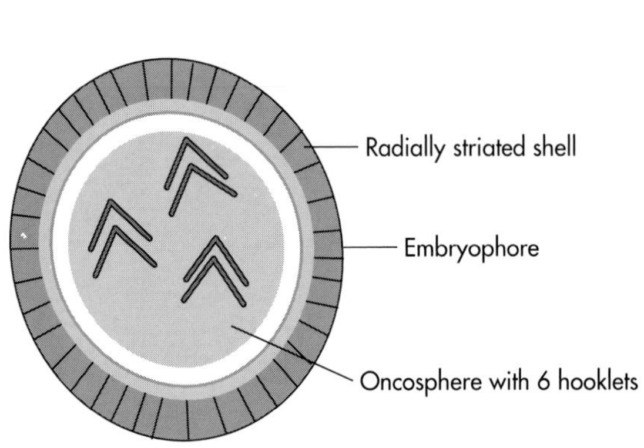

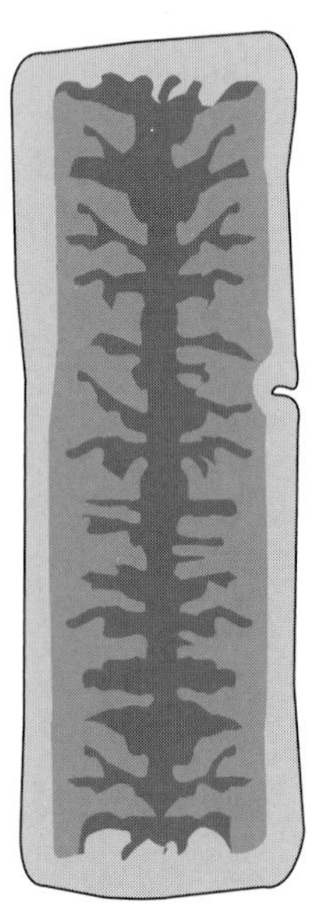

FIGURE 21–23
Life cycle and egg of *Taenia saginata.*

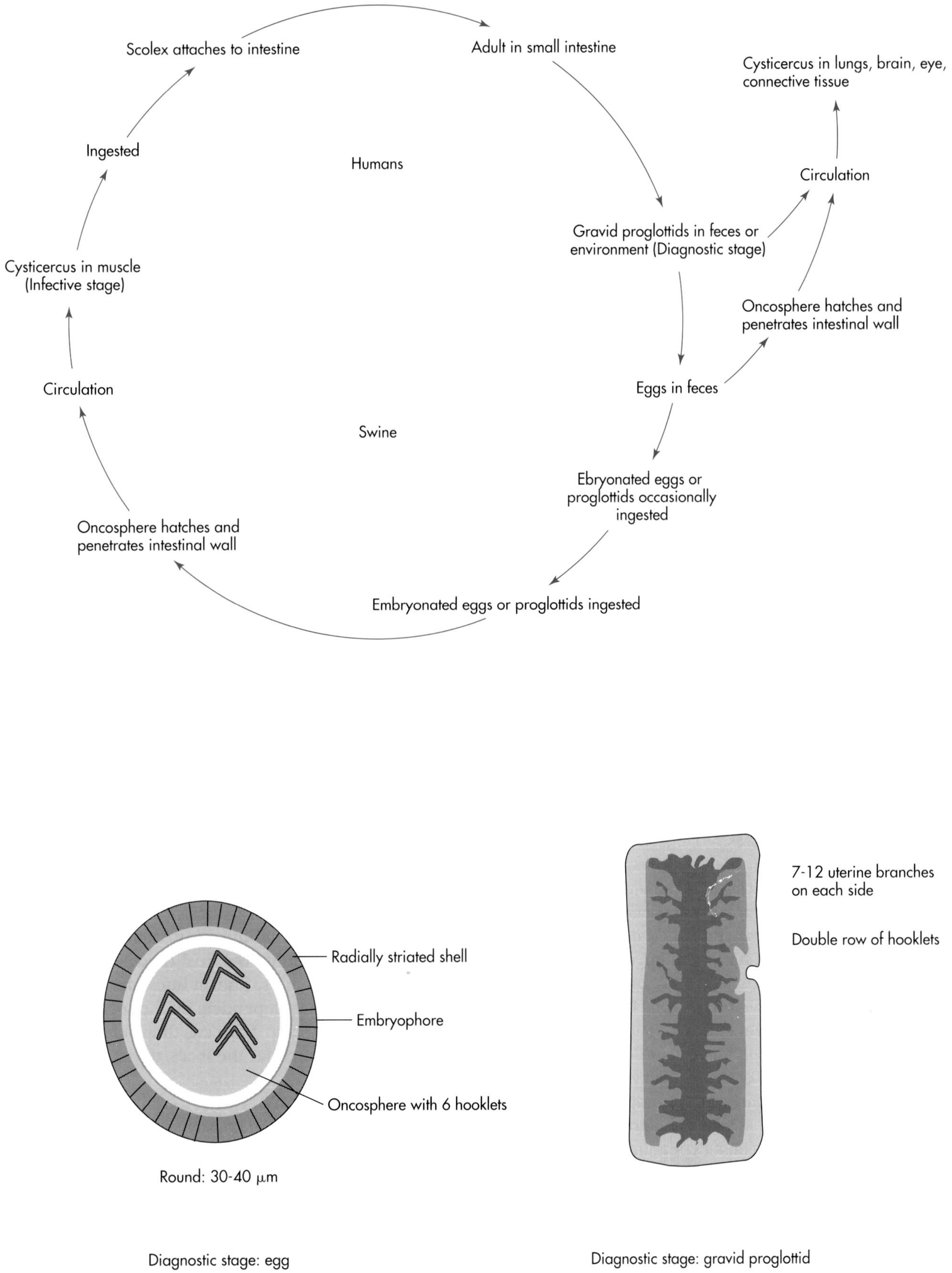

Scolex attaches to intestine

Adult in small intestine

Cysticercus in lungs, brain, eye, connective tissue

Ingested

Humans

Circulation

Gravid proglottids in feces or environment (Diagnostic stage)

Cysticercus in muscle (Infective stage)

Oncosphere hatches and penetrates intestinal wall

Circulation

Eggs in feces

Swine

Ebryonated eggs or proglottids occasionally ingested

Oncosphere hatches and penetrates intestinal wall

Embryonated eggs or proglottids ingested

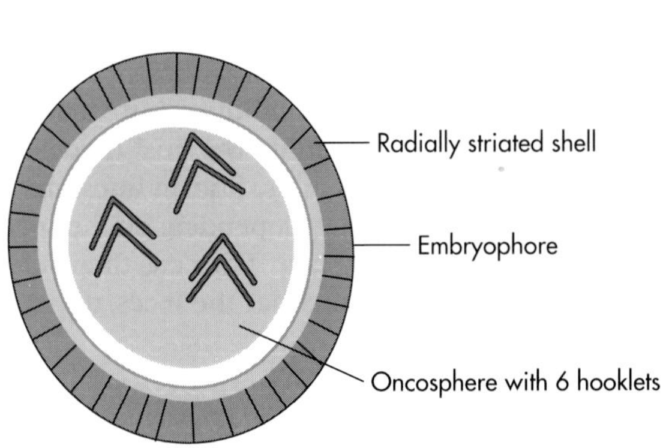

Round: 30-40 µm

Diagnostic stage: egg

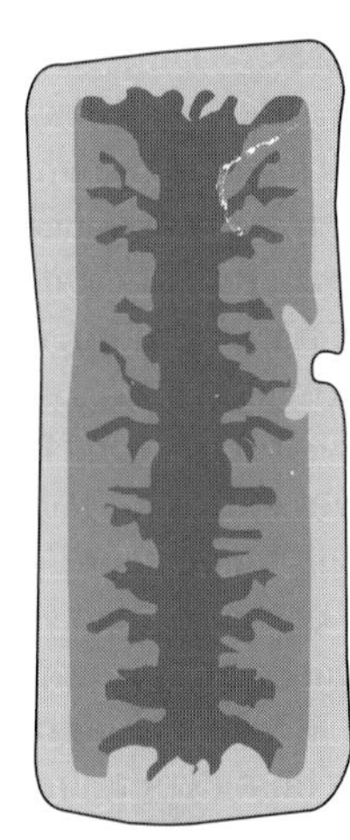

7-12 uterine branches on each side

Double row of hooklets

Diagnostic stage: gravid proglottid

FIGURE 21–24

Life cycle and egg of *Taenia solium.*

PROCEDURE
FORMALIN-ETHER CONCENTRATION
(Continued)

7. Add approximately 3 ml ethyl acetate, insert stopper, and shake vigorously for a minimum of 30 seconds. Carefully remove the stopper by holding tube away from yourself to avoid spraying as the stopper is removed and pressure is released.
8. Centrifuge at 500 g for 10 minutes. Four layers should result:
   1-Top layer of ethyl acetate
   2-Plug of fecal debris
   3-Layer of formalin
   4-Sediment with parasitic eggs, cysts, or larvae
9. Free the plug of debris from the sides of the tube with an applicator stick. Carefully decant the three layers. Use a cotton swab to clean debris from the walls of the tube to prevent it from settling down into the sediment.
10. Using a pipette, mix the remaining sediment with a small amount of the fluid that drains from the sides of the tube.
11. Mix the sediment well, and prepare a wet mount for examination.

Procedure for PVA-Preserved Specimens

1. Fixation time with polyvinyl alcohol (PVA) should be for at least 30 minutes. Mix one part stool to two to three parts PVA.
2. Pour 2 to 5 ml of this suspension into a flat-bottomed, waxed paper cup, carton, or 16 × 125 mm test tube. Add 10 ml saline. Filter suspension through funnel or paper cup with end cup off, lined with gauze or cheesecloth.

3. to 11. Follow as previously described.

Examination of Sediment

1. Prepare a saline mount by adding 1 drop sediment to 1 drop saline. Add a 22 × 22 mm coverslip. Scan the entire area under the coverslip under the 10× objective for eggs or larvae.
2. Add 1 drop iodine to the edge of the coverslip to assist in the observation of cysts. Examine under the high-dry objective (40 to 45×).

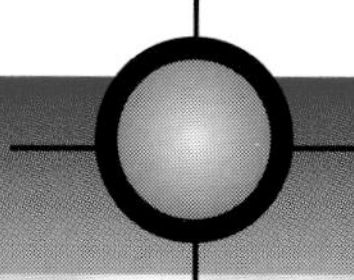

PROCEDURE

THICK AND THIN BLOOD FILMS

PURPOSE

Thick and thin blood films stained with Giemsa hematological stain permit the detection of blood parasites, including malarial parasites, trypanosomes, and microfilariae.

PRINCIPLE

The thick blood film permits the examination of a large amount of blood for the presence of parasites. Since the smear is not fixed with methanol, the red blood cells (RBCs) lyse, permitting better visualization of the organisms. The thin film allows for the observation of RBC morphology, inclusions, and intracellular and extracellular parasites. A larger area of the slide must be examined in the thin smear, although there is less distortion when compared with the thick smear.

MATERIALS

Microscope slides
Absolute methanol
Giemsa stock stain
Giemsa buffers 1 and 2
Triton-buffered water
Disodium phosphate

PROCEDURE

Stain Preparation

1. Giemsa stain may be purchased as a concentrated stock or prepared by grinding 1 g powdered Giemsa with 5 to 10 ml glycerol in a mortar. Add additional glycerol to a final total volume of 66 ml, and heat to 55°C in a water bath until stain is dissolved. Cool and add 66 ml absolute methanol. Allow to stand for 2 to 3 weeks. Filter and store in a brown bottle, protected from the light.
2. Prepare working Giemsa stain by mixing one part stock Giemsa stain to 10 to 50 parts triton-buffered water. The dilution chosen will determine the staining time. For example, if using a 1:50 dilution, stain for 50 minutes.
3. To prepare buffer 1, add 9.5 g 0.067 M Na_2HPO_4 (disodium phosphate) to 1000 ml distilled water.
4. To prepare buffer 2, add 9.2 g 0.067 M NaH_2PO_4; H_2O to 1000 ml distilled water.
5. Working buffer is prepared weekly and filtered before each use. Prepare the working buffer by adding 61.1 ml stock buffer 1 and 38.9 ml stock buffer 2 to 900 ml distilled water.

Thick Film

1. Prepare thick blood film by applying a free-flowing drop of blood, preferably without an anticoagulant, to a microscope slide cleaned with alcohol to remove any oil present.
2. Using the corner of a second slide, spread the film in a circle about the size of a dime. Avoid the formation of fibrin strands by spreading rapidly in a circular motion.

PROCEDURE

THICK AND THIN BLOOD FILMS

(Continued)

3. Allow to air-day overnight.
4. Place smears in a 1:50 dilution of stock Giemsa stain for 50 minutes. The lack of methanol fixation allows lysis or laking of the RBCs.
5. Rinse gently with triton-buffered water three times.
6. Drain slides in a vertical position and air-dry.

Thin Film

1. Clean a microscope slide with alcohol to remove any oil.
2. Touch the slide to 1 drop free flowing blood toward one end of the slide.
3. Holding a second slide at a 30-degree angle to the first slide, draw back into the drop, and allow it to spread into the edge of the spreader slide. Then quickly and evenly push the spreader slide forward, allowing the blood to spread out. There should be a "feathered edge" at the end of the smear and no holes, and the smear should cover one-half to two-thirds the slide.
4. Allow the slide to air-dry.
5. Fix the thin smear in absolute methanol for 30 seconds.
6. Place in working Giemsa stain for 50 minutes if using a 1:50 dilution. Staining time can be reduced by reducing the dilution of the stain. For example, when using a 1:20 dilution, staining time is reduced to 20 minutes.
7. Rinse gently with buffer for 2 minutes.
8. Dry vertically and examine under the 100× objective.

EXAMINATION OF SMEARS

1. Thick smear: examine 200 to 300 oil immersion fields for the presence of blood parasites.
2. Thin smear: examine the slide for a minimum of 30 minutes, and examine a minimum of 100 fields under the oil immersion objective.
3. Giemsa stains blood components as follows:

    Erythrocytes: pale gray-blue
    White blood cells: nuclei—purple
    cytoplasm—pale purple
    granules—eosinophils: bright red-purple; neutrophils: dark pink-purple

    Parasites stain blue to purple with red nuclei.

QUALITY CONTROL

Stain known positive blood smears or control slides periodically with patient samples.

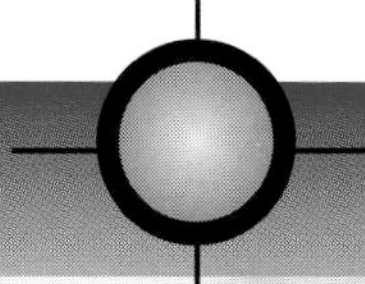

PROCEDURE

CELLOPHANE (CELLULOSE ACETATE) TAPE PREPARATION

PURPOSE:

To collect the eggs of pinworm, *Enterobius vermicularis,* as the female deposits the eggs at night on the perianal folds.

PRINCIPLE

Pinworm eggs will adhere to cellophane tape placed against the perianal folds. The tape is fixed to a microscope slide and examined microscopically.

MATERIALS

Cellophane tape
Microscope slides
Toluene or xylene

PROCEDURE

1. Place a strip of cellophane tape around the end of a tongue depressor so that the sticky side is out by looping the tape around the top edge of the depressor.
2. Spread the buttocks and apply the tape to the perianal folds. Press tape firmly against the left and right perianal folds and anal opening.
3. Remove the tape from the tongue depressor and place it sticky side down onto a microscope slide. Press firmly to remove all trapped air bubbles.
4. Lift one side of tape and apply 1 small drop of toluene or xylene to clear the tape. Press tape down onto slide.
5. Examine under low power (10×) with low light intensity. The entire area under the tape must be examined. Eggs are colorless and football shaped with one side flattened.
6. Generally, specimens should be collected on five consecutive mornings before a pinworm infection can be ruled out. The specimen is optimally collected before a bowel movement or bathing, since the eggs may otherwise not be detected.

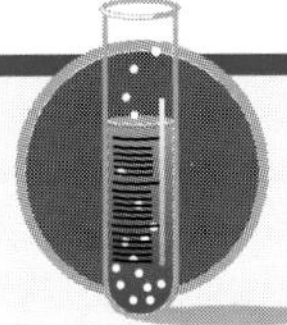

LABORATORY EXERCISES

1. Perform the modified zinc sulfate concentration procedure on the two stool specimens provided. Examine the slide and make a sketch of any significant findings, labeling it appropriately.

   Specimen # ______________________

   Observations:

   ____

   ____

   ____

   Specimen # ______________________

   Observations:

   ____

   ____

   ____

   ____

   State the principle of this procedure:

   ____

   ____

   ____

   Indicate which parasites this method is not suitable for:

   ____

   ____

2. Perform the formalin-ether concentration procedure on the two specimens provided. Examine your slides and make a sketch of any significant findings, labeling appropriately.

   Specimen # ______________________

   Observations:

   ____

   ____

   ____

   Specimen # ______________________

   Observations:

   ____

   ____

   ____

   State the principle of this procedure:

   ____

   ____

   Indicate what is present in the four layers that form after the addition of ethyl acetate:

   Top layer (first layer): ______________________________

   Second layer: ______________________________

   Third layer: ______________________________

   Bottom layer of sediment (fourth layer): ______________________________

LABORATORY EXERCISES

(Continued)

3. Examine the cellulose acetate preparation for the presence of pinworm eggs. Record your findings.

   Specimen # ______________________

   Observations:

   ____

   ____

   ____

4. Examine the prepared Giemsa- or Wright-stained smears for the presence of blood parasites. Make a sketch of each, labeling the significant findings.

   A. *Plasmodium falciparum*

   B. *Plasmodium ovale*

   C. *Trypanosoma* species:

LABORATORY EXERCISES
(Continued)

D. *Babesia* species:

4. Examine fixed, iodine-stained or trichrome-stained mounts of each of the following parasites. Sketch your findings. Alternatively, identify each from photographs or kodachromes.
   A. *Entamoeba histolytica*

   B. *Giardia lamblia*

   C. *Trichomonas* species

LABORATORY EXERCISES
(Continued)

D. Hookworm

E. *Ascaris lumbricoides*

F. *Trichuris trichiura*

G. *Taenia* species

LABORATORY EXERCISES
(Continued)

H. *Hymenolepsis nana*

I. *Schistosoma mansoni*

J. *Fasciolopsis* or *Fasciola*

K. *Paragonimus westermani*

REVIEW QUESTIONS

MATCHING

Match the parasite with its common name (responses may be used once or not at all):

1. ***Strongyloides stercoralis***
2. ***Necator americanus***
3. ***Enterobius vermicularis***
4. ***Ascaris lumbricoides***
5. ***Trichuris trichiura***
6. ***Taenia saginata***
7. ***Taenia solium***
8. ***Fasciolopsis buski***
9. ***Clonorchis sinensis***
10. ***Ancylostoma duodenale***

a. Large intestinal fluke
b. Old World hookworm
c. Pinworm
d. Whipworm
e. Broad or fish tapeworm
f. Threadworm
g. Chinese liver fluke
h. Lung fluke
i. Large roundworm
j. Dwarf tapeworm
k. New World hookworm
l. Pork tapeworm
m. Sheep liver fluke
n. Beef tapeworm

Correctly identify the parasitic eggs and proglottids shown. Use each response once. Choose from the following list.

11. **60 μm by 25 μm**

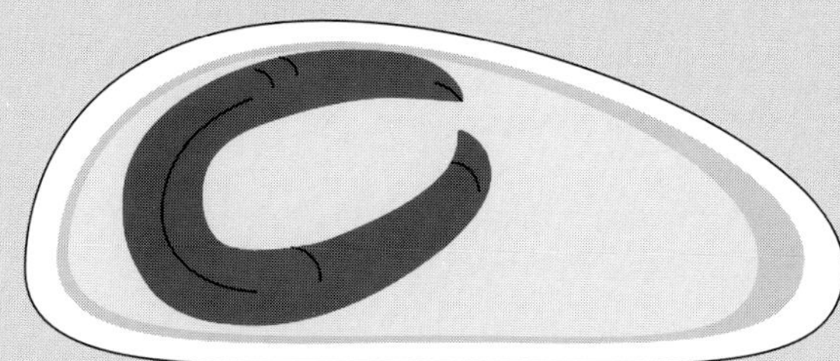

12. **60 μm by 40 μm**

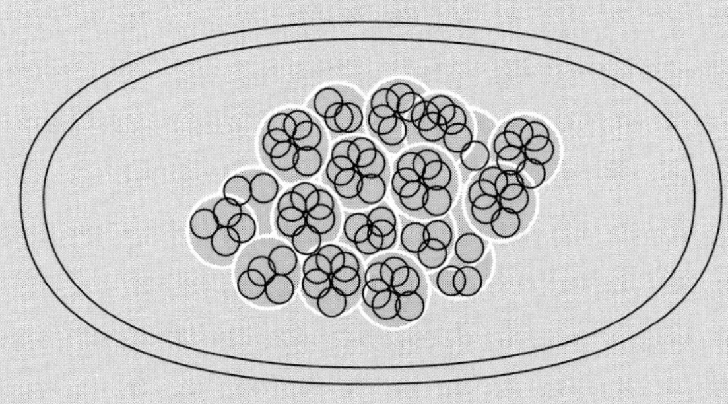

REVIEW QUESTIONS
(Continued)

13. 75 μm by 40 μm

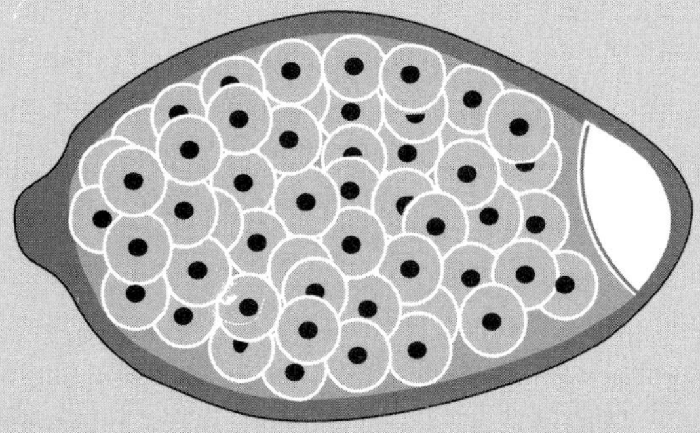

14. 50 μm by 40 μm

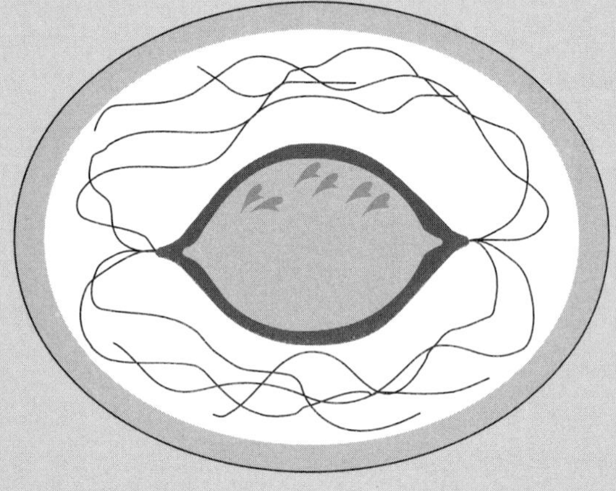

15. 100 μm by 50 μm

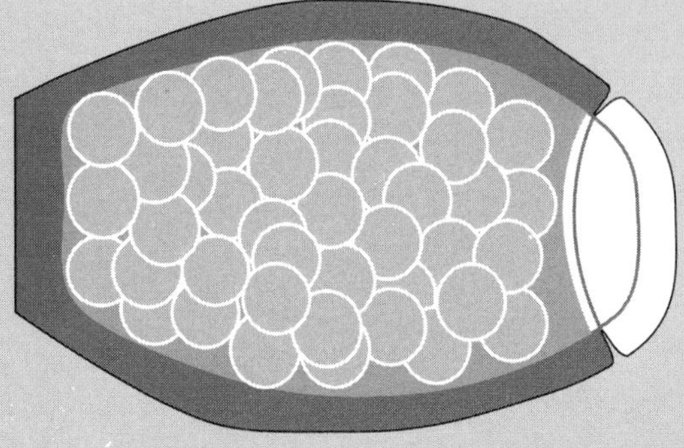

REVIEW QUESTIONS
(Continued)

16. **60 μm by 45 μm**

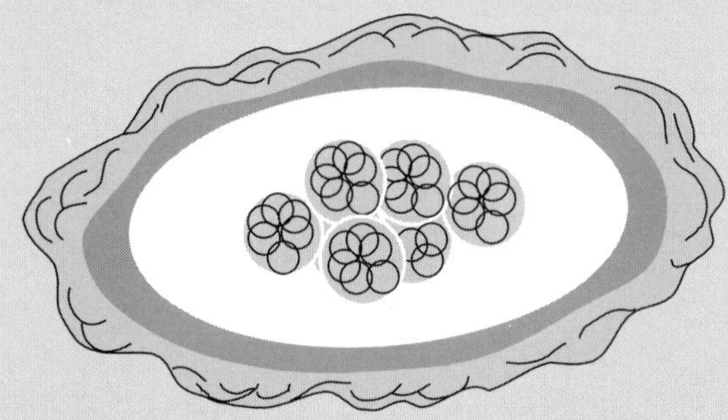

17. **55 μm by 20 μm**

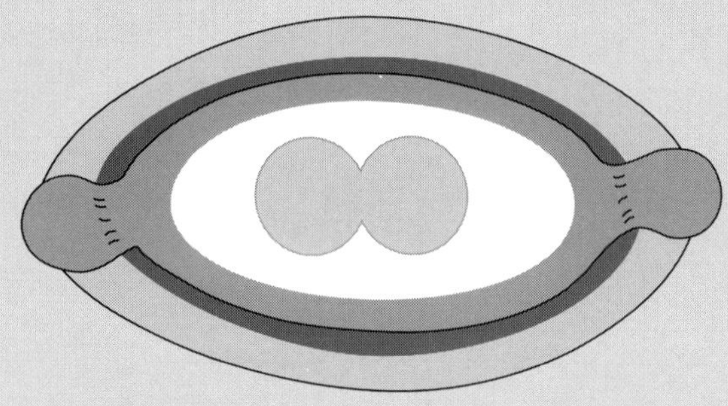

18. **35 μm diameter**

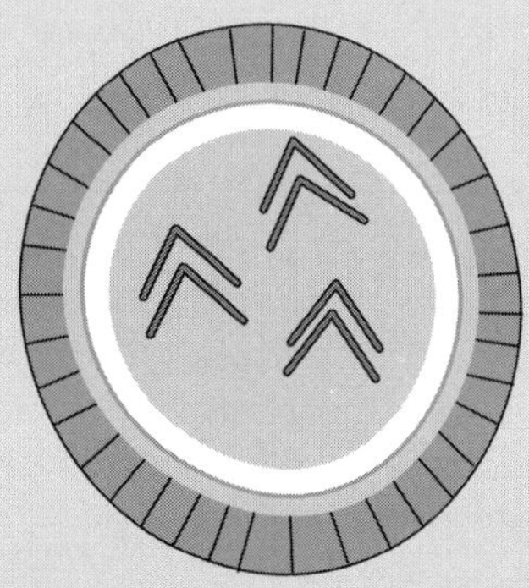

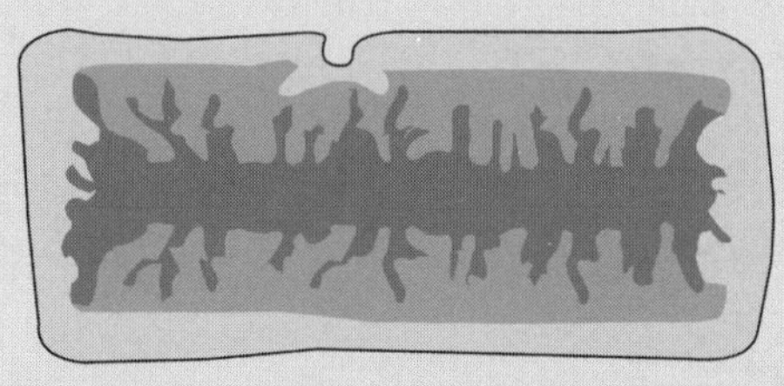

Lower Respiratory Tract Pathogens

Bacterial

Streptococcus pneumoniae: most comon cause in geriatric population; agent of community-acquired pneumonias; presence of capsule facilitates attachment and resistance to phagocytosis.

Klebsiella pneumoniae: agent is serious gram-negative pneumonia; produces "currant jelly" sputum; encapsulated; may be nosocomial. Other members of the Enterbacteriaceae associated with lower respiratory tract infections include *Serratia marcescens* and *Escherichia coli.*

Staphylococcus aureus: agent in community-acquired and nosocomial pneumonias; may be acquired through the aspiration route

Pseudomonas aeruginosa: agent in nosocomial pneumonias; acquired through aspiration and nonaspiration routes; mucoid strain associated with severe pneumonia in patients with cystic fibrosis

Haemophilus influenzae: agent of infections in nonimmunized infants and children and immunosuppressed adults; presence of capsule facilitates infection.

Mycobacterium tuberculosis: agent of chronic lung infections and tuberculosis

Legionella pneumophila: agent of Legionnaires' disease; acquired through inhalation of contaminated water aerosols; most often found in middle-aged males with an underlying medical problem

Mycoplasmal

Mycoplasma pneumoniae: agent of primary atypical pneumonia; most common cause of pneumonia in young adults

Viral

Myxoviruses (influenzae and parainfluenza viruses): agents of bronchitis and pneumonia; occur in endemics or epidemics

Respiratory syncytial virus: most often seen in children less than 5 years of age as cause of bronchitis and pneumonia

Fungal

Coccidioides immitis: agent of coccidioidomycosis

Histoplasma capsulatum: agent of histoplasmosis

Blastomyces dermatitidis: agent of blastomycosis

Cryptococcus neoformans: agent of cryptococcosis

The procedure for the sputum culture is described at the end of the chapter.

Other collection methods, which are more invasive but produce a less contaminated specimen, include bronchoalveolar lavage, in which saline is injected through a bronchoscope into the bronchi and then aspirated and cultured. Bronchial brushings use a catheter telescoped into the bronchi. The area is then "brushed" and the specimen collected. Invasive procedures include transtracheal aspiration, thin-needle aspiration, and open-lung biopsy. Transtracheal aspiration is a risky procedure that involves the insertion of a needle, connected to a catheter, into the trachea. Pleural fluid, collected through thoracentesis, is also suitable for the diagnosis of lower respiratory tract infection.

Figure 22-13 summarizes the identification of lower respiratory tract pathogens.

URINARY TRACT SPECIMENS

Urine from the ureters and bladder is sterile under normal conditions. When voided, urine passes over the superficial urogenital membranes and becomes contaminated by the normal flora of these areas. **Bacteriuria,** the presence of bacteria in the urine, is not necessarily indicative of a urinary tract infection (UTI) unless the number or colony count of the bacteria is significant. Types of UTIs include cystitis, urethritis, pyelonephritis, glomerulonephritis, and pyelitis.

UTIs may arise in three ways. The most common route is known as an ascending kidney infection, in which the bacteria reach the kidneys from the bladder through the ureters. A descending kidney infection results from hematogenous spread from the blood. The microorganisms are deposited by the blood in the kidneys, multiply there, and are shed in the urine. Finally, manipulation by devices, such as urinary catheters, that

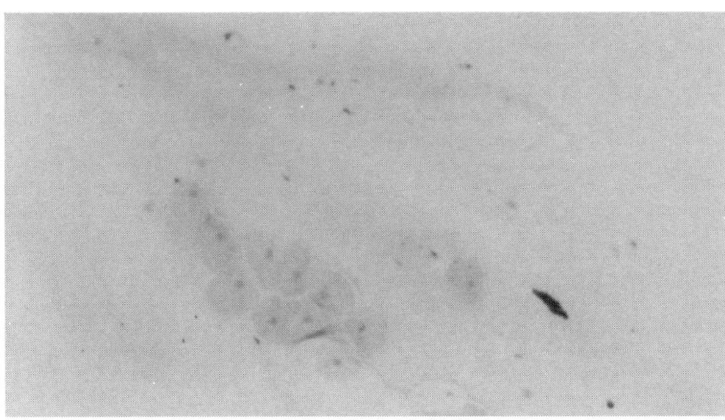

FIGURE 22–10
Gram stain of contaminated sputum showing squamous epithelial cells.

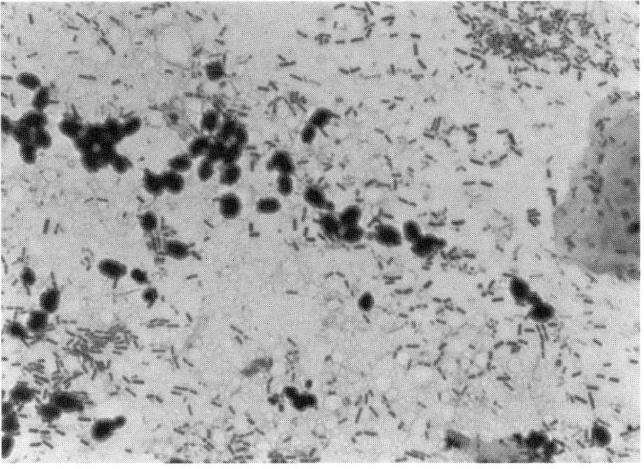

FIGURE 22–11
Gram stain of an acceptable sputum sample with gram-positive bacilli, gram-negative bacilli, and yeast. No WBCs are seen, which can be attributed to neutropenia or a diminished immune response.

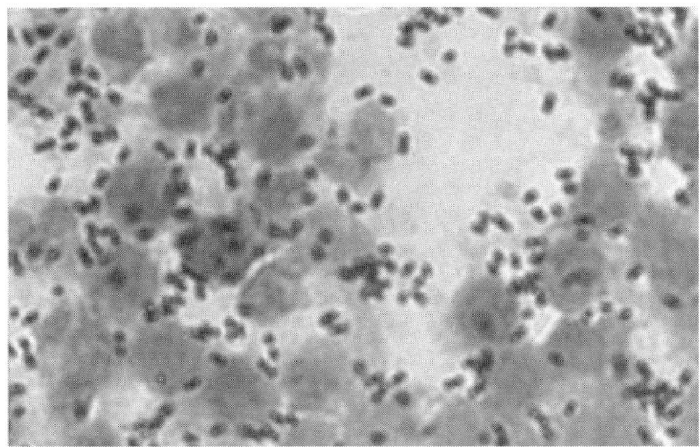

FIGURE 22–12
Gram stain of an acceptable sputum sample showing a moderate amount of gram-positive diplococci and segmented neutrophils.

become colonized with bacteria can initiate a bladder and kidney infection.

Predisposing factors associated with UTIs include urine retention or compromised urine flow caused by prostatic hypertrophy, tumors, kidney stones, or congenital defects; pregnancy because of hormonal and anatomical changes; and the use of urinary catheters. UTIs are frequent nosocomial infections.

The most common agent of UTIs in both ambulatory and hospitalized patients is the coliform *Escherichia coli,* which is found in the normal stool and thus is close to the external urethral surfaces. Other bacteria frequently associated with UTIs include *Klebsiella* species, *Enterobacter cloacae* and other species, *Proteus mirabilis* and other species, *Staphylococcus aureus* and *S. saprophyticus, Enterococcus faecalis, Pseudomonas aeruginosa,* and other members of the Enterobacteriaceae.

The specimen of choice for bacterial culture of urine is the clean-catch midstream sample. Specimens collected through a urinary catheter for urine culture should be requested only when the patient cannot produce a midstream specimen. Catheterized urine should be sterile.

Urine specimens should be preserved or refrigerated if not processed. Chemical preservatives include boric acid, glycerol, and formate. Urine samples can be screened using the Gram stain. One drop of the well-mixed sample is pipetted onto a microscope slide and allowed to air-dry. The smear is stained and examined for the presence of bacteria and WBCs At least 20 oil immersion fields should be examined, and the presence of at least one organism per field correlates with significant bacteriuria. Figure 22-14 (Color Plate 88) shows the Gram stain of an uncentrifuged urine specimen with moderate gram-negative bacilli. Figure 22-15 (Color Plate 89) shows a mixed infection of gram-negative bacilli and gram-positive cocci in a urine specimen.

Urine specimens with significant bacteriuria noted through the screening must be cultured. A colony count is performed on all samples to be cultured to determine the number of colony-forming units per milliliter (cfu/ml). The colony count is usually performed on sheep blood agar in the technique shown in Figure 22-16.

Most UTIs are caused by a single pathogen, but they may also be attributed to two different organisms. However, the isolation of three or more different species with a colony count in the range of 10^4 to 10^5 cfu/ml may indicate contamination. In such cases a repeat specimen should be requested. The isolation of a single species with a colony count of 10^4 cfu/ml may also be considered pathogenic. Explanations for this include a dilute urine sample, a partially treated UTI, dehydration, chronic pyelonephritis, or acute urethral syndrome.

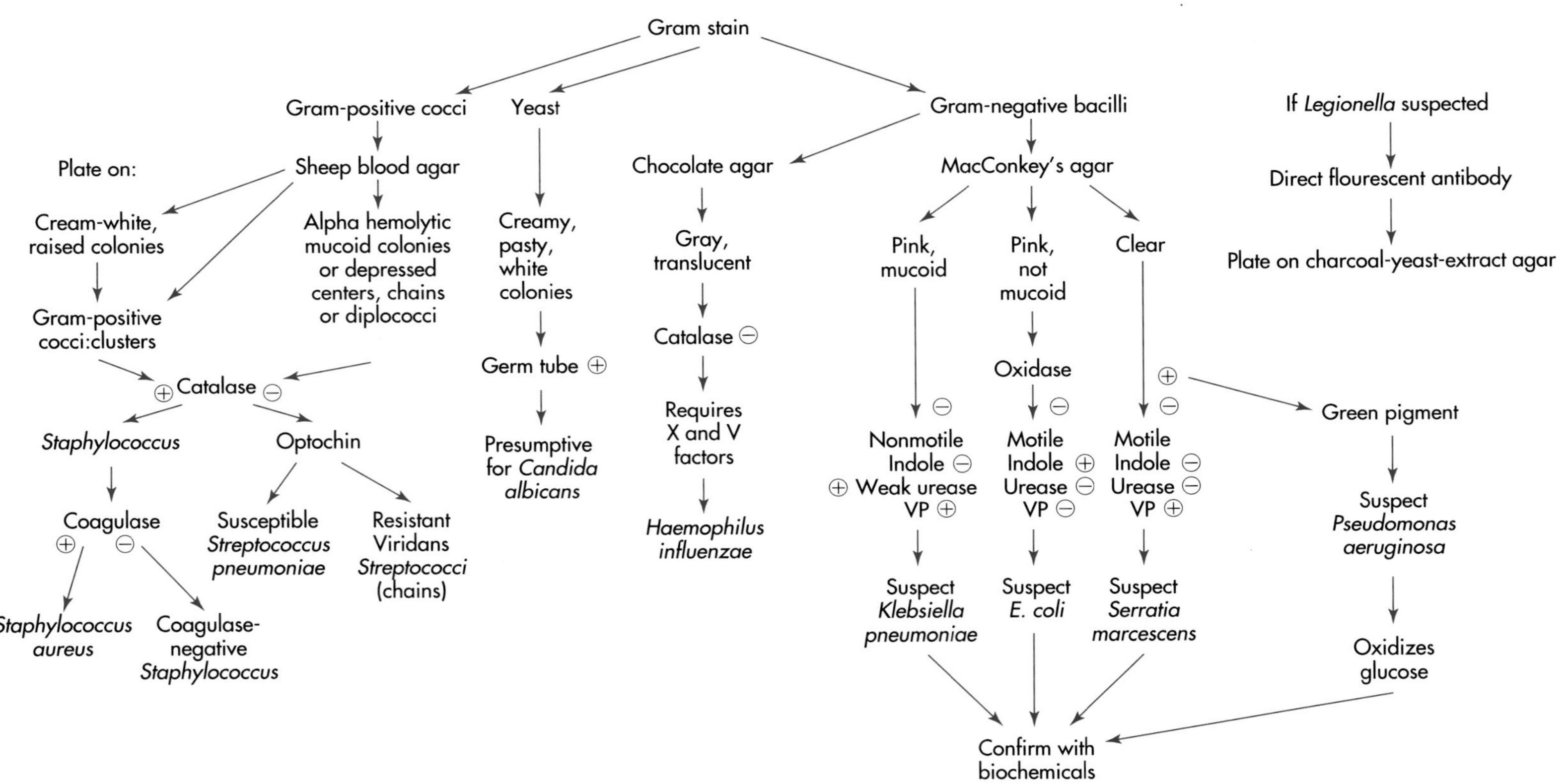

FIGURE 22–13
Identification scheme for common lower respiratory tract pathogens.

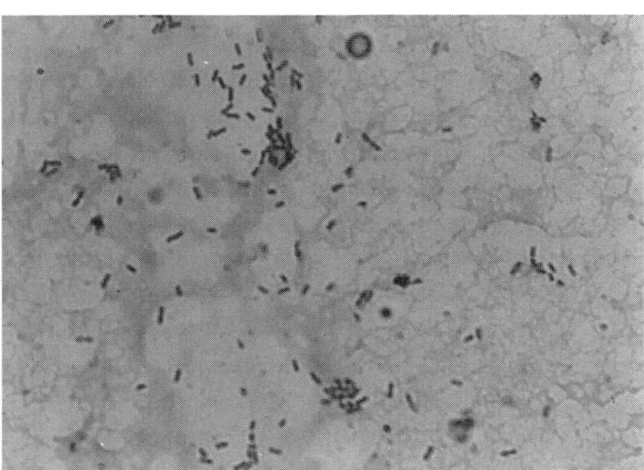

FIGURE 22–14
Gram stain of an uncentrifuged urine specimen showing gram-negative bacilli.

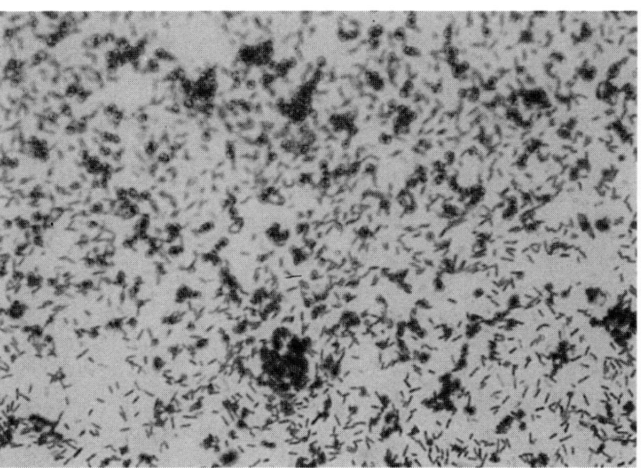

FIGURE 22–15
Gram stain of an uncentrifuged urine specimen showing mixed infection of gram-negative bacilli and gram-positive cocci.

After inserting calibrated loop vertically into the urine specimen, remove the loop vertically.

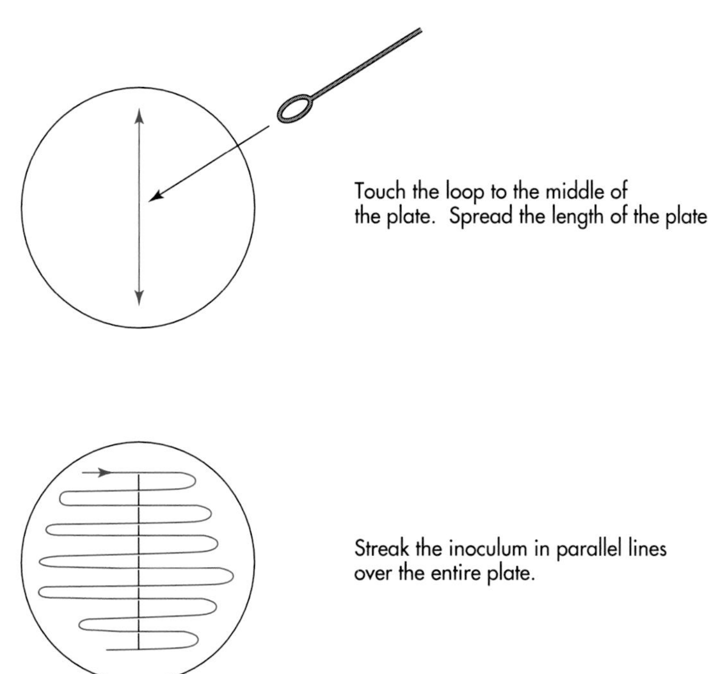

Incubate at 35°C for 18-24 hours. Count the isolated colonies. Multiply by 1000 if a 1 μl calibrated loop was used to determine CFU/ml of urine.

FIGURE 22–16
Colony count procedure and diagram.

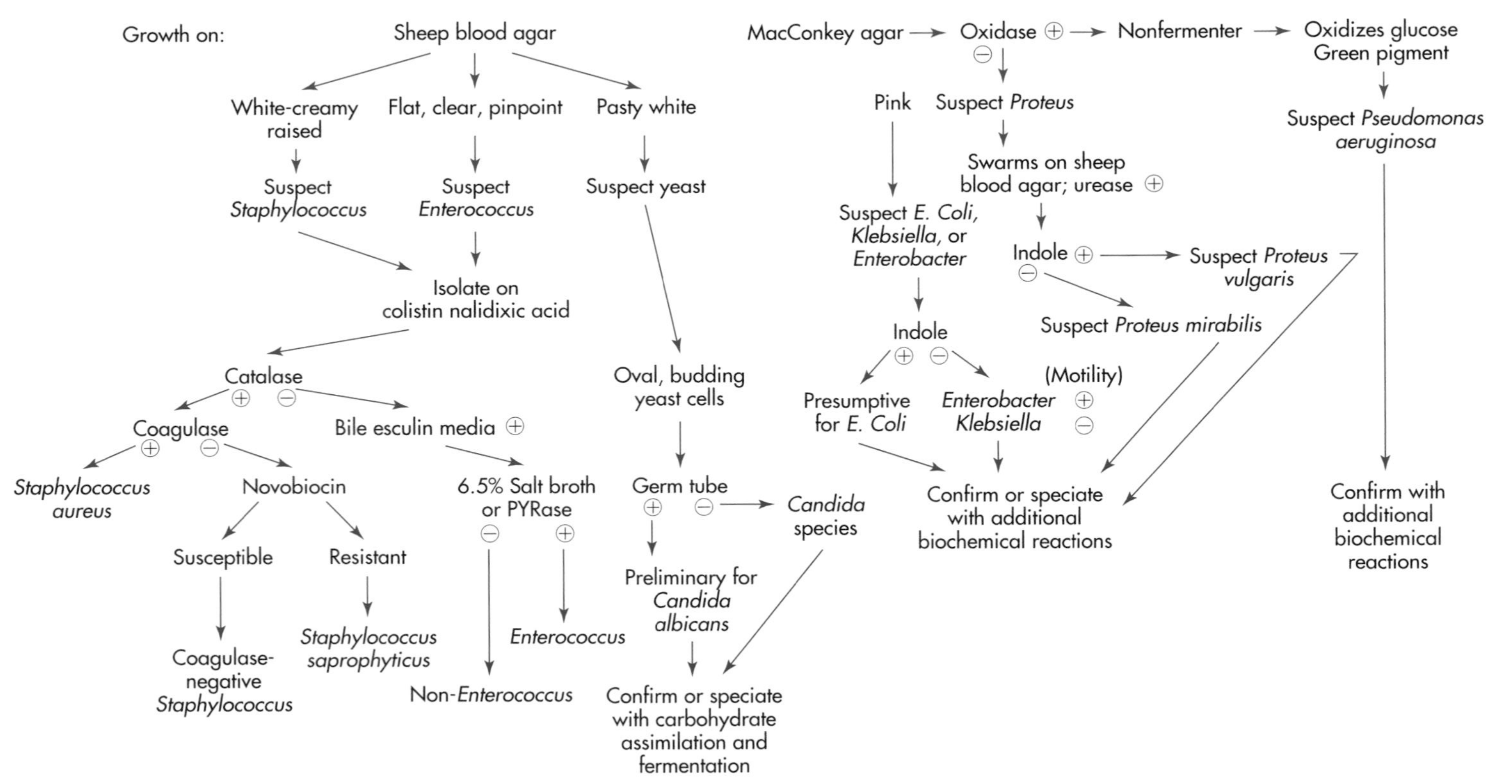

FIGURE 22–17

Identification scheme for common urinary tract pathogens.

Figure 22-17 depicts an identification scheme of common urinary tract pathogens. The procedure for urine culture is described at the end of the chapter.

GASTROINTESTINAL TRACT SPECIMENS

The gastrointestinal (GI) tract consists of the esophagus, stomach, small and large intestines, and anus.

Mechanisms that protect the GI tract from infection first include the acidic pH of the stomach. Normal flora in the small and large intestines also protects other bacteria from colonizing or establishing infection in the area. Although the upper small intestine harbors small numbers of normal flora, including *Streptococcus, Lactobacillus,* and yeast, the number of bacteria in the lower small intestine increases exponentially and includes members of the Enterobacteriaceae and *Bacteroides.* The large intestine contains immense numbers of normal flora bacteria, including the anaerobes *Bacteroides, Clostridium,* and *Peptostreptococcus; Escherichia coli* and other members of the Enterobacteriaceae, such as *Proteus, Klebsiella,* and *Enterobacter;* enterococci; and streptococci. Interestingly, anaerobes outnumber aerobes by a factor of 100 to 1000:1!

Microorganisms associated with **gastroenteritis** may establish infection in several ways, including production of toxins, such as the neurotoxin of *Clostridium botulinum,* the enterotoxins of *Staphylococcus aureus,* and the cytotoxin of *Clostridium difficile;* invasion of the mucosa by the enterotoxins of bacteria such as *Vibrio cholerae, Campylobacter,* and *Shigella;* and adherence to the mucosa. Routes of infection include ingestion of contaminated food or water, the fecal-oral route, person-to-person transmission, and animal-to-person transmission.

Stool specimens not processed within 2 hours of collection should be placed into transport media, such as Cary-Blair medium. When viruses are suspected, the specimen should be placed into a suitable viral transport medium. Rectal swabs are acceptable for culture when stools cannot be collected. Swabs should be plated immediately or placed into transport media to prevent drying of the specimen.

The method for the examination of stool cultures is described at the end of the chapter.

Stools can be examined directly by emulsifying in broth, saline, or water for the presence of *Campylobacter,* which exhibits a typical darting motility. A suspension is made on a microscope slide and a coverslip applied. Viral pathogens, such as *Rotavirus* and Norwalk agent, can be examined using electron microscopy. Since such methods are beyond the scope of many clinical microbiology laboratories, latex agglutination or ELISA for rotavirus can be performed directly on the specimen to detect the viral antigens.

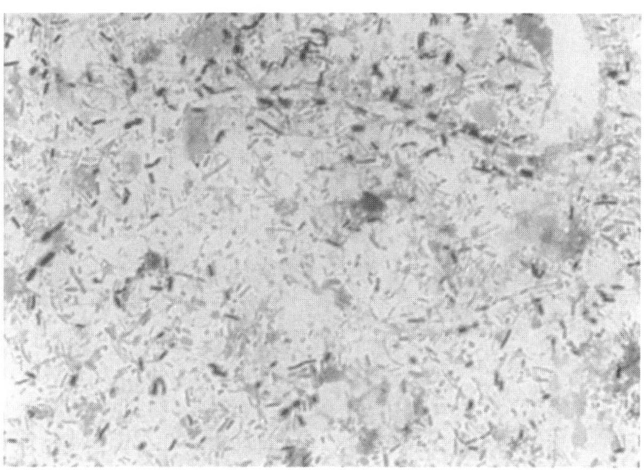

FIGURE 22–18

Gram stain of a normal stool specimen showing mixed flora of coliforms, gram-positive cocci, and anaerobic gram-negative bacilli.

Gram stains are prepared for the examination of fecal leukocytes, which may be indicators of infection and invasion of the intestinal mucosa. The smear can be examined for pathogens with unique morphologies, such as *Vibrio* and *Campylobacter,* which appear as curved gram-negative bacilli. The presence of neutrophils with aggregates of gram-positive cocci may suggest purulent enterocolitis. *C. difficile,* the agent of pseudomembranous colitis, can be observed in the Gram stain as a large, gram-positive bacilli. After prolonged antibiotic therapy, *C. difficile* appears in the stool, where the organism multiplies to large numbers. The organism produces a cytotoxin, which can also be detected in the stool. The predominance of yeast can also be detected through the Gram stain.

Figure 22-18 (Color Plate 90) shows the Gram stain of a normal stool.

Most laboratories routinely screen stool samples for *Salmonella, Shigella,* and *Campylobacter.* During epidemics, especially in infants, a procedure to detect rotavirus is also recommended. On request or when epidemiological information suggests, screening is also done for *Yersinia enterocolitica, Vibrio cholerae, Vibrio parahaemolyticus,* and verotoxic *E. coli.* For example, in eastern and southeastern U.S. coastal areas, agar for the detection of *Vibrio,* which is an occupational hazard for fishermen and a contaminant of shellfish, is suggested.

The diagnosis of lower intestinal tract infections is greatly facilitated by knowledge of the patient's medical history, of epidemiological considerations, and of any travel to foreign countries and if a similar infection occurred in family members or those who shared a meal.

Figure 22-19 presents an identification scheme for common lower intestinal tract pathogens.

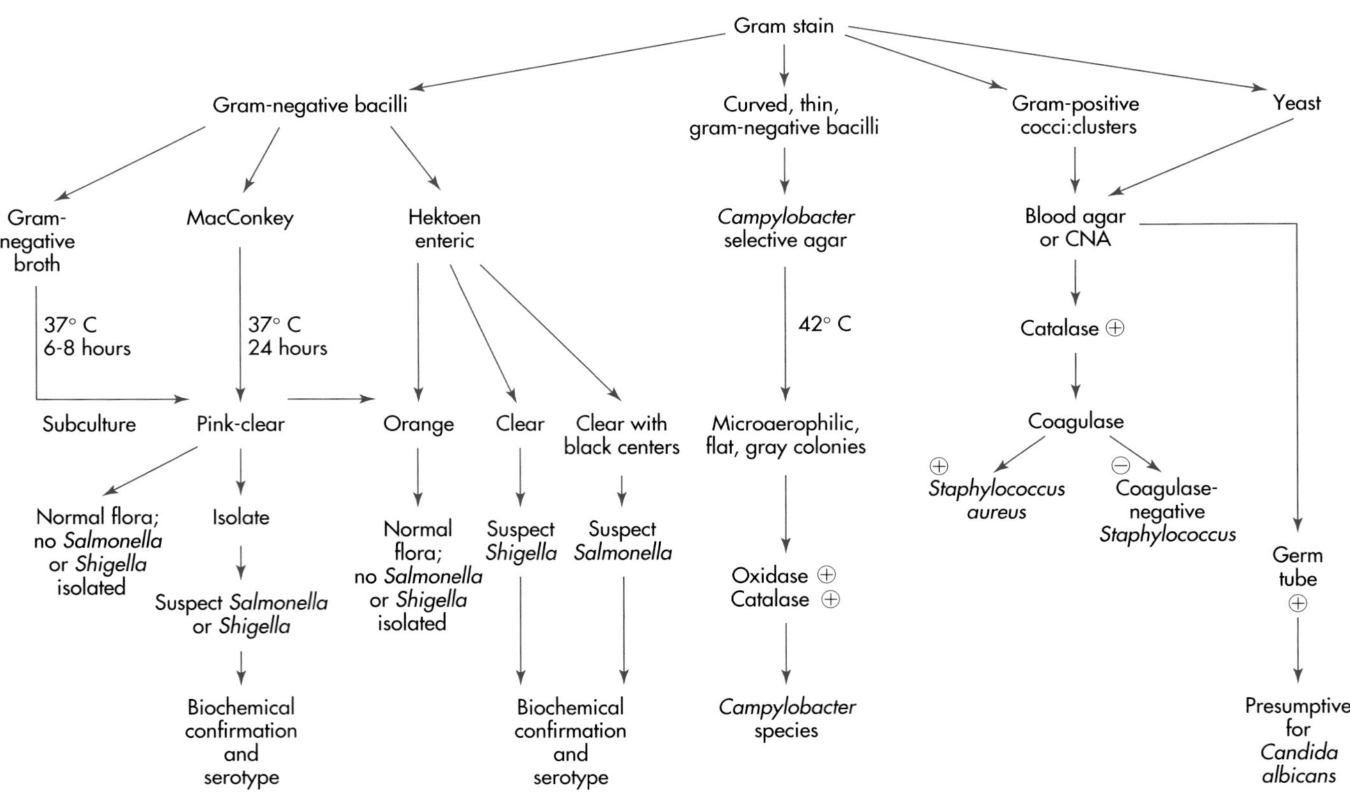

FIGURE 22–19
Identification scheme for common pathogens of the lower gastrointestinal tract.

GENITAL TRACT SPECIMENS

Genital tract specimens are cultured to determine the causative agents of urethritis, vaginitis, and cervicitis, as well as childbirth infections. Most often, genital tract specimens are collected to determine the presence of *Neisseria gonorrhoeae,* the agent of gonorrhea, and *Chlamydia trachomatis,* a common cause of cervicitis.

The mucosal surfaces of the female genital tract are normally colonized with several species of bacteria, which are usually considered to be normal flora and may even protect the host from the establishment of infection from pathogens. The normal flora of the female genital tract varies with age, hormonal levels, and pH. In adult females an acidic environment exists, and the normal flora includes Enterobacteriaceae, streptococci, staphylococci, *Peptococcus, Peptostreptococcus,* and anaerobic non-spore-forming bacilli, in addition to lactobacilli, which predominate. Yeasts, especially *Candida albicans,* are often isolated from the normal female genital tract. Approximately one fourth of all females carry group B streptococci as normal vaginal flora, which may cause pneumonia, meningitis, and septicemia in a neonate during delivery.

The normal flora in the penis includes small numbers of yeasts, corynebacteria, and coagulase-negative staphylococci. The normal flora of the urethra includes coagulase-negative staphylococci, corynebacteria, and some anaerobes.

Cervicitis, usually a sexually transmitted disease, may be caused by *C. trachomatis, N. gonorrhoeae,* herpes simplex virus (HSV), or the parasite *Trichomonas vaginalis.* **Urethritis** is most frequently caused by *N. gonorrhoeae* or *C. trachomatis,* with males having symptoms of urethral discharge and burning urination. Symptoms in females include a purulent vaginal discharge, burning urination, and lower abdominal pain, although some infections are asymptomatic.

The syndrome known as nonspecific vaginitis, which some now refer to as bacterial vaginosis, is frequently attributed to overgrowth by the organism *Gardnerella vaginalis,* a fixed flora of aerobes and anaerobes, and to a decrease in normal flora.

Pelvic inflammatory disease (PID) is a complication of infection caused by *N. gonorrhoeae* or *C. trachomatis* when the endometrium or fallopian tubes have been infected by vaginal or cervical pathogens.

Prostatitis may result from invasion of sexually transmitted pathogens or those transmitted through the urinary tract. These most often include members of the Enterobacteriaceae, *N. gonorrhoeae, C. trachomatis,* and *Pseudomonas aeruginosa.*

Infections of the external genitalia, characterized by the presence of lesions or chancres, include syphilis *(Treponema pallidum),* chancroid *(Haemophilus ducreyi),* and herpes genitalis (HSV type 2). Genital or venereal warts caused by papillomavirus are also an important sexually transmitted disease (STD) today.

Specimens collected from females with suspected genital infections most frequently are from the uterine cervix and urethra. To collect cervical specimens, the cervical mucus is first cleared with a swab, and then the sample is collected using a smaller swab with a Dacron or polyester tip and the aid of a speculum. The swab is rotated to collect cervical cells and exudate and is positioned to avoid touching the vaginal canal. Urethral specimens are obtained by either collecting the discharge or inserting a urogenital swab into the urethra and allowing it to remain for a few seconds to saturate the swab with exudate.

Endometrial specimens or aspirates from laparoscopy or culdoscopy are collected to diagnose PID.

For male patients the urethral exudate is usually collected. When there is insufficient material to collect, a narrow cotton, rayon, or Dacron swab on a plastic or aluminum shaft can be inserted into the urethra. The swab is left in place for a few seconds to saturate the fibers. For *Chlaymdia* the swab is rotated in a circular motion to collect some epithelial cells because *C. trachomatis* is an intracellular pathogen.

Because *N. gonorrhoeae* is very susceptible to temperature fluctuations, such as cooling, and does not sustain drying or low levels of CO_2 very well, it is imperative to smear, plate, and transport the specimen quickly. Direct smears for gonorrhea should be made immediately after collection. The specimen is then inoculated onto selective media, such as modified Thayer Martin or Martin-Lewis agar. Since some strains of *N. gonorrhoeae* are inhibited by these selective media, some laboratories prefer also to inoculate a chocolate agar plate. If immediate inoculation is not possible, the specimen should be placed into transport media and sent to the laboratory. The use of charcoal in transport systems neutralizes toxic materials in the specimen or on the swab. The use of agar plate transport systems, such as the Jem-Bec (Ames Co.) or Gono-Pak (Becton Dickinson Microbiology Systems), provides a medium selective for the *Gonococcus,* as well as a disposable, plastic zippered bag with a CO_2 activator. These plates are then incubated at 35° to 37°C in 5% CO_2 on receipt at the laboratory.

The Gram stain from male patients has a high degree of sensitivity for the diagnosis of gonorrhea. The presence and semiquantitation of the amount of gram-negative diplococci occurring intracellularly or extracellularly compared with the amount of segmented neutrophils are noted. However, because of normal flora of the female genital tract, including coccobacilli such as *Acinetobacter* and *Moraxella,* the Gram stain is less reliable. Figure 22-20 (Color Plate 91) illustrates a Gram stain showing the presence of many gram-negative diplococci occurring intracellularly and extracellularly

TABLE 22–2

Characteristics of Anaerobes Isolated from Wounds and Abscesses

ORGANISM	IMPORTANT CHARACTERISTICS
Bacteroides fragilis group	Gram-negative bacillus Grows on AB, PEA, and KV Enhanced growth in 20% bile Esculin hydrolysis positive No pigment produced
Prevotella melaninogenica	Gram-negative bacillus Grows on AB, PEA, and KV Inhibited by 20% bile Lactose fermented Esculin hydrolysis negative Brick-red fluorescence under ultraviolet light; older colonies brown to black
Fusobacterium nucleatum	Gram-negative bacillus with tapered ends Opalescent colonial morphology when viewed microscopically Grows on AB and PEA; may or may not grow on KV Indole positive, but basically biochemically inactive Lipase Glucose not fermented
Fusobacterium necrophorum	Gram-negative bacillus with tapered ends Grows on AB and PEA; may or may not grow on KV Indole positive Lipase positive Glucose fermented
Clostridium tetani	Gram-positive bacillus with round, terminal spores Rarely cultured from living wounds Diagnosis usually through clinical signs Unable to ferment most carbohydrates
Clostridium perfringens	Gram-positive bacillus; spores usually not observed Grows on AB and PEA Double-zone hemolysis on AB Lecithinase positive Ferments glucose, lactose, maltose, and fructose Reverse CAMP reaction positive
Clostridium ramosum	Gram-positive bacillus, but usually stains gram negative Grows on AB and PEA Grows well on 20% bile Esculin hydrolysis positive Lecithinase negative Lipase negative Very fermentative

AB, Anaerobic blood agar; PEA, phenylethyl alcohol agar; KV, kanamycin-vancomycin agar.

The Gram stain is very important in the initial identification of wound pathogens. For example, if a superficial wound reveals possible anaerobes, an anaerobic blood plate can be added to the initial isolation media. Table 22-2 summarizes the identification of common anaerobic pathogens found in wounds and abscesses.

Figure 22-22 (Color Plate 93) is a Gram stain of a wound showing gram-positive cocci that were identified as *S. aureus.* Figure 22-23 (Color Plate 94) is a Gram stain of an anaerobic gram-negative bacillus that was isolated from a peritoneal abscess and identified as *B. fragilis.*

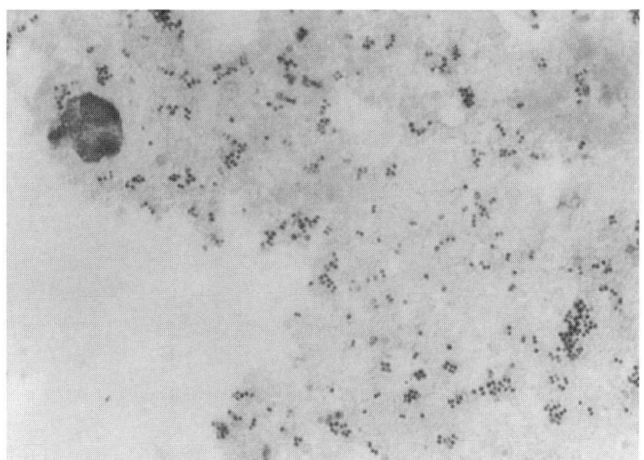

FIGURE 22–22
Gram stain of a wound aspirate showing gram-positive cocci in clusters, identified as *Staphylococcus aureus.*

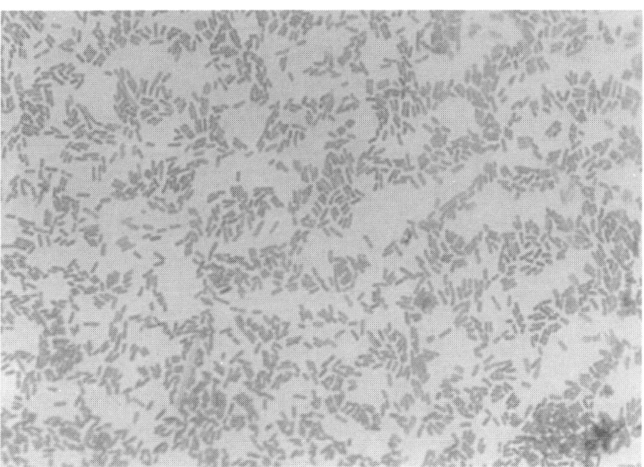

FIGURE 22–23
Gram stain of a pure isolate from a peritoneal abscess showing gram-negative bacilli that were subsequently identified as *Bacteroides fragilis.*

MISCELLANEOUS BODY FLUIDS: PLEURAL, PERITONEAL, PERICARDIAL, AND SYNOVIAL

Body fluids that are normally sterile are blood and cerebrospinal fluid, as discussed earlier, and pleural, peritoneal, pericardial, and synovial fluids. The accumulation of fluid in a cavity is known as an **effusion.** Effusions that have a low specific gravity and low levels of protein and cells are termed **transudates.** Effusions that have a high specific gravity, have higher levels of protein, and contain many cells are known as **exudates.** Transudates usually occur as a result of hepatic or renal disease and hemodynamic changes that lead to the accumulation of fluid in the cavity. Exudates may result from infection by bacteria and other microorganisms, as well as from malignancy, trauma, toxic compounds, and other sources of inflammation in the cavity itself.

These fluids are collected through percutaneous needle aspiration after a thorough disinfection of the skin. In some cases, multiple tubes are filled for analysis. Normal body fluids are clear and slightly yellow in color. A turbid or cloudy fluid often indicates inflammation. On receipt of the fluid in the laboratory, the color, transparency, and volume are recorded. Because the yield of microorganisms from body fluids may be low, a large volume of specimen is often needed to isolate the pathogen. For fluids that are visually purulent, a Gram stain is performed directly from the specimen. When the fluid is clear or if the volume is greater than 1 ml, the fluid should be centrifuged at 2500 rpm for 15 minutes. The sediment is resuspended in approximately 0.5 ml of supernatant, which is used to prepare the smear for the Gram stain and for culture.

Sterile fluids are routinely tested for protein and glucose values. In inflammatory states the protein is increased to more than 50% of the serum level, and the glucose level is decreased. Cell counts and differential WBC counts are also helpful in the diagnosis. Effusions with a predominance of segmented neutrophils often reflect a bacterial infection, whereas those with a predominance of lymphocytes often indicate a viral infection.

Pleural fluid lines the pleural space, which is between the lungs and chest cavity; normally, few cells are present. **Thoracentesis** is the collection of pleural fluid. Infections usually create an exudate. Pleural effusions may occur secondarily as a result of pneumonia; bacteria typically isolated as the pathogen include *Streptococcus pneumoniae, Staphylococcus aureus, Haemophilus influenzae, Pseudomonas aeruginosa,* various members of the Enterobacteriaceae, and several anaerobes. When associated with aspiration pneumonia, there is frequently a polymicrobic infection of aerobes and anaerobes.

Specimens are routinely plated on 5% sheep blood agar (SB), MacConkey agar (MC), anaerobic blood agar (AB), kanamycin-vancomycin blood agar (KV), and phenylethyl alcohol agar (PEA), as well as thioglycollate broth. If yeast or a dimorphic fungus such as *Coccidioides immitis* is suspected, a KOH preparation and inoculation onto brain-heart infusion agar (BHI) should also be done. In cases of suspected tuberculosis, an acid-fast smear is performed, and Löwenstein-Jensen and Middlebrook media are inoculated.

Peritoneal fluid surrounds the organs of the abdominal cavity, including the liver, kidneys, spleen, stomach, bladder, intestinal tract, pancreas, and ovaries. The accumulation of fluid secondary to systemic disease, such as hepatic disease, results in the formation of a transudate, known as ascitic fluid. Exudates are generally formed as a result of infectious disease, which may develop from surgery or trauma to the bowel or abdominal cavity, liver abscess, ruptured appendix, malignancy, obstruction, ulcerative colitis, or peritoneal or bowel abscess. The agents of **peritonitis** generally include *Escherichia coli, Bacteroides fragilis, S. aureus, Streptococcus, Enterococcus,* and other members of the Enterobacteriaceae. Since the normal bowel flora includes a high number of anaerobes, it is essential to collect and maintain the specimen free of oxygen. The collection of peritoneal fluid is known as a **paracentesis.** Peritoneal fluids are routinely plated on 5% SB, chocolate agar, MC, AB, KV, and PEA, as well as into thioglycollate broth.

Pericardial fluid fills the pericardial space, which is contained in the pericardium, the protective sac of the heart. The fluid is normally clear with a volume of 10 to 20 ml. The volume of fluid may accumulate because of hemodynamic changes, such as those caused by congestive heart failure or by systemic edema from hepatic or renal failure. Inflammation resulting from infection also leads to a pericardial effusion. Viruses are the most common infecting organisms of the pericardium, including coxsackieviruses A and B, echovirus, and influenza viruses. Bacteria are less frequently associated with pericarditis and include *S. aureus, S. pneumoniae,* members of the Enterobacteriaceae, *Mycobacterium tuberculosis,* various anaerobes, and *Nocardia* species.

Pericardial fluid is plated on the primary media SB, MC, AB, KV, and PEA, as well as into thioglycollate.

Synovial fluid, or joint fluid, is secreted by the synovial cells, which line the joints, and functions to lubricate the joint space. Infections typically involve one of the large joints, such as the knee, hip, elbow, wrist, ankle, or shoulder. Infections usually reach the joints from the blood. However, secondary infections from noninfectious arthritis may also occur. Rapid diagnosis of septic arthritis is essential, since destruction of the joint may occur quite rapidly.

Arthrocentesis, the collection of synovial fluid, is performed when an inflammatory response is present in the joint. Signs of inflammation include swelling, pain, redness, heat, and decreased mobility.

The Gram stain of the specimen is examined for bacteria and WBCs. Also, the cell count and a Wright-stained differential WBC smear provide information for the diagnosis. A WBC count of fewer than 200 cells/μl is considered normal, and counts less than 2000/μl are considered noninflammatory. WBC counts greater than 2000/μl are categorized as inflammatory and are generally associated with the infection septic arthritis. A predominance of segmented neutrophils suggests a bacterial infection.

The most common cause of septic arthritis is *S. aureus,* which accounts for more than half of all cases. Other gram-positive cocci, including *S. pneumoniae* and beta-hemolytic streptococcus, as well as Enterobacteriaceae, *Neisseria gonorrhoeae,* and the anaerobes *Fusobacterium* and *Bacteroides,* are also associated with septic arthritis.

Infections of prosthetic joints occur rarely, but the agents vary from those associated with other joint infections. The most common pathogens are coagulase-negative *Staphylococcus* and anaerobic bacilli, such as *Propionibacterium.* As normal skin flora, these organisms may be introduced during surgery.

Synovial fluid is routinely inoculated onto chocolate agar, AB, KV, and PEA and into thioglycollate broth. SB may also be added.

EYE AND EAR SPECIMENS

Eye infections may be caused by aerobic and anaerobic bacteria, fungi, viruses, and amebae. Eye infections may be characterized by conjunctival discharge, redness, ocular pain, or the presence of "pink eye." Examination of a swab or corneal scrapings may reveal the agent of the infection. If chlamydial infection is suspected, a direct antigen detection procedure is performed.

Bacterial agents of eye infection include *Haemophilus influenzae, Haemophilus aegyptius* (pink eye), *Moraxella, Neisseria gonorrhoeae,* and *Pseudomonas aeruginosa.* The free-living ameba of the genus *Acanthamoeba* is a cause of **keratitis** in soft contact lens wearers. It can be observed in a direct mount of the specimen.

Tympanocentesis, the puncture of the tympanic membrane with a needle to aspirate middle ear fluid, is reserved for complicated cases of ear infection. Because the infecting organisms are predictable in childhood ear infections and because the procedure for collection is complicated, most ear infections are treated by the physician without culture. *Streptococcus pneumoniae, H. influenzae,* and *Moraxella catarrhalis* account for most cases of acute otitis media in infants and children. Other bacteria less frequently associated with these infections include *Streptococcus pyogenes, Staphylococcus aureus, P. aeruginosa, Klebsiella pneumoniae,* and *Escherichia coli.* In complicated cases it may be necessary to identify the agent of recurrent, or chronic, otitis media through tympanocentesis. Nasopharyngeal and throat specimens are not suitable to isolate the invading pathogens for middle ear infections.

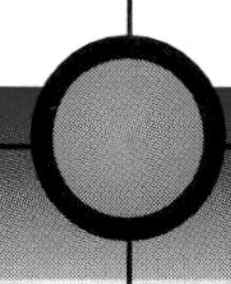

PROCEDURE
BLOOD CULTURES

COLLECTION OF BLOOD SPECIMEN

MATERIALS

70% alcohol swab
Povidone-iodine or 2% tincture of iodine
Gloves
Vacuum tube containing SPS or blood culture bottles (one aerobic and one anaerobic bottle)
Appropriate needle, syringe, or vacuum tube holder to perform phlebotomy; tourniquet

PROCEDURE

1. Observe universal precautions at all times during the procedure. Do not change needles at any time during the procedure.
2. Inspect both arms of the patient to select an appropriate vein.
3. Cleanse the patient's skin over the venipuncture site by wiping with 70% alcohol in a circular motion from the site outward. Allow the alcohol to air dry.
4. Using 2% tincture of iodine or povidone-iodine, vigorously wipe the site in a circular motion from the site outward. Allow the iodine to air-dry on the skin for at least 1 minute.
5. Optional: Cleanse the area again, this time with 70% alcohol in the method described. Alternatively, this can be done after the needle has been removed on completion of the phlebotomy.
6. Disinfect the stopper of the collection bottle(s) or tube(s) using povidone-iodine or tincture of iodine.
7. Apply the tourniquet, and have the patient make a fist. If the site must be probed again, disinfect the tips of the glove's fingers using the procedure described to prepare the site.
8. Insert the needle and collect the blood. Depending on the system being used, collect one SPS vacuum tube or an aerobic and anaerobic culture bottle.
9. Release the tourniquet, remove the needle, and apply pressure to the site.
10. Gently invert the tube(s) or bottle(s) to ensure anticoagulation. Label completely with patient's name, date and time of collection, and specific site of collection (such as right forearm). Apply a bandage to the site.
11. Immediately transport blood culture(s) to microbiology laboratory.

SPECIMEN ANALYSIS

MEDIA AND MATERIALS

Gram stain reagents
Clean microscope slides

Continued.

PROCEDURE
BLOOD CULTURES
(Continued)

List any tests used to identify the anaerobe. Describe your observations and interpret your results.

____

____

____

____

____

Identification: ________________________________

Rationale: ___________________________________

____

____

ANTIBIOTIC SUSCEPTIBILITY TESTING

ORGANISM	ANTIBIOTIC/CONCENTRATION/ZONE DIAMETER	INTERPRETATION

QUESTIONS

1. Explain why the skin preparations for blood cultures differs from those for routine phlebotomy. ____________________________

   ____

   ____

2. Compare the results obtained on the Gram stain with those obtained on the plated media. What conclusions can be made? __________________

   ____

   ____

3. Are the organisms isolated considered to be contaminants or pathogens? Justify your response. ____________________________

   ____

   ____

4. Why is it necessary to "vent" one bottle of the culture set when separate aerobic and anaerobic bottles are not used? __________________

   ____

   ____

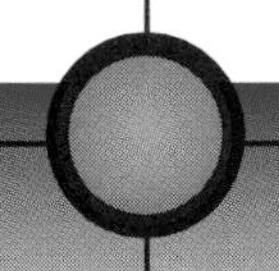

PROCEDURE
CEREBROSPINAL FLUID CULTURE

MEDIA AND MATERIALS

5% sheep blood agar
Chocolate agar
Thioglycollate broth
MacConkey agar
Gram stain reagents
Centrifuge
Autoclaved slides or slides dipped in alcohol and then flamed
Sterile Pasteur pipette or vortex

PROCEDURE

1. On receipt of the CSF, examine the specimen for volume, color, and transparency.
2. Centrifuge CSF tube no. 3 (if multiple tubes are collected). The specimen should be spun for 15 minutes at 1500 to 2000 g to concentrate the specimen if the volume is greater than 0.5 ml.
3. Decant the supernatant, leaving approximately 0.5 ml over the precipitate. The supernatant can be reserved for further testing.
4. Thoroughly mix the sediment either using a vortex or aspirating with a sterile Pasteur pipette.
5. Aspirate a large drop of the well-mixed CSF onto a sterile microscope slide. The slides are cleaned either by dipping into alcohol and flaming or by autoclaving. Do not flatten the drop or apply a coverslip. Allow the drop to air dry. Then heat-fix or fix with methanol.
6. Perform the Gram stain on the smear.
7. Examine the smear for the presence of bacteria, fungi, WBCs (neutrophils, lymphocytes), and RBCs. Record your observations.
8. Label all plates to be inoculated accurately and completely. Using the well-mixed or vortexed sediment, inoculate a sheep blood agar plate and a chocolate agar plate by pipetting several drops of the specimen onto the agar surfaces. Streak each plate for isolation. Incubate at 35° to 37°C under increased CO_2 for 72 hours. Examine plates daily for growth.
   a. Inoculate the thioglycollate broth with several drops of the sediment, and incubate with a loosened cap for 5 days at 35° to 37°C.
   b. If gram-negative bacilli are seen in the Gram stain, also inoculate a MacConkey agar plate and incubate in atmospheric oxygen at 35° to 37°C.
   c. If the Gram stain suggest anaerobes, inoculate an anaerobic blood agar plate and incubate in either an anaerobic jar or bag.
9. Examine all plates and broth daily for growth. Perform a Gram stain on any growth.
10. Perform appropriate identification procedures on each colony type.

Continued.

PROCEDURE

CEREBROSPINAL FLUID CULTURE

(Continued)

11. Perform the appropriate antibiotic susceptibility panel using the Kirby-Bauer method on all pathogens.
12. **Report any positive findings immediately to the physician.**

CSF CULTURE RESULTS

Specimen identification: ______

Number of tubes submitted: ______

Total volume of CSF: ______

Appearance (color/transparency): ______

______

Note any differences in appearance in tubes nos. 1, 2, and 3: ______

______

Gram stain results: ______

______

______

______

GROWTH CHARACTERISTICS

MEDIA	COLONY TYPE DESCRIPTION/NUMBER	GRAM STAIN	POSSIBLE ORGANISMS	ADDITIONAL TESTING
Blood				
Chocolate				
Thioglycollate				
Other:				

Perform and interpret all necessary tests to identify any pathogens present.

TESTS	OBSERVATIONS/INTERPRETATION	POSSIBLE ORGANISMS

PROCEDURE
CEREBROSPINAL FLUID CULTURE
(Continued)

Identify any pathogens present in the specimen: ______________________

____

Rationale: ______________________________________

____

ANTIBIOTIC SUSCEPTIBILITY TESTING

ISOLATE	ANTIBIOTIC/ CONCENTRATION	ZONE DIAMETER	INTERPRETATION

QUESTIONS

1. Compare the results of the Gram stain with those obtained in culture.

   ____

   ____

2. What would you expect to see in a Wright-stained smear of CSF in which gram-positive cocci were observed in the Gram stain? ______________

   ____

   ____

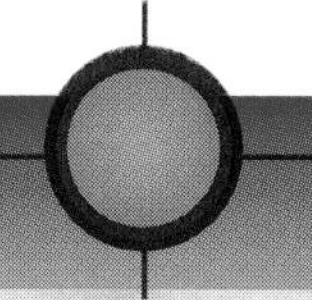

PROCEDURE
THROAT CULTURE

MEDIA AND MATERIALS

5% sheep blood agar
Chocolate agar (if patient is less than 5 years old or if request for *Haemophilus*)
Loeffler agar slant and cystine-tellurite agar (if request for *Corynebacterium diphtheriae*)
Modified Thayer-Martin agar (if request for *Neisseria gonorrhoeae*)
Sterile tongue depressors
Sterile Dacron swabs
Sterile latex gloves

PROCEDURE

1. Identify patient correctly.
2. Wearing sterile latex gloves, press patient's tongue with a sterile tongue depressor and have patient say, "Ah." This will expose the posterior pharynx.
3. Swab areas of inflammation or irritation over the posterior pharynx. Swab any red or swollen sites, as well as any exudate. Avoid touching the tongue, lips, and sides and roof of mouth. Collect two swabs in this manner if direct antigen testing is to be performed.
4. Label swab(s) and transport to laboratory in a Culturette or in transport media if plates are not to be inoculated at this time.
5. For routine throat cultures, streak one sheep blood agar plate for isolation. Make three to five stabs into the growth so that subsurface hemolysis can be noted.
6. Streak any additional media for special requests for isolation.
7. Incubate blood agar at 35°C for 24 hours. Incubate all chocolate agar plates in increased CO_2. Some laboratories prefer to incubate the blood agar in increased CO_2 as well.
8. Examine plates for growth and hemolysis at 24 hours' incubation. Note the presence of any beta-hemolytic streptococci. Also, determine if normal flora is present. Describe each type of colony (size, color, hemolysis) present on the blood agar plate, and estimate the number of each. Perform a Gram stain on each colony type.
9. Perform the bacitracin (and sulfamethoxazole-trimethoprim [SXT] if desired) susceptibility test on any colonies suggestive of group A streptococci.
10. Determine a possible genus and species for the other organisms present.
11. If the direct antigen test was performed, correlate these results with those observed on the culture plate.

THROAT CULTURE RESULTS

Specimen identification: ______________________________
Date and time of collection: ______________ Collected by: ______________
____

PROCEDURE
THROAT CULTURE
(Continued)

	PATIENT	POSITIVE CONTROL
Direct antigen testing		

CHARACTERISTICS ON SHEEP BLOOD AGAR

	PRESENT/ABSENT	DESCRIPTION	POSSIBLE ORGANISMS
Beta-hemolytic streptococci			
Normal flora			

COLONY TYPES ON SHEEP BLOOD AGAR

CHARACTERISTICS OF COLONY	GRAM STAIN	NORMAL FLORA OR PATHOGENS	POSSIBLE ORGANISMS

BACITRACIN AND SXT SUSCEPTIBILITY TESTS

COLONY TYPE	ZONE DIAMETERS AND INTERPRETATIONS			
	BACITRACIN		SXT	
	DIAMETER (mm)	SUSCEPTIBLE/RESISTANT	DIAMETER (mm)	SUSCEPTIBLE/ RESISTANT

QUESTIONS

1. Identify any pathogens present in the throat culture. __________
2. Is this a "normal throat?" Explain. __________

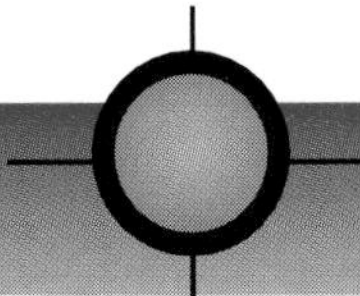

PROCEDURE
SPUTUM CULTURE

MEDIA AND MATERIALS

5% sheep blood agar
Chocolate agar
MacConkey agar
Gram stain reagents

PROCEDURE

1. Working in a biological safety cabinet, prepare a Gram stain smear from the specimen.
2. Examine the slide under the low-power (10×) objective for the presence of SECs and WBCs. Specimens containing less than 10 SECs/LPF or more than 25 WBCs/LPF are considered to be acceptable.
3. Switch to the oil immersion objective, and examine the smear to determine the morphology and Gram stain reaction of any bacteria present. Describe your observations.
4. Correctly and completely label all plates to be inoculated. Dip a swab in the sputum sample, and roll over the surface of the blood, chocolate, and MacConkey agar plates. Streak each plate for isolation; stab the blood agar.
5. Incubate the blood and chocolate agar plates at 35°C under increased CO_2. Incubate the MacConkey agar plate in atmospheric oxygen at 35°C.
6. Examine the plates after 24 hours' incubation. Determine if normal flora is present, absent, or decreased. Describe the various colony types, noting the color, size, and type of hemolysis.
   a. Perform a Gram stain on each colony type. Record your results.
   b. Note any mucoid colonies or those with depressed centers, which are alpha hemolytic and may indicate *Streptococcus pneumoniae.*
7. Prepare a flow chart to identify all pathogenic isolates. Perform the required tests to identify any pathogen. The optochin susceptibility test should be performed on any colony suspected to be *S. pneumoniae.*
8. Perform the appropriate antibiotic panel on all pathogens using the Kirby-Bauer method.
9. Record all results.

SPUTUM CULTURE RESULTS

Specimen identification: ______________________________

Date and time of collection: __________ Collected by: ____________________

Gram Stain Screening

SECs/LPF: ______________________________

WBCs/LPF: ______________________________

Interpretation: ______________________________

____

PROCEDURE
SPUTUM CULTURE
(Continued)

Gram Stain Observations (Oil Immersion Objective)

DESCRIPTION OF ORGANISM (GRAM STAIN REACTION, MORPHOLOGY)	POSSIBLE IDENTIFICATION

Colonial Morphology

MEDIA	COLONIAL MORPHOLOGY	GRAM STAIN	POSSIBLE ORGANISMS	TESTS TO IDENTIFY

Perform the optochin susceptibility test on any organism suspected to be *S. pneumoniae.* Record your results.

COLONY TYPE	OPTOCHIN SUSCEPTIBILITY	ZONE DIAMETER (mm)	INTERPRETATION

Perform the germ tube test on any yeast if it is the predominant organism or present in large numbers. Record your results. Any yeast that is germ tube positive can be presumptively identified as *Candida albicans.*

COLONY TYPE	GERM TUBE RESULT	INTERPRETATION

Continued.

PROCEDURE
URINE CULTURE
(Continued)

c. Convert the number to scientific notation; for example, if 150 colonies were counted and a 1 ml loop was used, the count would be 150,000, or 1.5×10^5, cfu/ml urine.
d. Colony counts greater than 10^5 cfu/ml are considered to be positive for UTIs. Those in the range of 10^4 to 10^5 cfu/ml may be contaminated or may indicate a partially treated UTI. Dehydration, chronic pyelonephritis, and low urine specific gravity may also produce counts in this range in the presence of infection. Counts in the area of 10^3 cfu/ml are usually considered to be negative.

8. Examine the other plates for growth. Determine if gram-positive or gram-negative bacteria are present. Give possible species for each colony type.
9. Perform all necessary tests to identify any pathogen(s) present.
10. Perform the appropriate antibiotic panel using the Kirby-Bauer method on all pathogens.
11. Record all results.

URINE CULTURE RESULTS

Specimen identification: ______________________

Specimen type: ______________________

Date and time of collection: ______________ Collected by: ______________

Gram stain results: ______________________

____

MEDIA	TYPE OF COLONIES/ ESTIMATE OF NUMBER	POSSIBLE ORGANISMS (GENUS)	FURTHER TESTS INDICATED
Blood			
Colony count: ________ cfu/ml			
MacConkey			
CNA			

ANTIBIOTIC SUSCEPTIBILITY TESTING

ANTIBIOTIC/CONCENTRATION	ZONE DIAMETER (mm)	INTERPRETATION

PROCEDURE
URINE CULTURE
(Continued)

IDENTIFICATION OF PATHOGEN

Specimen Identification: ______________________________

TESTS PERFORMED	OBSERVATIONS	INTERPRETATION

Identification: ______________________________

Rationale: ______________________________

____

____

QUESTIONS

1. Correlate the results of the Gram stain with your observations on the primary isolation medium. ______________________________

____

____

2. A urine specimen submitted to the laboratory by a patient who collected the sample at home produced 59 colonies when using a 1 μl calibrated loop. On sheep blood agar, three distinct colony types were noted. What is your action? ______________________________

____

____

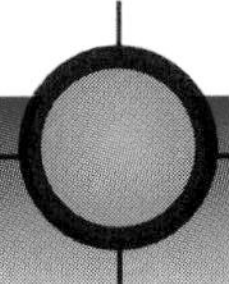

PROCEDURE
STOOL CULTURE

MEDIA AND MATERIALS

MacConkey agar (or eosin–methylene blue)
Hektoen enteric (HE) agar (or *Salmonella-Shigella* or xylose-lysine-desoxycholate)
Gram-negative (GN) broth (or selenite broth)
Campylobacter blood agar
5% sheep blood agar
Gram stain reagents
Optional media
- Cefsulodin-irgasan-novobiocin (CIN) medium (if *Yersinia enterocolitica* suspected)
- Sorbitol-MacConkey agar (if verotoxic *Escherichia coli* suspected)
- Thiosulfate-citrate–bile salts–sucrose (TCBS) agar (if *Vibrio* suspected)
- Cycloserine-cefotixin-fructose–egg yolk (CCF) agar (if *Clostridium difficile* suspected)
- Brilliant green (BG) or bismuth sulfite (BS) agar (if *Salmonella typhi* suspected)

PROCEDURE

1. Insert a swab into the stool culture and prepare a smear. Allow it to air dry, and then fix using heat or methanol. Perform the Gram stain on the smear.
2. Examine the smear for the presence of WBCs, RBCs, and any abnormal bacterial forms, including curved gram-negative bacilli, which may indicate *Vibrio* or *Campylobacter*. A normal stool contains numerous gram-negative bacilli, some gram-positive cocci, and gram-positive bacilli. Record your observations.
3. Insert another swab into the specimen, and roll it over the surfaces of the blood agar, MacConkey agar, HE agar, and *Campylobacter* blood agar plates. Streak each plate for isolation. Insert the swab into the GN broth and cap the tube. Streak any other optional plates for isolation if indicated.
4. Incubate all plates, except the *Campylobacter* blood agar, and the broth at 35° to 37°C for 24 hours. The *Campylobacter* blood agar is incubated at 42°C in a microaerophilic environment, such as in a *Campylobacter* bag.
5. At 6 to 8 hours' incubation, subculture the GN broth to fresh MacConkey and HE plates.
6. At 24 hours' incubation, examine the plates for growth.
   a. Examine the MacConkey plate for the presence of normal flora, which appears as pink lactose fermenters. Scan the plate closely to detect any colorless, non–lactose fermenters that are likely pathogens.
   b. Note the inhibition of the normal flora on the HE plate. Examine the plate for any colorless colonies with or without a black pigment, which indicate a pathogen.
   c. Record all results.

PROCEDURE
STOOL CULTURE
(Continued)

7. Examine the blood agar plate for growth. Note the number of colonies that are not members of the Enterobacteriaceae. In particular, examine the plate for yeast and *Staphylococcus aureus*.
8. Examine the *Campylobacter* blood agar for flat, gray colonies typical of *Campylobacter*. Perform a Gram stain and the oxidase and catalase tests on any suspicious growth. *Campylobacter* appears as a thin, curved, gram-negative bacillus; it is oxidase and catalase positive.
9. Reincubate any plates without growth for another 24 hours.
10. Examine the plates after 48 hours' incubation, as well as those subcultured from the GN broth. Record your results.
11. Prepare a flow chart for the identification of any pathogens that are isolated.
12. After consulting with your instructor, perform all tests that are necessary to identify the pathogen(s).
13. Perform the Kirby-Bauer antibiotic susceptibility test on all pathogens identified.

STOOL CULTURE RESULTS

Specimen identification: ______________________________

Date and time of collection: __________ Collected by: ______________

Gram stain results: ______________________________

____

____

COLONIAL MORPHOLOGY

PLATES	COLONY TYPE AND NUMBER	REACTIONS LACTOSE	H_2S	OTHER	POSSIBLE ORGANISMS	NORMAL FLORA/PATHOGENS
Blood						
MacConkey						
HE						
MacConkey (subculture)						
HE (subculture)						
Other						

Compare your observations on the Gram stain with the growth on the agar plates. Perform a Gram stain on each distinct colony type. Record your results.

____

____

____

Continued.

PROCEDURE
STOOL CULTURE
(Continued)

PLATE	COLONY TYPE	GRAM STAIN	POSSIBLE ORGANISM

Perform all necessary tests to identify any pathogen(s).

TESTS/MEDIA	OBSERVATIONS/INTERPRETATION	POSSIBLE ORGANISM(S)

Based on colonial morphology on the various plates and results to tests performed, identify any pathogen(s) present.
Identification: ____________________

Explain your reasoning for identification: ____________________

ANTIBIOTIC SUSCEPTIBILITY TESTING

ISOLATE	ANTIBIOTIC/ CONCENTRATION	ZONE DIAMETER (mm)	INTERPRETATION

QUESTIONS

1. Contrast the growth on the MacConkey plate with that on the HE plate. What differences do you note? ____________________
   Why do these occur? ____________________
2. Contrast the growth on the MacConkey plate streaked from the swab from that streaked from the subculture from the GN broth. Are there any differences? ____________________
   Explain why or why not ____________________
   State the purpose of enrichment broth. ____________________

CASE STUDIES AND REVIEW QUESTIONS

CASE STUDY 1

A 65-year-old male is admitted to the hospital with high fever, shaking chills, nausea, and vomiting. His medical record indicates that he has a history of emphysema and has been a heavy cigarette smoker since he was a teenager.

A complete blood cell count, differential, and chemistry profile are ordered by the physician. The CBC reveals a WBC of 15,000/μl, with 40% bands, 46% segmented neutrophils, 11% lymphocytes, and 3% monocytes.

Breathing was labored, and a chest x-ray film revealed consolidation of the upper part of the lung. Sputum and blood cultures were performed.

1. **The Gram stain from the sputum specimen revealed numerous segmented neutrophils, many gram-negative bacilli, and few gram-positive cocci. An occasional squamous epithelial cell was seen. What can be said about the quality of this specimen?**
   a. It is suitable for culture and does not seem to be contaminated.
   b. It is unsuitable for culture and definitely contaminated; it should be re-collected.
   c. Its quality cannot be determined until the specimen is plated, incubated, and the growth examined.
   d. None of the above
2. **Which of the following indicate the most appropriate plating media for the sputum specimen?**
   a. 5% sheep blood agar, MacConkey agar, chocolate agar, anaerobic blood agar
   b. Chocolate agar, Bordet-Gengou, MacConkey agar, thioglycollate
   c. 5% sheep blood agar, MacConkey agar, chocolate agar, CNA
   d. 5% sheep blood agar, MacConkey agar, anaerobic blood agar, CNA
3. **Examination of the plates at 24 hours' incubation reveals heavy growth of a mucoid lactose fermenter on the MacConkey plate. A few alpha hemolytic colonies are observed on the CNA plate. Which statement most likely describes these observations?**
   a. The colonies on MacConkey and CNA are both pathogens.
   b. The colonies on MacConkey and CNA are both normal flora.
   c. The colonies on MacConkey should be considered to be pathogenic, and those on CNA, normal flora.
   d. The colonies on CNA should be considered to be pathogenic, and those on MacConkey, normal flora.
4. **Which of the following tests are most appropriate in the identification of the pathogen(s)?**
   a. Catalase, coagulase, optochin
   b. Indole, motility, decarboxylase patterns
   c. Indole, urease, deaminase
   d. Oxidase, catalase, porphyrin
5. **The blood cultures were positive. What do you think a Gram stain performed on a subculture of the blood culture would reveal?**
   a. Gram-positive diplococci
   b. Gram-positive cocci in clusters
   c. Gram-negative diplococci
   d. Gram-negative bacilli

CASE STUDY 2

A 26-year-old female patient reports to her obstetrician during her seventh month of pregnancy for a routine visit. She has no concerns, except that she has experienced painful, burning, and frequent urination for the past few days. The routinely voided urine sample yielded positive results for nitrate and leukocyte esterase.

6. **What can be said about the quality of the specimen for culture?**
   a. A pathogen is obviously present, so there is no need to be concerned about normal flora or contaminants—it is a suitable specimen.
   b. A Gram stain should be performed to see if normal flora contaminants are present in order to determine if it is suitable.

CASE STUDIES AND REVIEW QUESTIONS

(Continued)

c. Normal flora contaminants are causing the positive nitrate and esterase reactions. Re-collect for a clean-catch midstream specimen.
d. A clean-catch midstream specimen should be collected to determine the presence of a urinary tract infection.

Upon receipt of the specimen in the laboratory, a colony count is performed using a 1 μl calibrated inoculating loop on 5% sheep blood agar; a MacConkey agar plate is also inoculated. At 24 hours, heavy growth of a lactose fermenter is observed on the MacConkey plate. The colonies are counted on the blood agar plate, revealing 140 colonies, which are flat, grayish, and nonhemolytic.

7. Determine the colony count per ml of urine.
a. 1.4×10^2/ml
b. 1.4×10^3/ml
c. 1.4×10^4/ml
d. 1.4×10^5/ml
e. 1.4×10^6/ml

8. A rapid indole test is performed on the lactose fermenter, with a positive result. This organism can be presumptively identified as:
a. *Enterobacter cloacae*
b. *Klebsiella pneumoniae*
c. *Escherichia coli*
d. *Proteus mirabilis*
e. *Enterococcus*

9. Which of the following tests are most helpful in the final identification of this organism?
a. VP, citrate, motility
b. Urease, deaminase, motility
c. Lysine decarboxylase, VP, urease
d. Glucose fermentation, citrate, deaminase

CASE STUDY 3

A 9-month-old infant boy is brought to the emergency room by his mother. She states that the child has been listless and hasn't been interested in eating or taking his bottle for the last 2 days. She says the baby has been sleeping long hours and that she has difficulty waking him from his nap. The baby has had a low-grade fever, which she was treating with acetaminophen. While taking the medical history, the physician notes that the baby has not received any immunizations.

A CBC and differential are performed, revealing a WBC of 14,500/μl with 90% neutrophils, including 35% bands. The infant's condition worsens, and a cerebrospinal fluid collection is performed. The Gram stain reveals few gram-negative coccobacilli and 3-4 segmented neutrophils/oil immersion field. A tentative diagnosis of meningitis is made.

10. Which of the following should be considered as the possible pathogen?
a. *Streptococcus pneumoniae* or *Neisseria meningitidis*
b. *Haemophilus influenzae* or *Staphylococcus aureus*
c. *E. coli* or *Neisseria meningitidis*
d. *Haemophilus influenzae* or *Neisseria meningitidis*

11. The specimen was plated on 5% sheep blood agar, chocolate agar, CNA, MacConkey agar, and anaerobic blood, and into thioglycollate. After 48 hours' incubation, growth was observed only on the chocolate agar. Which of the following tests are most appropriate in the identification?
a. Oxidase, X and V factors, porphyrin
b. Oxidase, carbohydrate utilization tests
c. Oxidase, indole, VP, motility
d. Catalase, coagulase, optochin

CASE STUDIES AND REVIEW QUESTIONS
(Continued)

CASE STUDY 4

A 60-year-old male diabetic patient received a puncture wound on his finger with a screwdriver while repairing his car. He cleaned the wound with soap, water, and peroxide; he then applied a local antibiotic. Three days later, he noticed the area was red, hot, and swollen. He also developed a low-grade fever, and he decided to call his physician.

The physician noted the development of cellulitis; he cultured the site using a needle and syringe and debrided the site. He also prescribed an oral broad-spectrum antibiotic.

Upon receipt in the laboratory, the specimen was Gram stained and plated onto sheep blood agar and MacConkey agar, which were incubated at 35°C; anaerobic blood, PEA, KV, and thioglycollate samples were inoculated and incubated anaerobically.

The Gram stain revealed the presence of many gram-positive cocci in clusters, moderate gram-positive bacilli, and many segmented neutrophils.

12. The aerobic plates revealed a moderately heavy growth of a medium-sized, creamy white colony with narrow zone beta hemolysis on the blood agar plate. No growth was seen on the MacConkey agar. Which of the following is the most appropriate action to identify this organism?

a. Perform Gram stain and catalase
b. Plate on CNA to isolate anaerobic gram-positive cocci
c. Re-collect the specimen since normal skin flora have been isolated
d. Perform CAMP and bacitracin tests to speciate

13. To differentiate normal skin flora from the pathogenic *Staphylococcus,* which of the following tests is most appropriate?

a. Novobiocin
b. Coagulase
c. Bile esculin hydrolysis
d. Bacitracin

14. Growth was evident on the anaerobic blood agar and PEA plates; no growth was observed on the KV. Growth was observed in the lower third of the thioglycollate tube, and a foul odor was very evident in this tube. Which group of anaerobes can be eliminated as the possible infecting organism?

a. Gram-negative cocci
b. Gram-positive cocci
c. Gram-negative bacilli
d. Gram-positive non–spore-forming bacilli
e. Gram-positive spore-forming bacilli

15. Lombard-Dowell quadplates were inoculated, with the following results obtained:

Indole	−
Esculin hydrolysis	+
Catalase	−
Lecithinase	+
Starch hydrolysis	−
Milk digested	−
DNAse	+
Gelatinase	+

Glucose and lactose fermented

This anaerobe is most likely:

a. *Bacteroides fragilis*
b. *Clostridium tetani*
c. *Clostridium perfringens*
d. *Peptostreptococcus anaerobius*
e. *Fusobacterium nucleatum*

16. What observation of the anaerobic blood agar would have been an important clue to this bacterium's identification?

a. Brown to black pigmentation
b. Wide zone of beta hemolysis
c. Pearly, opalescent growth
d. Double zone of hemolysis

CASE STUDIES AND REVIEW QUESTIONS

(Continued)

CASE STUDY 5

A 34-year-old female is transported to the emergency room by ambulance after reporting that she was severely burned. It is determined that she leaned over the flame of the burner of her gas stove while cooking, and the sleeve of her blouse caught fire. Examination by the emergency room physician reveals second- and third degree burns to her forearm and upper arm. The burns are cleansed and dressed, and the patient is immediately given intravenous antibiotics. She is admitted to the hospital. A specimen is obtained from the burn site for culture and susceptibility testing. After 3 days of hospitalization, an exudate is observed at the burn site. Although no pathogens were isolated from the specimen, the burn remains red and painful and does not seem to be improving. The attending physician questions the initial culture results, and another specimen from the site is sent to the laboratory. The Gram stain of the second specimen reveals many gram-negative bacilli.

17. How do you account for the discrepancy between the first and second specimens?
   a. Poor culture technique was used for the initial specimen.
   b. Second specimen is contaminated with normal skin flora.
   c. Patient developed an infection while in the hospital.
   d. All of the above are possible explanations.

The second specimen revealed the presence of a nonlactose fermenter and a lactose fermenter on MacConkey agar. The CNA plate showed no growth, and no anaerobes were isolated.

18. The nonlactose fermenter produced a bluish-green pigment on MacConkey agar and may be presumptively identified as:
   a. *Serratia marcescens*
   b. *Pseudomonas fluorescens*
   c. *Pseudomonas aeruginosa*
   d. *Flavobacter meningosepticum*

19. Which of the following biochemical profiles most likely correlates with the correct identification of the nonlactose fermenter?

	Oxidase	Growth at 42°C	Glucose/ Oxidized	LDC	ADH	ODC
a.	+	−	+	−	+	−
b.	+	+	+	+	−	+
c.	+	−	+	−	−	+
d.	+	+	+	−	+	−
e.	−	+	+	−	+	−

20. The lactose fermenter was determined to be indole negative by the spot indole test. Which of the following organisms are not possible choices for identification of this isolate?
   a. *Enterobacter cloacae*
   b. *Enterobacter aerogenes*
   c. *Klebsiella pneumoniae*
   d. *E. coli*
   e. Responses a, b, and c

21. The following biochemical profile was obtained for the lactose fermenter:

VP +	Citrate +	Motile
LDC −	ADH +	ODC +
Urease −		

Fermented sucrose, manitol, sorbitol, arabinose, raffinose
Failed to ferment dulcitol and adonitol

It can most likely be identified as:
   a. *Klebsiella pneumoniae*
   b. *Enterobacter aerogenes*
   c. *Enterobacter cloacae*
   d. *Pantoa (Enterobacter) agglomerans*
   e. *Escherichia coli*

CASE STUDIES AND REVIEW QUESTIONS

(Continued)

CASE STUDY 6

A 68-year-old male is examined in the hospital emergency room with complaints of a fever and worsening shortness of breath. He had been diagnosed a few years earlier with chronic obstructive pulmonary disease. His vital signs showed a temperature of 100°F, pulse of 92 beats/minute, respiration of 22/minute, and a blood pressure of 124/78 mm Hg. Chest x-ray films revealed small infiltrates in both upper lobes and in many small cavities. A sputum specimen was collected for culture and acid-fast bacilli.

The Gram stain yielded more than 25 neutrophils/LPF, a rare squamous epithelial cell, moderate gram-positive cocci, a few gram-negative bacilli, and a few corynebacteria. The acid-fast stain revealed approximately 10-12 acid-fast bacilli on the entire slide. The patient was prescribed a therapy of isoniazid and ethambutol.

22. The sputum specimen:

a. Appears to be contaminated
b. Indicates the presence of one or more pathogenic organisms
c. Reflects the normal oropharyngeal flora
d. More than one response applies

23. Based on the patient's history and the findings in the smears, which of the following are the most appropriate media for primary plating?

a. Sheep blood agar, MacConkey agar, chocolate agar, and Middlebrook
b. Sheep blood agar, MacConkey agar, chocolate agar, thioglycollate
c. CNA, MacConkey agar, anaerobic blood, selective Middlebrook
d. CNA, MacConkey agar, chocolate agar, Sabauraund's dextrose agar

24. The routine culture showed a mixed flora of a moderate amount of viridans *Streptococcus,* a few *Haemophilus,* and a few corynebacteria. What is the next step toward working up this culture?

a. Speciate *Streptococcus* and *Haemophilus*
b. Speciate *Haemophilus* and corynebacteria
c. Report findings that suggest normal mixed bacterial flora
d. Report, "No organisms isolated."

25. The acid-fast bacillus grew in 5 days when incubated in the dark at 35°C as tan to buff-colored colonies. The plate was exposed to direct light from a 100 watt light for 5 hours, then reincubated. Within 48 hours, the colonies all developed an orange to yellow pigment.

Which of the following are possible species for this *Mycobacterium?*

a. *M. kansasii*
b. *M. marinum*
c. *M. gordonae*
d. *M. tuberculosis*
e. More than one is correct

26. This mycobacterium is classified as a

a. Photochromogen
b. Scotochromogen
c. Nonphotochromogen
d. Rapid grower

27. The mycobacterium produced the following results:

Heat stable catalase +
Nitrate reduction +
Tween 80 hydrolysis +
Niacin accumulation −

It can be most likely identified as:

a. *M. gordonae*
b. *M. tuberculosis*
c. *M. simiae*
d. *M. marinum*
e. *M. kansasii*

CASE STUDIES AND REVIEW QUESTIONS

(Continued)

CASE STUDY 7

A 55-year-old male patient recovering from surgery for a bowel obstruction had redness, swelling, pain, and tenderness at the surgical incision. The patient had been recovering well up to that time from the surgery, which was successfully performed 4 days earlier. A low-grade fever was noted and both aerobic and anaerobic cultures were collected from the incision. Several hours later, the patient's condition worsened as the fever increased and shaking chills occurred. A stat complete blood cell count was performed, and blood cultures were collected. Results revealed the presence of moderate gram-positive cocci and gram-negative bacilli in the Gram stain from the cultures taken earlier in the day. The CBC revealed a WBC of 16,500/μl with 85% neutrophils (60% segmented and 25% banded). Subculture of the aerobic blood culture bottle at 8 hours' incubation revealed a moderate number of gram-positive cocci. The blood culture was subsequently subcultured to both blood and chocolate agar and incubated at 35°C. At 18 hours' incubation, heavy growth was noted of flat, gray, nonhemolytic colonies, which were determined to be catalase negative.

28. Which of the following tests are most needed to identify this isolate?
   a. CAMP, bacitracin, bile esculin, 6.5% salt broth
   b. Optochin, bile esculin, and PYRase
   c. Coagulase, bile esculin, and optochin
   d. CAMP, bile esculin, and PYRase

29. If the organism is bile esculin positive, it can be classified as:
   a. Group D *Streptococcus*
   b. *Enterococcus*
   c. Group D *Streptococcus*—non-*Enterococcus*
   d. Viridans *Streptococcus*

30. The gram stain morphology of this isolate will most probably show gram-positive:
   a. Cocci in clusters
   b. Cocci in chains
   c. Diplococci
   d. Coccobacilli

31. Tubudity and hemolysis were noted in the anaerobic blood culture vial at 18 hours' incubation. A Gram stain revealed many gram-negative bacilli. You would expect this anaerobe to grow on/in which of the following anaerobic media?
   a. Anaerobic blood only
   b. Anaerobic blood and thioglycollate
   c. Anaerobic blood, thioglycollate, and PEA
   d. Anaerobic blood, thioglycollate, PEA, and KV

32. Appropriate anaerobic media were inoculated and incubated. Lombard Dowell media were inoculated from colonies growing on the anaerobic sheep blood agar. At 48 hours, the following results were observed on the LD plates:

Indole −	Enhanced growth on 20% bile
Esculin hydrolysis +	Glucose and lactose fermented
Catalase +	Starch hydrolysis −
Lecithinase −	Gelatin hydrolysis −
Lipase −	

The anaerobic growth is most likely
   a. *Fusobacterium nucleatum*
   b. *Clostridium perfringens*
   c. *Bacteroides fragilis*
   d. *Prevotella melaninogenica*
   e. *Porphyromonas asaccharolyticus*

33. The source of this pathogen is most likely:
   a. Nosocomial infection acquired from health care environment
   b. Nosocomial infection acquired from health care providers
   c. Endogenous infection from patient's normal flora
   d. Exogenous infection from unsterile wound dressings

BIBLIOGRAPHY

Bartlett RC: Making optimum use of the microbiology laboratory. Part II. Urine, respiratory, wound, and cervicovaginal exudate, *JAMA* 247:1336, 1982.

Centers for Disease Control: Recommendations for Collection of laboratory specimens associated with outbreaks of gastroenteritis, *Lab Med* 22:623, 1991. (Reprinted from U.S. Department of Health and Human Services, Public Health Services, CDC, Atlanta, 1990, *MMWR* 39:No RR-14, 1-13.)

Colmer J, Sodeman TM: Contemporary pathogens of the genitourinary system, *Lab Med* 21:730, 1990.

Crowe HM, Craven DE: Preventing and managing nosocomial pneumonia, *J Resp Dis* 9:96, 1988.

Daly JA: Nonautomated rapid methods for bacteriuria detection, *J Med Tech* 2:759, 1985.

Detection of septicemia, Cleveland Clinic Foundation Symposium, JA Washington, Course Director; FP Koontz and LB Reller, Faculty; 1992.

Finegold S: Aspiration pneumonia, *Rev Infect Dis* 13:(Suppl 9)S:737, 1991.

Gilligan P: Laboratory diagnosis of diarrheal disease, Clinical microbiology update 1993, Western Pennsylvania Society for Clinical Microbiology Symposium, 1993.

Gray LD, Fedorko DP: Laboratory diagnosis of bacterial meningitis, *Clin Microbiol Rev* 5:130, 1992.

Gross PA, Flower M, Barden G: Polymicrobic bacteriuria: significant association with bacteremia, *J Clin Microbiol* 3:246, 1976.

Hall GS: Newer infectious diseases, 1994, Ohio Society for Clinical Laboratory Science.

Isenberg HD, Washington JA II, Balows A, and Sonnenwirth AC: Specimen collection and handling. In Lennette EH, editor: *Manual of clinical microbiology,* ed 4, 1985, American Society for Clinical Microbiology.

Kellogg JA, Ferrentino FL, Liss J et al: Justification and implementation of a policy requiring two blood cultures when one is ordered, *Lab Med* 25:323, 1994.

Kwa B, Pentella M: Sexually transmitted diseases: risks, transmission, and laboratory diagnostic update, *Clin Lab Sci* 6:85, 1993.

Levine MM: *Escherichia coli* that cause diarrhea: enterotoxigenic, enteropathogenic, enteroinvasive, enterohemorrhagic, and enteroadherent, *J Infect Dis* 155:377, 1987.

Lipsky BA, Ireton RC, Fihn SD et al: Diagnosis of bacteriuria in men: specimen collection and culture interpretation, *J Infect Dis* 155:847, 1987.

Murray PR, Traynor P, and Hopson D: Critical assessment of blood culture techniques: analysis of recovery of obligate and facultative anaerobes, strict aerobic bacteria, and fungi in aerobic and anaerobic blood culture bottles, *J Clin Microbiol* 30:1462, 1992.

Palac DM: Urinary tract infections in women: a physician's perspective, *Lab Med* 17:25, 1986.

Phillips SE, Milan JC: Reassessment of microbiology protocol for cerebrospinal fluid specimens, *Lab Med* 22:619, 1991.

Ramsey MK: *Gardnerella vaginalis:* clinical implications and laboratory identification, *Clin Lab Sci* 2:48, 1989.

Reimer LG: The diagnosis of urinary tract infections, *J Med Tech* 2:754, 1985.

Schumann GB: Clinical utility of body fluid analysis: an overview, *Clin Lab Sci* 7:28, 1994.

Smith SV, Forman DT: Laboratory analysis of cerebrospinal fluid, *Clin Lab Sci* 7:32, 1994.

Sodeman TM, Colmer J: Microbiology of the respiratory tract, *Lab Med* 14:96, 1983.

Tenney JH, Reller LB, Mirret S, Wang W, and Weinstein WP: Controlled evaluation of the volume of blood cultured in detection of bacteremia and fungemia, *J Clin Microbiol* 15:558, 1982.

Washington JA II: Blood cultures: principles and new approaches, *J Med Tech* 1:604, 1984.

Washington JA II, Illstrup DM: Blood cultures: issues and controversies, *Rev Infect Dis* 8:792, 1986.

Washington JA II, White CM, Laganiere M, and Smith LH: Detection of significant bacteriuria by microscopic examination of urine, *Lab Med* 12:294, 1981.

Watanakunakorn C: Community-acquired pneumonia, *Curr Ther Infect Dis* 130, 1986.

Weinstein MP, Reller LB, Murphy JR, and Lichtenstein KA: The clinical significance of positive blood cultures: a comprehensive analysis of 500 episodes of bacteremia and fungemia in adults. Part I. Laboratory and epidemiologic observations, *Rev Infect Dis* 5:35, 1983.

Weinstein MP, Reller LB, Mirrett S, Wang W, and Alcid DV: Clinical comparison of an agar slide blood culture bottle with tryptic soy broth and a conventional blood culture bottle with supplemented peptone broth, *J Clin Microbiol* 21:815, 1985.

Werner V, Kruger RL: Value of the bacterial antigen test in the absence of CSF fluid leukocytes, *Lab Med* 22:787, 1991.

York MK: Rapid, cost-effective testing in microbiology, *Clin Microbiol Newsletter* 12:10, 1990.

GLOSSARY

acid-fast bacilli (AFB) name given to bacteria in the genus *Mycobacterium* due to the ability of these bacteria to retain stain even after acid decolorization.

acquired immunity resistance due to prior exposure to the infectious agent; may be actively acquired from the actual infection or from vaccination or passively acquired, as from mother to fetus.

acquired immunodeficiency syndrome AIDS; disease characterized by loss of immune compentency; opportunistic infections such as *Pneumocystis carinii* infections, cryptococcosis, candidiasis, and unusual malignancies such as Kaposi's sarcoma and non-Hodgkin's lymphomas; caused by the retrovirus Human Immunodeficiency Virus, and transmitted by the exchange of body fluids, including semen or blood or through the transfusion of contaminated blood or blood products.

acquired resistance ineffectiveness of an antimicrobial agent against a particular microorganism that results from prior exposure of the organism to the agent; may result from chromosomal mutations or effects of bacterial enzymes.

actinomycosis infection characterized by thick, lumpy abscesses or granulomas that drain a thin granular pus through multiple sinuses, usually in the cervicofacial, thoracic, or abdominal areas in humans; attributed to infection by *Actinomyces israelii.*

acute phase specimen serum specimen to determine specific antibody levels; serum is collected early in infection when antibody levels are generally low.

additive effect two antimicrobial agents produce effects equal to the combined effect of the drugs when administered separately.

adsorption first step in the establishment of a viral infection, which involves the attachment of the virus to the host receptor site.

aerotolerance method to determine oxygen preference of a microorganism by determining its ability to grow on aerobic blood agar in the presence of oxygen and on anaerobic blood agar in the absence of oxygen.

agglutination clumping or adhering of bacterial, viral, or fungal antigens to corresponding antibody evidenced by aggregation of the antigen and antibody; antibody may be tagged for visualization of reaction with latex beads (latex agglutination) or red blood cells (hemagglutination).

alginate mucoid polysaccharide found in certain strains of *Pseudomonas aeruginosa* that may protect the organism from phagocytosis.

amastigote leishmanial or intracellular form of the hemoflagellates that is small and oval, containing a kinetoplast and nucleus but lacking an undulating membrane and external flagellum; generally found in the host reticuloendothelial tissue.

anaerogenic E. coli non-gas producing strains of *Escherichia coli.*

antagonistic effect effect of one antimicrobial agent opposes that of the second such that the resulting action is significantly less than the action of each agent alone.

anthrax infectious disease of farm animals, such as cattle, goats, pigs, and sheep, that is caused by the gram-positive bacillus *Bacillus anthracis* and may be transmitted to humans through direct contact or inhalation; also known as pulmonary anthrax or Woolsorter's Disease.

antibacterial antimicrobial agents that prevent the growth of bacteria.

antibiogram unique pattern of susceptibility and resistance of a microorganism to a group of antibiotics; useful in epidemiology.

antibiotic a chemical derived from a microorganism that inhibits the growth of another microorganism; some are chemically modified.

antibiotic media agar that contains antibiotics as inhibitory agents that may suppress the normal flora or other bacteria and enhance the isolation of a particular organism or group of bacteria; for example, colistin nalidixic acid inhibits gram-negative bacteria; Modified Thayer-Martin is selective for *N. gonorrhoeae.*

antibody protein that is induced by the introduction of antigen into the host and that reacts specifically with the antigen; the following immunoglobulins comprise the immune response: IgG, IgM, IgA, IgD, and IgE.

antibody titer amount of antibody present in a serum sample; the inverse of the highest dilution at which the antibody is detected.

antifungal antimicrobial agent that inhibits or prevents the growth of fungi.

antigen foreign compound capable of stimulating the production of antibody.

antimicrobial agents that inhibit the growth or action of microbes.

antiviral antimicrobial agent that inhibits or prevents the growth of viruses.

arthrocentesis puncture of a joint, with the withdrawal of synovial fluid for diagnositic purposes, such as the diagnosis of infectious disease.

ascospore type of specialized spore involved in sexual reproduction of some fungi in which two to eight spores are contained in a sac-like ascus.

assimilation ability of microorganisms to utilize nutrients that are useful in the classification of yeasts and used to determine if the yeast can grow in the presence of either an individual carbohydrate or nitrate.

asymptomatic carrier an individual who harbors a microorganism without any harmful effects who may transmit the infection to others.

autonomous effect antibiotic interaction in which the combined effect of both drugs is equal to the result of the most effective drug used alone.

auxotype gonococcal strains that require specific nutrients for growth; for example: AHU auxotypes require arginine, hypoxanthine, and uracil for growth.

bacitracin susceptibility selective inhibition of group A *Streptococcus* to 0.02-0.04 units of bacitracin; used in the identification of streptococci.

bacteremia the presence of bacteria in the blood.

bacterial vaginosis nonspecific vaginosis; mixed vaginal flora of anaerobes and aerobes with an absence of lactobacilli and white blood cells.

bacteriocidal antimicrobial agents that cause the death of bacteria.

bacteriostatic antimicrobial agents that inhibit the growth of bacteria without killing.

bacteriuria the presence of bacteria in the urine; the presence of more than 100,000 CFU per milliliter of urine is generally diagnostic for a urinary tract infection.

Bartlett's classification scheme used to determine suitability of sputum specimens by a numerical comparison based on the amount of neutrophils and squamous epithelial cells observed in a Gram-stained smear prepared from the specimen.

basidiospore type of specialized spore involved in sexual reproduction of some fungi; the spores are contained in a club-shaped basidium.

beta lactamase bacterial enzymes that destroy the beta-lactam ring of penicillins and cephalosporins leading to bacterial resistance; penicillinase.

bile esculin media used to select group D *Streptococcus* and *Enterococcus* based on their ability to grow in 40% bile and to hydrolyze esculin.

biohazard laboratory dangers that may be a source of infection to laboratory workers; examples include exposure to microorganisms through the airborne route, ingestion, direct inoculation, mucous membrane contact, or through arthropod vectors.

biological false positives conditions that produce a false reaction for *T. pallidum* in nontreponemal screening tests for syphilis including autoimmune diseases and infections that cross-react, producing a positive reaction in nontreponemal tests, such as the RPR (Rapid Plasma Reagin), but a negative reaction in the treponemal tests.

biosafety level four levels of protocol to be followed when working with potentially pathogenic microorganisms; protocol may include protective gloves, laboratory coats, biological safety cabinets, warning signs, and barrier controls.

blastomycosis infectious disease caused by the dimorphic fungus *Blastomyces dermatitidis,* which may infect the skin, lungs, kidneys, central nervous system, and bones and is most commonly found in North America, especially in the southeastern United States. The disease is characterized by cough, dyspnea, chills, and fever; also known as Gilchrist's disease.

botulism often fatal form of food poisoning caused by the anaerobic spore-forming bacillus *Clostridium botulinum* and the ingestion of the powerful botulism toxin, which acts as a neurotoxin, causing eventual respiratory paralysis.

bound coagulase clumping factor; enzyme produced by *Staphylococcus aureus* that converts fibrinogen to fibrin and is useful in the identification of the organism.

bradyzoite slowly replicating trophozoites of the parasite *Toxoplasma gondii;* they are intracellular and encyst in the host tissue.

brightfield microscopy type of microscopy in which the field is illuminated with a light source; specimen appears dark against a light background; useful in examining stained smears.

broad-spectrum antibiotic type of antimicrobial agent that has a range of effectiveness against several types of bacteria, including both gram-positive and gram-negative microorganisms.

bronchitis acute or chronic inflammation of the tracheobronchial tree characterized by cough and fever and caused by any of several bacterial or viral pathogens.

Brown's classification scheme to identify *Streptococcus* that is based on the organism's type and pattern of hemolysis; types of hemolysis include alpha, beta, alpha prime, and nonhemolytic.

CAMP reaction synergistic hemolysis observed between beta-hemolytic *Staphylococcus aureus* and group B streptococci; named for Christie, Atkins, and Munch-Peterson.

capnophilic microorganisms that prefer an incubation environment with increased carbon dioxide (3%-10% CO_2).

capsid protein covering of the virus particle.

capsomer protein subunits that form the protein coat (capsid) of a virion or virus particle.

carbohydrate fermentation ability of microorganisms to utilize carbohydrates in the absence of oxygen; anaerobic breakdown of carbohydrates, such as glucose, into carbon compounds, such as pyruvic acid.

cell-mediated immunity type of acquired immunity associated with T lymphocytes involved in resistance to infectious disease caused by viruses and some bacteria; cell-mediated immunity is also involved in delayed hypersensitivity reactions, graft rejection, and certain autoimmune diseases.

cellulitis an infection of the skin or connective tissue characterized by local heat, redness, pain, and swelling.

cercaria stage of the trematode life cycle with a body and a tail that develops from germ cells in the sporocyst or rediae; this is the final stage that develops in the snail host.

cervicitis acute or chronic inflammation of the mucous membranes of the cervix characterized by redness, edema, and pain.

chancroid very contagious local veneral ulcer caused by *Haemophilus ducreyi.*

choleragen cholera enterotoxin that is associated with the loss of electrolytes and fluids.

chromoblastomycosis type of subcutaneous fungal infection caused by the dematiaceous fungi, which are dark, slow-growing fungi such as *Fonsacaea* species, *Phialophora verrucosa, Cladosporium carrionii, Exophiala* species, and *Wangiella dermatitidis;* these fungi are found on vegetation and in the soil, and infection is generally transmitted through a puncture wound or skin trauma involving fungally contaminated vegetation.

clue cell adherence of small bacilli, usually *Gardnerella vaginalis* to squamous vaginal epithelial cells; significant in the diagnosis of bacterial vaginosis.

coagulase-negative staphylococci (CONs) those species of *Staphylococcus* that do not produce coagulase, including *S. epidermidis* and *S. saprophyticus.*

coccidioidomycosis infectious fungal disease caused by the inhalation of spores of the dimorphic fungus, *Coccidioides immitis,* characterized by respiratory symptoms and later a low-grade fever, anorexia, weight loss, dyspnea, and pain in the joints and bones, and most commonly found in the hot, dry climates of the southwestern United States and Central and South America; also known as desert fever, San Joaquin fever, and valley fever.

cold agglutinins nonspecific immunoglobulin M (IgM) antibodies that may be produced in response to *My-*

coplasma pneumoniae infection that agglutinate human type O red blood cells at 4° C but not at 37° C; useful in the diagnosis of *Mycoplasma pneumoniae* infection when present in high titer or if a four-fold increase is noted between the acute and convalescent titers.

colonization presence and multiplication of a microorganism in or on a host without signs of infectious disease.

colony count colony-forming units per milliliter (cfu/ml) of urine determined by using a calibrated inoculating loop; counts equal to or greater than 10^5/ml are diagnostic for urinary tract infections.

colorimetry quantitative analysis through comparison of the color development in an unknown sample with that of a known standard; color absorbance is directly proportional to the concentration of the substance to be measured.

conidia asexual spores produced by some fungi either singly or multiply in long chains or clusters by specialized hyphae known as conidiophores.

conidiogenesis conidia formation exhibited by some fungi.

convalescent phase specimen serum sample collected to determine antibody level later in the infection when the antibody response is high; generally collected at least 2 weeks after the acute phase specimen.

coracidium free-living larval stage of the cestode *Diphyllobothrium latum* that hatches in fresh water and is ingested by the first intermediate host, crustaceans or copepods of the genus *Diaptomus.*

counterimmunoelectrophoresis solid-phase system that uses electricity and the precipitin reaction to detect antigen or antibody; antigen and antibody move in opposite directions in an electrical field and form precipitates in the area where their concentrations meet in optimal proportions.

cyst form immotile form of the protozoan parasites that is protected by a cyst wall and may be transmitted to another host.

cytopathogenic effect CPE; alteration, disruption, or damage to the cells of a cell monolayer resulting from virus infection.

darkfield microscopy form of microscopy in which the specimen appears light against a black background since the field is illuminated by a peripheral light source; technique is used to examine spirochetes, including *Treponema, Borrelia,* and *Leptospira.*

definitive host the host in which the sexual reproductive phase of a parasite occurs.

delta-aminolevulinic acid (delta-ALA) used in the procedure that determines the ability of members of the genus *Haemophilus* to convert delta-ALA to porphyrins.

dematiaceous fungi a group of dark, slow-growing fungi that are found on vegetation and are associated with subcutaneous mycoses, including the development of chronic, warty, tumor-like lesions of the feet and lower legs; examples include *Fonsacaea fedrosoi, F. compactum, Phialophora verrucosa, Cladosprorum carrionii, Exophilia species,* and *Wangiella dermatitidis.*

deuteromycetes division in botanical taxonomy that includes most medically important fungi; characterized by septate hyphae and asexual reproduction.

differential media class of primary isolation media that selects for a particular group of bacteria and also permits the classification of the organism based on distinct growth characteristics; example is MacConkey agar, which selects for gram-negative bacteria by inhibition of gram-positive bacteria and also permits characterization of lactose-fermenting bacteria by a pink color.

digenetic sexual cycle of the trematodes in which distinct patterns of reproduction occur in alternate generations.

dimorphic those fungi that possess both a yeast phase that grows at 35°-37° C and a mold or mycelial phase that grows at 25°-30° C.

diphtheroid pleomorphic morphology of some gram-positive bacilli, including *Corynebacterium,* characterized by club-shaped or branching forms that resemble "Chinese letters."

diploid cell lines type of cell culture that must have at least 75% of the cells with the same karyotype from the normal cells from which the cell line was derived; examples include MRC-5, HDF, and WE-38 cell lines.

direct immunofluorescence microscopic method to determine presence of an antigen by exhibition of fluorescence when the specimen is reacted with a fluorescein-labeled antibody.

disinfection the process of destroying pathogenic organisms or causing inhibition of their activity.

eclipse stage in the establishment of viral infection in which replication and expression of genetic material occur as the viral nucleic acid acts as a template for production of messenger RNA, which directs the synthesis of viral proteins.

ectoparasite parasite that lives on or in the external area of the host.

ectothrix fungal infection of the hair involving the outside of the hair shaft.

effusion escape of fluid from the blood vessels or lymphatics, usually into a body cavity; may be associated with circulatory, hepatic, or renal disorders or from infection, malignancy, or other inflamatory states.

ELISA enzyme-linked immunosorbent assay; system to detect antigen or antibody; uses an enzyme that can react with a substrate to form a colored end product; the antigen (or antibody) is bound to an enzyme, such as horseradish peroxidase or alkaline phosphatase.

encephalitis inflammation of the brain, usually resulting from a viral infection.

endemic syphilis bejel; nonvenereal syphilis caused by the spirochete *Treponema pallidum* subspecies *endemicum,* which is transmitted through poor sanitation or poor personal hygiene.

endoparasite parasite that lives within the body of its host.

endothrix fungal infection of the hair involving the inside of the hair shaft.

endotoxin phosopholipopolysaccharide macromolecules that comprise the gram-negative bacterial cell wall; released only on cell lysis when the bacterium dies.

enrichment broth media used to enhance the growth of certain bacteria or groups of bacteria; for example, gram-negative broth that destroys gram-positive bacteria and inhibits the early multiplication of coliforms, thioglycollate that permits the differentiation of bacteria based on oxygen requirements.

enterohemorrhagic *E. coli* (EHEC) verotoxic *E.coli;* serotypes of *E.coli* that produce verotoxin that may result in mild diarrhea, nonbloody diarrhea, hemorrhagic colitis, or hemolytic uremic syndrome; most frequently identified serotype is O:157H:7, although more than fifty serotypes of verotoxic *E.coli* are known.

enteroinvasive *E. coli* (EIEC) diarrhea-producing serotypes of *E.coli* that invade the intestinal mucosal epithelial cells, resulting in a form of dysentery.

enteropathogenic *E. coli* (EPEC) serotypes of *E.coli* that attach to intestinal epithelial cells and are associated with acute diarrhea, especially in infants and children less than 2 years of age.

enterotoxigenic *E. coli* (ETEC) serotypes of *E.coli* associated with diarrhea and traveler's diarrhea that result from the ingestion of the organism's heat-labile toxin and heat-stable toxin.

enterotoxins cytotoxins that generally attack the cells of the mucous membranes of the small intestine; for example, enterotoxin A produced by *Staphylococcus aureus.*

envelope outer membrane composed of a phospholipid bilayer, glycoproteins, and matrix proteins that surrounds the nucleocapsid of some viruses.

envelope antigen antigenic determinant possessed by some members of the Enterobacteriaceae, which are capsular polysaccharides, surround the cell wall, and are heat labile; envelope or K antigens are possessed by *Salmonella, Klebsiella, E.coli,* and some *Citrobacter* species.

epimastigote crithidial, extracellular hemoflagellate form that is long and thin with an undulating membrane extending from the flagellum to the small kinetoplast located near the larger nucleus; found in the arthropod host.

erysipelas infectious skin disease usually caused by *Streptococcus pyogenes* and characterized by redness, swelling, vesicular rash, fever, pain, and lymphoadenopathy.

erythema chronicum migrans characteristic skin lesion of Lyme Disease, a tick-borne borreliosis caused by *Borrelia burgdorferi.*

examthem subitum "sixth disease" or roseola; viral disease of infants and children characterized by a rapid onset of fever and a fine macular rash caused by Human Herpesvirus Type 6 (HHV-6).

exoerythrocytic schizogony preerythrocytic cycle of the malarial parasite *Plasmodium,* which occurs outside of the erythrocyte and is characterized by repeated nuclear division followed by cytoplasmic division into daughter cells or merozoites.

exotoxin intracellular toxin generally released into the environment by living gram-positive bacteria.

exotoxin A exotoxin produced by virulent strains of *Pseudomonas aeruginosa* that inhibits protein synthesis and is associated with tissue destruction.

exudate type of effusion resulting from an infection, malignancy, or other inflammatory state; exudates generally contain many cells and have high specific gravities and protein levels.

facultative anaerobe having the ability to adapt to more than one oxygen level in the environment; organisms are able to grow in the presence and absence of oxygen.

facultative parasite an organism that lives on or in a host, but may also survive independently.

fastidious bacteria that possess very complex or extensive nutritional requirements.

febrile agglutinin test bacterial agglutination test to determine presence of antibodies in serum; useful in the diagnosis of disease in which the agent is difficult to culture, such as *Brucella* and *Francisella.*

fermentative ability of a microorganism to utilize a carbohydrate in the absence of oxygen.

fibrinolysin plasmin; proteolytic enzyme that lyses fibrin; includes staphylokinase produced by *Staphylococcus aureus* and streptokinase produced by *Streptococcus pyogenes.*

flagellar antigen antigenic determinant possessed by some motile members of the Enterobacteriaceae that are heat labile, composed of protein, and located in the flagellum.

fluorescent microscopy examination with a fluorescent microscope, which uses ultraviolet light to examine specimens that have been stained with a fluorescent dye.

fluorometric measurement of fluorescence emitted by compounds when exposed to ultraviolet radiation; useful in certain automated identification methods in microbiology.

free coagulase an extracellular enzyme produced by *Staphylococcus aureus* that converts fibrinogen into fibrin.

fungemia the presence of fungi in the blood.

fungi imperfecti the imperfect fungi; those fungi that do not exhibit a sexual phase and produce spores asexually from the mycelium.

gas-liquid chromatography method for separating and analyzing gaseous and chemical end products of metabolism through differences in their absorbency; used in the identification of anaerobes, which produce specific organic acids as end products of metabolism.

gastroenteritis inflammation of the stomach and intestines, resulting from various gastrointestinal disorders attributed to bacterial enterotoxins or invasion by viruses or bacteria.

general isolation media media, such as trypticase soy agar or trypticase soy broth, that supports the growth of most nonfastidious bacteria.

genetic probe method of identification in which sequences of deoxyribonucleic acid (DNA) or ribonucleic acid (RNA) form hybrids with the specific complementary strand of nucleic acid.

germ tube a hyphal-like extension of a yeast cell showing no constriction at the point of origin; useful in the identification of *Candida albicans.*

glanders an infection caused by *Pseudomonas mallei,* which may be transmitted to humans from horses or other animals, such as sheep, goats, or dogs, and is associated with inflammation of the mucous membranes, ulcerating skin nodules, lymphadenopathy, pneumonia, or septicemia.

gonorrhea sexually transmittable disease that most often affects the genitourinary tract and less frequently the pharynx, conjunctiva, or rectum; infection results from direct contact with the causative organism, *Neisseria gonorrhoeae.*

Gram stain commonly used differential staining method used to classify bacteria as gram-positive or gram-negative; gram-positive bacteria retain the primary stain crystal violet and appear purple whereas gram-negative bacteria lose the primary stain and retain the secondary stain of Safranin O and appear pink.

gravid proglottid mature segments of a tapeworm that have fully developed reproductive structures and a uterus containing eggs.

***Haemophilus influenzae* serotype b** capsular serotype of *H.influenzae* that is the most frequent cause of *H. influenzae* infections.

halophilic requiring increased chloride ions for growth.

Hansen's disease leprosy; chronic, communicable disease caused by *Mycobacterium leprae,* characterized by a thickening of the cutaneous nerves and round, saucer-shaped skin lesions or widespread plaques and nodules in the skin, eye, or bone.

hemagglutinin antigen viral surface antigen possessed by the influenza viruses and some parainfluenza viruses that permits the virus to attach to glycoprotein on the surface of red blood cells and respiratory epithelial cells.

hematin hemin; degradation product of hemoglobin in red blood cells that is a nutrient requirement for several fastidious bacteria, such as *Haemophilus* and *Neisseria.*

hemolysins substances that lyse or dissolve red blood cells; produced by various bacteria, including certain staphylococci and streptococci.

hepatitis inflammation of the liver characterized by fever, nausea, vomiting, jaundice, and necrosis of liver cells caused by one of the following hepatitis viruses: hepatitis A virus, hepatitis B virus, or hepatitis C virus.

hermaphroditic containing both male and female reproductive organs; the mature proglottids of tapeworms are hermaphroditic.

heteroploid cell lines cell cultures whose cells contain more than 25% cells with an abnormal karyotype when compared with the normal cells of the primary culture; heteroploid cell lines are derived from malignant tissue or other transformed cells. Examples include HeLA, Hep-2, and KB.

histoplasmosis fungal infection caused by inhalation of spores in soil contaminated with excreta from birds infected with the dimorphic fungus *Histoplasma capsulatum;* the disease is characterized by fever, malaise, cough, and lymphadenopathy, which may disseminate to ulcerations in the mouth and nose; enlargement of the spleen, liver, and lymph nodes; and severe lung infiltration. Most commonly found in the Ohio and Mississippi Valleys.

humoral immunity type of defense mechanism against foreign antigen and tissue associated with the production of antibodies produced by the immunoglobulins; humoral immunity includes antibody production against bacterial and viral antigens.

hyphae tubular filaments that are the microscopic units of the fungi and intertwine to form the mycelium.

immunoglobulin classes of humoral antibodies produced in response to foreign antigens; five classes, IgA, IgD, IgE, IgG, and IgM exist; IgM is involved in the primary immune response, whereas IgG is found in the secondary immune response.

immunoserology diagnosis of infectious disease through analysis of antibody levels or titers in patient sera; generally, acute phase and convalescent phase specimens are obtained and the titers compared.

immunosuppressive disease, irradiation, or use of chemical, pharmacologic, or physical agents that depress the immune system, often resulting in an increased host susceptibility to infectious disease.

impetigo highly contagious skin infection generally attributed to *Streptococcus pyogenes*, which begins as an erythema and progresses to lesions, erosions, and crusts.

incidental host accidental host; infection of a host that is not considered to be the normal host such that the life cycle of the parasite may or may not be completed.

indirect immunofluorescence microscopic technique to detect the presence of antibody by permitting an antibody to react with its substrate and then adding a second fluorescein-labeled antibody that will bind to the first antibody in a positive reaction.

infection invasion of a host by multiplying microorganisms.

infectious disease structural or functional harm caused to a host by the effects of microorganisms that have multiplied and established disease.

inflammatory process protective response of the body to irritation or injury caused by a physical, chemical, or biologic agent; consists of complex cellular and histologic reactions in the local blood vessels and adjacent tissues; cardinal signs of inflammation are *rubor* (redness), *calor* (heat), *tumor* (swelling), and *dolor* (pain).

innate immunity natural immunity; inborn resistance in an individual not immunized by previous infection or vaccination that is nonspecific and not stimulated by a particular antigen.

intermediate host the host in which the asexual reproductive or larval phase of the parasite occurs.

intrinsic resistance ability of a genus or species to remain unaffected by a particular antimicrobial agent; may delineate the antibiotic spectrum or be used as an identification tool; for example, *Staphylococcus saprophyticus'* resistance to novobiocin.

Kauffman-White classification method of classifying *Salmonella* species according to the presence of particular O, H, and Vi antigens; more than 2200 different serovars of *Salmonella* exist using this method.

Lancefield grouping method to classify streptococci based on the type-specific cell wall carbohydrate or "C" substance.

late (slow) lactose fermenters those bacteria that possess beta-galactosidase, but not lactose permease, which results in the delayed or slow degradation of lactose; late lactose fermenters are detected using the ONPG reaction.

latent viral infections viral infections that can become reactivated after months or years of dormancy; associated with the viral family Herpetoviridae; viruses remain dormant in the white blood cells or peripheral nerves, and infection may reactivate in periods of physical stress or illness.

Legionnaire's disease severe type of legionellosis, an acute bacterial pneumonia and multisystemic disease caused by the gram-negative bacillus *Legionella pneumophilia.*

leptospirosis acute infectious disease caused by the spirochete *Leptospira interrogans,* which is transmitted in the urine of both wild and domestic animals; humans may acquire the infection by direct contact with the animal's infected tissues or urine. The disease is characterized by fever, chills, jaundice, muscle ache, or hemorrhage into the skin.

leukocidan exotoxin produced by *Staphylococcus aureus* that inhibits or lyses white blood cells.

listeriosis infectious disease caused by the gram-positive bacillus *Listeria monocytogenes* and may be transmitted to humans by contact with vegetation, food, or water infected with the organism; the disease is characterized by shock, endocarditis, hepatosplenomegaly, and meningitis or encephalitis.

Lyme disease acute, recurring inflammatory disease involving the joints; may progress, causing neurological effects caused by the spirochete *Borrelia burgdorferi,* generally acquired through the bite of an infected tick.

lymphogranuloma venereum LGV; sexually transmitted disease caused by specific strains of *Chlamydia trachomatis* that is characterized by ulcerative genital lesions, swelling of the lymph nodes in the groin, headache, fever, and malaise.

macroconidia large, multicellular, club-, oval-, or spindle-shaped asexual fungal spores that are usually septate.

macrogamete mature female sex cell that produces zygotes once fertilized by the male microgamete in the genus *Plasmodium* and the intestinal coccidia; macrogametes develop from macrogametocytes.

melioidosis pneumonia-like disease caused by *Pseudomonas pseudomallei,* most commonly seen in Southeast Asia; also transported to the west by Asian immigrants and returning Vietnam war veterans. Acquired through inhalation or direct contact through breaks in the skin.

meningitis infection or inflammation of the membranes covering the brain or spinal cord, usually purulent and involving the subarachnoid space.

meningococcemia the presence of the meningococci *(Neisseria meningitidis)* in the blood.

merogony schizogony; asexual life cycle of the sporozoan protozoa characterized by nuclear division followed by cytoplasmic division; the dividing cell is known as the schizont and the daughter cells, merozoites.

merozoite trophozoite released from the host red blood cells or hepatic cells on maturation during the asexual life cycle of *Plasmodium.*

mesophilic pertaining to a microorganism with an optimal growth temperature between 25° C and 40° C; most human pathogens are mesophilic.

metacercaria infective stage of trematodes for humans, occuring when the cercaria loses its tail and encysts on water plants or a second intermediate host.

metachromatic granules Babes-Ernst bodies; irregularly staining granules believed to function as strorage depots in *Corynebacterium* species; they appear as beads in the methylene blue stain.

microaerophilic microorganisms that grow only under reduced oxygen tension and are unable to grow either aerobically or anaerobically.

microconidia small, unicellular, round, elliptical, or piriform asexual fungal spores.

microgamete mature male sex cell that fertilizes the female macrogamete, producing zygotes in the malarial parasite *Plasmodium* and the coccidian protozoans; microgametes develop from microgametocytes.

minimal bacteriocidal concentration (MBC) the lowest concentration of an antimicrobial agent that produces 99.9% killing or a reduction of 99.9% of the viable colony-forming units.

minimal inhibitory concentration (MIC) the lowest concentration of an antimicrobial agent that prevents visible growth; the lowest concentration of antimicrobial agent showing no visible growth in macrobroth or microbroth dilution procedure.

miracidium first-stage larva of the trematodes, which is released from the egg and is ciliated and free swimming; is able to penetrate the snail tissue to continue its life cycle.

moderately obligate anaerobe those anaerobes that can grow at oxygen levels of 2%-8%.

mold phase mycelial phase of a dimorphic fungus that is usually observed on Sabaroud's Dextrose Agar at 25° C to 30° C; the saprophytic phase is generally observed in nature.

monoclonal antibody antibody produced by the offspring of a single hybrid cell; large amounts of antibodies of one molecule type are produced that react with a single epitope.

MRSA methicillin-resistant *Staphylococcus aureus.*

multi-drug resistant *Mycobacterium tuberculosis* (MDRTB) those strains of *Mycobacterium tuberculosis* that are resistent to two or more antimycobacterial agents used to treat tuberculosis infection.

multitest systems commercially available identification methods using several biochemical reactions and an identification index.

mumps acute viral disease characterized by swelling of the parotid glands and caused by a *Paramyxovirus.*

mycelium intertwining structure of fungi, composed of tubular filaments or hyphae.

mycetoma chronic granulomatous infection of the cutaneous and subcutaneous tissue and bone characterized by tumorlike deformities of the subcutaneous tissue with abscesses, draining sinuses, and granulomatous pus and caused by members of the aerobic *Actinomyces* or several septate fungi, such as *Aspergillus, Exophiala, Pseudoallescheria,* and *Curvularia.*

***Mycobacterium* other than *tuberculosis* (MOTT)** method of classification proposed by Runyan for species of *Mycobacterium* other than tuberculosis that groups these atypical mycobacterial species based on growth rate and pigment production.

mycoses fungal infections.

myonecrosis gas gangrene; irreversible damage to muscle tissue frequently caused by anaerobic bacteria such as *Clostridium* species and characterized by pain, tenderness, the accumulation of gas within the muscle tissue, and blackish-green colorization of the muscle tissue.

narrow-spectrum antibiotic antibiotic that is useful for treating a limited group of microorganisms, such as either gram-positive or gram-negative bacteria.

nephelometry quantitative method based on determining the amount of turbidity by measuring light scattering.

neuraminidase antigen possessed by the *Influenza* viruses and some *Parainfluenza* viruses that permits the virus to enter the host cell.

nicotinamide-adenine dinucleotide (NAD) coenzyme I; compound produced by certain bacteria, such as *Staphylococcus aureus,* and yeast, that is a nutrient requirement for certain fastidious bacteria, such as *Haemophilus.*

nonphotochromogen those mycobacteria that do not form a pigment even in the presence of a constant light source; Runyan Group III.

nonsaccharolytic asaccharolyic; inability of a microorganism to use carbohydrates even in the presence of oxygen.

nonselective media enriched media; primary isolation media that contain a nutrient supplement; for example, chocolate agar or sheep blood agar.

nontreponemal tests nonspecific screening tests, such as the RPR (Rapid Plasma Reagin) and VDRL (Veneral Disease Research Laboratory) for syphilis that detect reagin; positive nontreponemal tests must be confirmed with a treponemal test.

normal flora microorganisms that are found in or on a particular body site and usually do not cause infectious disease; for example, viridans streptococci in the oral cavity.

nosocomial of or pertaining to the health care setting; a nosocomial infection is one acquired in the hospital or other health care setting.

nucleic acid hybridization binding of a single-stranded nucleic acid probe with its DNA complement in an unknown sample.

nucleocapsid virus particle consisting of the viral nucleic acid (DNA or RNA) with its protein coat (capsid).

obligate aerobe microorganism that requires oxygen for growth and cannot grow in the absence of oxygen.

obligate anaerobe microorganism that cannot grow in the presence of oxygen, growing only in conditions with very little or no oxygen present.

obligate parasite a parasite that requires a host, depending on it for survival.

oocyst encysted form of the motile zygote of *Plasmodium* species that is formed when the microgamete fertilizes the macrogamete; the oocyst encysts in the stomach wall of the *Anopheles* mosquito.

oospore sexual reproductive spore in some fungi that involves the fusion of cells from two separate, nonidentical hyphae.

ophthalmia neonatorum gonococcal conjunctivitis of the newborn acquired from infected maternal secretions during delivery.

opportunistic normally nonpathogenic microorganisms that are capable of causing infection in an immunosuppressed host.

opportunistic mycoses fungal infections that are observed in immunocompromised individuals and include candidiasis, zygomycosis, and aspergillosis.

optochin susceptibility procedure to differentiate *Streptococcus pneumoniae* from other alpha-hemolytic streptococci; *Streptococcus pneumoniae* is inhibited by optochin (ethylhydrocupreine hydrochloride), whereas other alpha-hemolytic streptococci are resistant to optochin.

osteomyelitis infection of the bone or bone marrow usually caused by bacteria introduced by trauma, surgery, extension of a nearby infection, or from the blood; most commonly caused by *Staphylococcus aureus.*

oxidative ability of a microorganism to utilize a carbohydrate only in the presence of oxygen.

paracentesis removal of ascitic or peritoneal fluid from the abdominal cavity.

paracoccidioidomycosis chronic fungal infection caused by the dimorphic fungus *Paracoccidioides brasiliensis* and characterized by ulcers of the mouth and nose, enlarged, draining lymph nodes, cough, dyspnea, weight loss, and skin lesions; it occurs primarily in Mexico and South and Central America and is acquired through inhalation of fungal spores; also called South American blastomycosis.

parasitism relationship between two different organisms in which the smaller lives on or in the larger with a dependence on the larger host for survival.

partially acid fast ability of the genus *Nocardia* to retain carbolfuchsin during mild acid decolorization due to the presence of unusual long-chain fatty acids in the cell wall; other gram-positive branching bacilli cannot retain the stain.

pasteurellosis local wound infection caused by the gram-negative bacillus *Pasturella multicida,* which may be acquired through the bite or scratch of an infected animal, usually a cat.

pathogen any microorganism capable of causing infection.

peak and trough specimens serum specimens collected to determine the level of a pharmaceutical agent, such as an antibiotic; peak specimens, which represent the highest level of the agent in the blood, are generally collected one half hour after the dose is given intravenously or intramuscularly; trough specimens represent the lowest level of the agent and are collected approximately one half hour before the next dose.

penetration stage in establishment of viral infection in which the viral genetic material enters the host cell, either through fusion, phagocytosis, or injection.

penicilliosis an acute fungal infection of the lungs, bone marrow, and other organs in immunosuppressed individuals; it is caused by the dimorphic fungus *Penicillium marneffei* and is found primarily in Southeast Asia, China, India, and Hong Kong.

pertussis acute, highly contagious respiratory disease characterized by paroxysmal coughing that may end in a whooping inspiration; caused by the gram-negative bacillus *Bordetella pertussis.*

phaeohyphomycosis opportunistic fungal infections other than mycetoma and chromoblastomycosis caused by the dematiaceous or darkly pigmented molds.

phagocytosis process of engulfing and destroying of microorganisms by neutrophils, monocytes, and macrophage.

phase-contrast microscopy form of microscopy using a special condenser and objective with a phase-shifting ring that permits viewing of small differences in the refractive index and differences in intensity; useful in viewing unstained specimens that appear transparent.

photochromogen those mycobacteria that are nonpigmented in the dark but produce a yellow pigment on constant exposure to light; Runyan Group I.

piedra fungal disease of the hair characterized by the presence of several small black or white nodules: white piedra is caused by *Trichosporon beigelii,* and black piedra is caused by *Piedria hortae.*

pili short, hair-like projections on the bacterial cell that are involved in attachment, bacterial conjugation, and transfer of genetic material.

pinta ulcerative skin disease caused by the spirochete *Treponema carateum,* characterized by flat, red, nonulcerating skin lesions and spread through direct contact with infected lesions.

pityriasis versicolor tinea versicolor; a superficial fungal infection characterized by brownish or scaly areas on light skin and irregular patches of nonpigmented areas on dark skin and caused by the fungus *Malassesia furfur.*

plasmid extrachromosomal DNA that determines traits not necessary for the bacterium's survival but may aid its adaptation to adverse conditions; certain plasmids enable the microorganism to resist particular antimicrobial agents.

plerocercoid second larval stage of the cestode *Diphyllobothrium latum* that develops in the second intermediate host, the fresh water fish, and is the infective form for humans if ingested.

pneumolysin virulence factor produced by *Streptococcus pneumoniae* associated with cytolysis.

pneumonia acute inflammation of the lungs attributed to infection by bacteria, commonly *Streptococcus pneumoniae,* viruses, or fungi characterized by fever, chills, headache, cough, and chest pain.

polio poliomyelitis; acute inflammation of the gray matter of the spinal cord caused by the *Poliovirus* in the enterovirus family; asymptomatic, mild, and paralytic forms of the disease occur.

polymerase chain reaction (PCR) procedure used to detect bacterial or viral nucleic acid in specimen using DNA polymerase to copy a DNA strand between two primer ends resulting in amplification of the original DNA strand.

polymicrobic infections containing more than one pathogenic organism, for example, an abscess that contains both an aerobe and an anaerobe.

PPNG penicillinase-producing *Neisseria gonorrhoeae* those strains of *Neisseria gonorrhoeae* that are resistant to the effects of penicillin through the production of penicillinase or beta lactamase.

precipitin formation of an insoluable complex between an antibody and a specific soluable antigen.

primary atypical pneumonia acute, systemic disease involving the lungs; caused by *Mycoplasma pneumoniae* and characterized by fever and cough but relatively few physical symptoms.

primary cell culture cell lines derived directly from parent tissue; cells in primary culture must have the same karyotype and chromosome number as the original tissue; examples include HEK, RK, and PMK.

procercoid the fist larval stage that develops from the coracidium stage of *Diphyllobothrium latum;* it develops in the body of the first intermediate host, either crustaceans or copepods of the genus *Diaptomus.*

proglottid a segment of a tapeworm containing both male and female reproductive organs when mature.

promastigote leptomonal hemoflagellate form, which is long and thin and is found extracellularly in the midgut or pharynx of the arthropod host; this form resembles the epimastigote form except that the kinetoplast is located anteriorly and there is no undulating membrane.

psittacosis ornithosis; infectious disease of psittacine birds, including parrots and parakeets, caused by *Chlamydia psittaci,* which may be transmitted to humans and is characterized by headache, nausea, and fever preceeded by chill; commonly known as "parrot fever."

pyocyanin a blue or blue-green water-soluble pigment that may be extracted with chloroform and is produced by *Pseudomonas aeruginosa.*

pyogenic pus-forming; those bacteria associated with pus-forming infections.

pyogenic exotoxin extracellular toxin secreted by *Streptococcus pyogenes* that may be associated with fever and the development of renal failure, respiratory distress, and necrosis.

pyoverdin a yellow pigment produced by some strains of *Pseudomonas aeruginosa.*

rabies an acute, usually fatal disease of the central nervous system transmitted from wild animals, such as skunks, bats, foxes, dogs, and raccoons infected with the *Lyssavirus* in the family Rhabdoviridae through an infected bite; the virus travels along nerves to the brain and other organs and incubates for days to months; incubation is followed by fever, malaise, paresthesia, myalgia, and later severe encephalitis, delirium, muscle spasms, paralysis, and usually death.

rapid grower saprophytic mycobacteria that grow within 3 to 5 days; Runyan Group IV.

reactivation tuberculosis form of secondary tuberculosis that recurs due to the activation of a dormant endogenous infection; reactivation may result from a diminished immune status, hormonal changes, poor nutrional status, or other debilitating states.

redia the elongated, sac-like second or third larval stage of the trematode that develops in the sporocyst and matures into many cercariae.

relapsing fever an acute infectious disease caused by the spirochete *Borrelia recurrentis* and spread through the bite of an infected tick that feeds on rodents and other animals.

resistant the ability of a microorganism to remain unaffected by an antimicrobial agent such that the organism is not inhibited by the agent.

retrovirus RNA-containing viruses characterized by possessing RNA-dependent DNA polymerases or reverse transcriptases such as the Human T Cell Lymphotrophic Viruses (HTLV-1 and HTLV-2) and the Human Immunodeficiency virus (HIV-1 and HIV-2).

rostellum the anterior, protruding portion of the scolex of a tapeworm that may be armed with a row or several rows of hooklets.

rubella contagious viral infection occuring primarily in nonimmunized children and characterized by fever, upper respiratory infection, enlarged lymph nodes, arthralgia, and a fine, diffuse, red maculopapular rash; caused by the genus *Rubivirus* in the family Togaviridae and transmitted by infected respiratory droplets; also called German measles or three-day measles since the symptoms generally last for three days.

rubeola measles; acute, contagious viral infection occuring primarily in nonimmunized children involving the respiratory tract and characterized by a spreading maculopapular rash and caused by a *Paramyxovirus* and transmitted through infected respiratory droplets.

salt tolerant the ability of certain bacteria to withstand and grow well in high concentrations of sodium chloride; for example, *Enterococcus* can sustain 6.5% NaCl.

satellitism phenomenon of colonies of *Haemophilus* growing about beta-hemolytic colonies of *Staphylococcus aureus* due to the latter's production of NAD and the presence of hematin.

schizogony merogony; form of asexual multiple fission seen in sporozoan protozoa in which the nucleus divides many times before the cytoplasm divides into as many parts as there are nuclei; the dividing cell is known as the schizont and the daughter cells, merozoites.

schizont sporozoan trophozoite that reproduces by schizogony to form daughter cells known as merozoites.

scolex the head or anterior end of a tapeworm, which enables the worm to attach by suckers and frequently by hooks on the rostellum to the intestinal wall.

scotochromogen those mycobacteria that are pigmented yellow to orange in the dark and on exposure to light intensify to an orange or orange-red color; Runyan Group II.

selective media primary isolation media that enhances the growth of a bacterium or group of bacteria while inhibiting the growth of another group or groups of bacteria; for example, Hektoen enteric agar is selective for *Salmonella* and *Shigella* while inhibiting the normal flora coliforms.

septicemia systemic disease associated with the presence of pathogenic microorganisms and toxins in the blood; characterized by fever, chills, pain, prostration, and nausea.

serum bacteriocidal test Schlichter test; the lowest dilution of a patient's serum that kills a standard inoculum of an organism isolated from the patient.

shigellosis bacillary dysentery; acute, bacterial infection of the bowel, characterized by diarrhea, fever, and abdominal pain caused by bacteria in the genus *Shigella*.

smallpox highly contagious viral infection characterized by fever, prostration, and a vesicular, pustular rash caused by the *Smallpox* or *Variola* virus in the family Poxviridae; smallpox was eradicated and the world declared free of smallpox in 1979 by the World Health Organization.

somatic antigen antigenic determinant possessed by members of the Enterobacteriaceae that is present in the cell wall and is associated with lipopolysaccharide; somatic (body) antigens are heat stable and are important in the serotyping of *E. coli, Shigella,* and *Salmonella*.

sporangiospores asexual fungal spores contained in a sac or sporangium that are produced terminally on sporangiophores or aseptate hyphae.

sporogony form of sexual reproduction whereby sporozoites from during the sexual stage of the life cycle of a sporozoan, primarily the malarial parasite, *Plasmodium;* the sex cells fuse in the body of the invertebrate host, the female *Anopheles* mosquito, where the ensysted zygote divides and gives rise to sporozoites.

sporotrichosis chronic, subcutaneous fungal infection caused by *Sporothrix schenckii* and characterized by skin ulcers and subcutaneous nodules along the lymphatics; it is usually transmitted through a thorn prick or puncture wound from decaying vegetation, flowers, or soil.

sporozoite the form of the malarial parasite *Plasmodium* that develops in the sporocyst by mutiple fission of the zygote in the oocyst of the female *Anopheles* mosquito during the sexual reproductive phase of the parasite; after release from the oocyst, the sporozoites migrate to the mosquito's salivary glands, where they may be transmitted to humans.

sterilization method to destroy microorganisms in or on an object through heat, steam, chemicals, gas, or radiation.

streptokinase extracellular enzyme produced by streptococci that cleaves plasminogen into plasmin, resulting in the lysis of a fibrin clot.

streptolysin S and O hemolysins produced by streptococci; streptolysin S is oxygen stable and nonantigenic whereas streptolysin O is oxygen labile and antigenic.

strict obligate anaerobe those anaerobes that cannot grow in the presence of even 0.5% oxygen and are thus unable to grow on the surface of agar.

strobila chain of developing segments or proglottids of a tapeworm.

subcutaneous mycoses fungal infections of the subcutaneous tissue, which usually do not disseminate and include sporotrichosis, mycetoma, chromoblastomycosis, and phaeohyphomycosis.

superficial (cutaneous) mycoses fungal infections of the skin, hair, and nails, including dermatophytic infections, piedra, and tinea versicolor.

superinfection an infection that occurs as a result of the antimicrobial therapy for another infection; it results from a change in the normal flora that permits the multiplication of other microorganisms; for example, infection with *Candida albicans* resulting from penicillin treatment for streptococcal pharyngitis.

susceptible effectiveness of an antimicrobial agent against a particular microorganism indicated by inhibition of growth of the organism around the antibiotic disk.

SXT trimethoprim-sulfamethoxazole susceptibility test used to differentiate beta-hemolytic streptococci; Lancefield groups A and B are resistant to SXT, whereas groups C, F, and G are susceptible.

synergistic antibiotic response in which the combined effect of two antibiotics is greater than the total of the individual effects.

systemic mycoses fungal infections of the lung and other organs that generally disseminate and include histoplasmosis, coccidioidomycosis, histoplasmosis, and paracoccidioidomycosis.

tachyzoite the crescent-shaped, rapidly dividing, intracellular trophozoite form of *Toxoplasma gondii.*

tetanospasmin exotoxin produced by *Clostridium tetani;* the lethal neurotoxin that produces painful muscle spasms resulting in lockjaw, laryngeal spasm, and tonic spasm of all muscles in the body.

tetanus acute, often fatal disease of the central nervous system caused by infection by *Clostridium tetani,* which enters the body through a puncture wound, laceration, burn, or through the umbical cord stump in a newborn. The disease is characterized by headache, fever, painful spasms of the muscles, and eventually tonic spasms of all muscules.

thallophytes those members of the plant family that possess true nuclei, lack stems and roots, do not possess chlorophyll, and absorb nutrients from the environment; the fungi are classified as thallophytes.

thoracentesis aspiration of pleural fluid for diagnostic purposes.

tinea ringworm; fungal skin, hair, and nail diseases caused by the dermatophytes and characterized by itching, scaling, and erythema of the skin; crumbling and destruction of the nails, and erythema, scaling, and crusting of the hair.

trachoma chronic, contagious infection of the conjunctiva caused by specific strains of *Chlamydia trachomatis* and characterized by inflammation, pain, photophobia, lacrimation, and if untreated, blindness.

transposons "jumping gene"; genetic material that may move from one plasmid to another or from plasmid to chromosome.

transudate type of effusion that contains few cells, has a low specific gravity and protein level, and generally develops from renal, hepatic, or circulatory disorders.

treponemal tests specific tests for syphilis, such as the Fluorescent Treponemal Antibody (FTA), that detect antigens to the spirochete *Treponema pallidum* and are used to confirm positive non-treponemal tests.

trophozoite form the motile stage of the protozoans that feeds and multiplies.

trypanomastigote trypanosomal hemoflagellate form that is long and thin, with an undulating membrane and free flagellum; found extracellularly in the arthropod host.

tuberculosis chronic, granulomatous infection caused by the organism *Mycobacterium tuberculosis,* which is transmitted through inhalation of infected droplets. Generally affecting the lung, although other organs may be infected; tuberculosis is characterized by pulmonary hemorrhage, dyspnea, purulent sputum, tubercles, and caseates in the lungs.

tularemia infectious disease of animals caused by the gram-negative bacillus *Francisella tularensis,* which may be transmitted by insect vectors or direct contact to humans causing lymph node enlargement, fever, skin ulcerations, or pneumonia.

tympanocentesis puncture of the tympanic membrane with a needle to aspirate middle ear fluid.

uncoating stage in the establishment of viral infection in which the virus loses its protein coat or capsid, exposing the viral nucleic acid, which will then be replicated and expressed in the eclipse stage.

undulant fever brucellosis; disease caused by gram-negative bacilli in the genus *Brucella;* primarily a disease of goats, pigs, and cattle and may be transmitted to humans through a break in the skin or ingesting contaminated animal products.

universal precautions set of safety regulations stating that blood, serum, or any body fluid or secretion containing blood should be handled as if it were capable of transmitting infectious disease.

urethritis inflammation or infection of the urethra; characterized by dysuria.

varicella chickenpox; acute, highly contagious viral disease occuring primarily in children caused by the *Varicella zoster* virus of the family Herpetoviridae and characterized by crops of pruritic vesicular skin eruptions and transmitted either through contaminated respiratory droplets or direct contact with the skin lesions.

vector carrier, usually an arthropod that transmits a pathogenic microorganism, such as a parasite, from an infected to a noninfected host.

venereal syphilis sexually transmittable disease caused by the spirochete *Treponema pallidum* subspecies *pallidum;* usually transmitted through the sexual or congenital route. The disease usually consists of primary, secondary, latent, and tertiary stages.

viremia the presence of viruses in the blood.

viridans *Streptococcus* term applied to several species of streptococci that are alpha-hemolytic and make up the normal oropharyngeal flora.

virion elementary virus particle consisting of a central nucleic acid core of either DNA or RNA that is surrounded by a protein coat or capsid.

Weil-Felix reaction method of whole-cell agglutination that uses various *Proteus* surface antigens to detect cross-reacting antibodies to species of *Rickettsia;* useful in the speciation of *Rickettsia.*

yaws chronic, nonvenereal disease of the skin and bones caused by the spirochete *Treponema pallidum* subspecies *pertenue* and transmitted by direct contact with infected lesions.

yeast phase tissue or invasive phase of a dimorphic fungus that is observed in vivo and grows on enriched media at 35°-37° C.

zoonoses diseases of animals that may be transmitted to humans from the primary animal host; examples include pasturellosis, rabies, Lyme disease, and tularemia.

zygomycosis opportunistic fungal infection caused by the zygomycetes *(Rhizopus, Absidia, Mucor)* and found in immunocompromised hosts and associated with infections of the nasal mucosa, sinuses, face, lung, liver, spleen and brain.

zygospore sexual reproductive spore of some fungi that involves the fusion of two identical cells arising from the same hypha.

ANSWERS TO REVIEW QUESTIONS

Chapter 1

1. e
2. a
3. b
4. c
5. d
6. d
7. a
8. c
9. b
10. d
11. a
12. a
13. d
14. c
15. d
16. e

Chapter 2

1. c
2. c
3. a
4. b
5. b
6. c
7. a
8. b
9.
   - Identify hazardous areas with biohazard label.
   - No food, beverages, or smoking are permitted in the laboratory.
   - Protective eyewear must be worn when using chemicals or infectious agents.
   - Laboratory coats or gowns must be worn in the laboratory.
   - Frequent and thorough handwashing is essential.
   - Eye-wash stations must be plumbed in and functional.
   - Mouth pipetting is prohibited.
   - Dispose of sharp objects and infectious articles in suitable containers.
   - Report all accidents to the instructor.
   - Adhere to universal precautions.
   - Use a biological safety cabinet when appropriate.
   - Decontaminate laboratory benches with 70% ethanol or a 10% solution of bleach.
10. Correctly identify the listed items in the laboratory.

Chapter 3

1. e
2. d
3. b
4. c
5. a
6. b
7. a
8. b
9. a
10. c
11. b
12. b
13. c
14. d
15. b
16. d
17. b
18. a
19. c
20. c
21. d

Chapter 4

1. c
2. d
3. b
4. a
5. d
6. b
7. c
8. d
9. b
10. b
11. a
12. c
13. c

Chapter 5

1. a
2. b
3. c
4. a
5. d
6. a
7. d
8. a
9. a
10. b
11. d
12. d

13. b
14. b
15. c

Chapter 6

1. d
2. a
3. g
4. b
5. h
6. c
7. e
8. i
9. f
10. A
11. A
12. A
13. B
14. B
15. B
16. b
17. b
18. d
19. I
20. I
21. I
22. C
23. I
24. c
25. c
26. b
27. c
28. b
29. d
30. c

Chapter 7

1. c
2. e
3. d
4. a
5. b
6. b
7. b
8. b
9. b
10. a
11. b
12. c
13. d

Case Studies

I. Media inoculated: sheep blood agar, CNA, anaerobic blood or PEA

Biochemical tests: catalase, coagulase, mannitol salt agar

II. *Staphylococcus saprophyticus;* CC = 7.5×10^4/ml

Chapter 8

1. c
2. e
3. b
4. d
5. h
6. a
7. d
8. f
9. h
10. b
11. b
12. d
13. a
14. a
15. a
16.

SPECIES	BACITRACIN	SXT	CAMP
S. pyogenes	S	R	Neg
S. agalactiae	R	R	Pos
Groups C, F, and G	R	S	Neg

SPECIES	OPTOCHIN	BEA	SALT BROTH (6.5%)	PYRASE
Enterococcus	R	Pos	Pos	Pos
Non-Enterococcus	R	Pos	Neg	Neg
S. pneumoniae	S	Neg	Neg	Neg
Viridans *Streptococcus*	R	Neg	Neg	Neg

Chapter 9

1. d
2. d
3. c
4. b
5. a
6. d
7. b
8. b

9. b
10. b
11. c
12. a
13. b
14. c
15. c
16. b
17. c
18. d
19. b

Chapter 10

1. e
2. d
3. c
4. a
5. b
6. b
7. d
8. a
9. e
10. c
11. b
12. b
13. c
14. b
15. c
16. b
17. c
18. d
19. b
20. b

Chapter 11

1. a
2. c
3. b
4. d
5. e
6. b
7. a
8. d
9. c
10. a
11. c

Chapter 12

1. b
2. a
3. e
4. b
5. c
6. b
7. c
8. c
9. d
10. b
11. b
12. c

Chapter 13

1. e
2. a
3. d
4. b
5. d
6. e
7. c
8. b
9. d
10. b
11. a
12. c
13. d
14. a
15. c
16. c
17. b
18. d

Chapter 14

1. d
2. c
3. f
4. a
5. b
6. a
7. c
8. b
9. a
10. c
11. d
12. d
13. c
14. a

15. b
16. a
17. c
18. c
19. c

Chapter 15

1. c
2. b
3. c
4. c
5. d
6. b
7. b
8. c

Chapter 16

1. a
2. b
3. d
4. e
5. c
6. c
7. d
8. a
9. b
10. b
11. A
12. U
13. A
14. U
15. A
16. U
17. A
18. U
19. b
20. d
21. b
22. c
23. b
24. d
25. b
26. c
27. b
28. c
29. a
30. d
31. c

Chapter 17

1. b
2. d
3. c
4. a
5. e
6. d
7. a
8. b
9. c
10. d
11. e
12. c
13. b
14. a
15. c
16. a
17. b
18. d
19. c
20. d
21. d
22. IV
23. II
24. I
25. II
26. none
27. none
28. II
29. I
30. III
31. a
32. a
33. b
34. d
35. b
36. c

Chapter 18

1. b; A
2. d; E
3. f; B
4. c; A, D
5. a; C
6. c
7. d
8. d
9. b
10. a
11. b
12. c
13. b
14. d

Chapter 19

1. e
2. b
3. c
4. a
5. c
6. i
7. l
8. b
9. d
10. m
11. n
12. j
13. p
14. g
15. o
16. f
17. k
18. e
19. a
20. h
21. d
22. b
23. a
24. d
25. c
26. b
27. b
28. d
29. b
30. a
31. d
32. c
33. d
34. 4
35. 1
36. 2
37. 5
38. 3
39. RNA
40. DNA
41. DNA
42. DNA
43. RNA
44. RNA
45. DNA
46. DNA

Chapter 20

1. a
2. e
3. d
4. c
5. b
6. b
7. c
8. e
9. a
10. d
11. b
12. a
13. a
14. d
15. b
16. d
17. c
18. c
19. c
20. b
21. b
22. a
23. c
24. b
25. c
26. d

Chapter 21

1. f
2. k
3. c
4. i
5. d
6. n
7. l
8. a
9. g
10. b
11. d
12. f
13. g
14. k
15. m
16. e
17. a

18. i
19. l
20. b
21. h
22. c
23. j
24. b
25. e
26. a
27. d
28. c
29. c
30. c
31. b
32. c
33. b
34. b
35. a
36. b
37. c

	PRIMARY	SECONDARY	INFECTIVE STAGE	DIAGNOSTIC STAGE
38.	None	None	Filariform larva	Rhabidiform larva
39.	None	None	Filariform larva	Egg
40.	None	None	Embryonated egg	Egg
41.	Crustaceans	Fresh water fish	Plerocercoid Second larval stage	Egg
42.	None	None	Embryonated egg	Embryonated egg
43.	Cattle Herbivores	None	Cysticercus in herbivore muscle	Egg and gravid proglottid
44.	Snails	Crustaceans	Metacercaria in crustacean	Unembryonated egg

45. b
46. b
47. a

Chapter 22

1. a
2. c
3. c
4. b
5. d
6. d
7. d
8. c
9. a
10. d
11. a
12. a
13. b
14. c
15. c
16. d
17. c
18. c
19. d
20. d
21. c
22. b
23. a
24. c
25. e
26. a
27. e
28. d
29. a
30. b
31. d
32. c
33. c

INDEX

C

G

Q

R